DISCARD

BIOCHEMISTRY OF ALCOHOL AND ALCOHOLISM

ELLIS HORWOOD SERIES IN CHEMICAL SCIENCE

KINETICS AND MECHANISMS OF POLYMERIZATION REACTIONS: Applications and Physicochemical Systematics
P.E.M. ALLEN, University of Adelaide, Australia and
C.R. PATRICK, University of Birmingham
ELECTRON SPIN RESONANCE
N. ATHERTON, University of Sheffield
METAL IONS IN SOLUTION
J. BURGESS, University of Leicester
ORGANOMETALLIC CHEMISTRY - A Guide to Structure and Reactivity
D.J. CARDIN and R.J. NORTON, Trinity College, University of Dublin
STRUCTURES AND APPROXIMATIONS FOR ELECTRONS IN MOLECULES
D. D.B. COOK, University of Sheffield
LIQUID CRYSTALS AND PLASTIC CRYSTALS
Volume I, Preparation, Constitution, and Applications
Volume II, Physico-Chemical Properties and Methods of Investigation
Edited by W. GRAY, University of Hull and
A. WINSOR, Shell Research Ltd.
POLYMERS AND THEIR PROPERTIES: A Treatise on Physical Principles and Structure
J.W.S. HEARLE, University of Manchester Institute of Science and Technology
BIOCHEMISTRY OF ALCOHOL AND ALCOHOLISM
L.J. KRICKA and P.M.O. CLARK, University of Birmingham
STRUCTURE AND BONDING IN SOLID STATE CHEMISTRY
M.F.C. LADD, University of Surrey
METAL AND METALLOID AMIDES: Synthesis, Structure, and Physical and Chemical Properties
M.F. LAPPERT, University of Sussex
A.R. SANGER, Alberta Research Council, Canada
R.C. SRIVASTAVA, University of Lucknow, India
P.P. POWER, Stanford University, California
BIOSYNTHESIS OF NATURAL PRODUCTS
P. MANITTO, University of Milan
ADSORPTION
J. OSCIK, Head of Institute of Chemistry, Marie Curie Sladowska, Poland
CHEMISTRY OF INTERFACES
G.D. PARFITT, Tioxide International Limited and
M.J. JAYCOCK, Loughborough University of Technology
METALS IN BIOLOGICAL SYSTEMS: Function and Mechanism
R.H. PRINCE, University Chemical Laboratories, Cambridge
APPLIED ELECTROCHEMISTRY: Electrolytic Production Processes
A. SCHMIDT
CHLOROFLUOROCARBONS IN THE ENVIRONMENT
Edited by T.M. SUGDEN, C.B.E., F.R.S., Master of Trinity Hall, Cambridge and
T.F. WEST, former Editor-in-Chief, Society of Chemical Industry
HANDBOOK OF ENZYME BIOTECHNOLOGY
Edited by A. WISEMAN, Department of Biochemistry, University of Surrey

BIOCHEMISTRY OF ALCOHOL AND ALCOHOLISM

L. J. KRICKA and P. M. S. CLARK
Department of Clinical Chemistry,
University of Birmingham

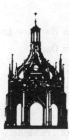

ELLIS HORWOOD LIMITED
Publishers   Chichester

Halsted Press: a division of
JOHN WILEY & SONS
New York - Chichester - Brisbane - Toronto

First published in 1979 by
ELLIS HORWOOD LIMITED
Market Cross House, Cooper Street, Chichester, West Sussex, PO19 1EB, England

The publisher's colophon is reproduced from James Gillison's drawing of the ancient Market Cross, Chichester

Distributors:

Australia, New Zealand, South-east Asia:
Jacaranda-Wiley Ltd., Jacaranda Press,
JOHN WILEY & SONS INC.,
G.P.O. Box 859, Brisbane, Queensland 40001, Australia.

Canada:
JOHN WILEY & SONS CANADA LIMITED
22 Worcester Road, Rexdale, Ontario, Canada.

Europe, Africa:
JOHN WILEY & SONS LIMITED
Baffins Lane, Chichester, West Sussex, England.

North and South America and the rest of the world:
HALSTED PRESS, a division of
JOHN WILEY & SONS
605 Third Avenue, New York, N.Y. 10016, U.S.A.

© 1979 L.J. Kricka and P.M.S. Clark/Ellis Horwood Ltd.

British Library Cataloguing in Publication Data
Kricka, L.J.
Biochemistry of alcohol and alcoholism
(Ellis Horwood Series in Chemical Science)
1. Alcohol in the body
I. Title II. Clark, P.M.S.
615.9'51'31   QP801.A3   79-40252
ISBN 0-85312-131-1 (Ellis Horwood Ltd., Publishers)
ISBN 0-470-26712-7 (Halsted Press)
Typeset in Press Roman by Ellis Horwood Ltd.,
Printed in Great Britain by Biddles of Guildford.

Table of Contents

Preface 11

Abbreviations 13

Chapter 1   Definitions of Alcoholism
1.1   Introduction 15
1.2   Alcohol Dependence and Alcohol-related Disabilities 19
1.3   Conclusions 20
1.4   References 21

Chapter 2   Incidence and Diseases Associated with Alcohol Abuse
2.1   Historical Aspects 22
2.2   Incidence of Alcoholism 23
2.3   Diseases Associated with Alcoholism 26
2.4   Summary 29
2.5   References 29

Chapter 3   Absorption, Excretion and Metabolism of Ethanol
3.1   Introduction 30
3.2   Absorption of Ethanol 31
3.3   Factors Influencing Ethanol Absorption 32
3.4   Endogenous Ethanol 35
3.5   Distribution of Ethanol in Body Fluids 35
3.6   Excretion of Ethanol 37
3.7   Hepatic Metabolism of Ethanol 37
      3.7.1   Alcohol Dehydrogenase 38
      3.7.2   Microsomal Ethanol Oxidising System 40
      3.7.3   Catalase 40
3.8   Factors Influencing Elimination and Metabolism of Ethanol 40
3.9   Summary 45
3.10 References 46

Chapter 4   Congeners in Alcoholic Beverages
    4.1   Introduction. 54
        4.1.1   Definitions. .54
        4.1.2   Origins 55
        4.1.3   Analysis. 55
        4.1.4   Metabolism 55
        4.1.5   Blood and Urine Levels. 56
        4.1.6   Pharmacology and Toxicity. 57
        4.1.7   Pathology 60
        4.1.8   Behaviour 60
    4.2   The Higher Alcohols 61
        4.2.1   Absorption and Metabolism. 61
        4.2.2   Metabolic Effects 61
        4.2.3   Toxicity and Pharmacology. 61
    4.3   Methanol. 62
        4.3.1   Absorption and Metabolism. 62
        4.3.2   Blood Levels. 63
    4.4   Acetaldehyde 64
        4.4.1   Metabolism 64
        4.4.2   Blood Levels and Excretion. 66
        4.4.3   Metabolic Effects 70
        4.4.4   Organ Effects 71
        4.4.5   Miscellaneous Effects 71
    4.5   References. 71

Chapter 5   Biochemical Effects of Alcohol Abuse
    5.1   Introduction. 87
    5.2   Extent and Duration of Ethanol Intake and Previous Experience
           of Ethanol 87
    5.3   Time of Testing. 93
    5.4   Type of Alcoholic Beverage and Congeners. 93
    5.5   Solubility and Solvent Effect of Ethanol 93
    5.6   Nutritional Status 93
    5.7   Endocrine Effects of Ethanol. 100
    5.8   Stress Due to Intoxication. 100
    5.9   Disease Due or Secondary to Alcohol Abuse. 100
    5.10   Genetic Factors. 100
    5.11   Analytical Interferences 100
    5.12   Summary. 100
    5.13   References. 100

Chapter 6 Biochemical Tests for the Detection and Assessment of Alcohol Abuse
6.1   Introduction. 111
6.2   Blood Ethanol and Serum Osmolality 111
6.3   Tests Based on the Altered Hepatic NADH/NAD Ratio. 113
    6.3.1   Blood Lactate/Pyruvate Ratio 113
    6.3.2   Galactose Tolerance Test 114
    6.3.3   Biogenic Amine Metabolites 114
    6.3.4   Steroids. 116
6.4   Plasma Alpha-aminobutyric Acid/leucine Ratio. 116
6.5   Enzymes 119
    6.5.1   Gamma-Glutamyl Transferase (Transpeptidase). 119
    6.5.2   Delta-Aminolaevulinic Acid Dehydratase 124
    6.5.3   Glutamate Dehydrogenase. 124
6.6   Biochemical Profiling Coupled with Pattern Analysis 124
6.7   Serological Markers 128
6.8   Mean Corpuscular Volume 129
6.9   D-Glucaric Acid 130
6.10 Miscellaneous Tests . . . . : . . 130
6.11 Summary. 131
6.12 References. 132

Chapter 7 Effects of Alcohol Intake on Individual Biochemical Parameters
7.1   Introduction. 138
7.2   Water and Electrolytes 138
    7.2.1   Water 138
    7.2.2   Sodium, Potassium and Chloride 139
    7.2.3   Osmolality. 146
    7.2.4   Magnesium. 146
    7.2.5   Calcium. 147
    7.2.6   Zinc 147
    7.2.7   Copper 148
    7.2.8   Phosphate 148
    7.2.9   Iron 150
    7.2.10 Acid Base. 152
7.3   Enzymes 154
    7.3.1   Aspartate and Alanine Aminotransferase 163
    7.3.2   Gamma-Glutamyl Transferase 163
    7.3.3   Alkaline Phosphatase 166
    7.3.4   Creatine Phosphokinase 166
    7.3.5   Lactate Dehydrogenase. 167

7.4　　Proteins. 167
　　　7.4.1　Albumin and Pre-albumin 172
　　　7.4.2　Globulins and Immunoglobulins. 172
　　　7.4.3　Alpha-Foetoprotein. 174
　　　7.4.4　Caeruloplasmin. 174
　　　7.4.5　Carcinoembryonic Antigen 174
　　　7.4.6　Haptoglobin 175
　　　7.4.7　Transferrin. 176
　　　7.4.8　Fibrin 176
　　　7.4.9　Protein Metabolism 176
7.5　　Amino Acids 177
7.6　　Non-Protein Nitrogenous Compounds 179
　　　7.6.1　Urea and Creatinine. 179
　　　7.6.2　Uric Acid. 179
7.7　　Peptide Hormones. 180
　　　　　　Adenohypophyseal Hormones. 182
　　　7.7.1　Growth Hormone 182
　　　7.7.2　Prolactin 184
　　　7.7.3　Follicle-Stimulating Hormone 184
　　　7.7.4　Luteinising Hormone 185
　　　7.7.5　Adrenocorticotropin, Thyrotropin, and Melanocyte-
　　　　　　Stimulating Hormone. 185
　　　　　　Neurohypophyseal Hormones 186
　　　7.7.6　Antidiuretic Hormone 186
　　　7.7.7　Oxytocin. 186
　　　　　　Thyroid and Parathroid Hormones 186
　　　7.7.8　Thyroid Hormones, Parathyroid Hormone and Calcitonin . . .186
　　　　　　Pancreatic Hormones. 186
　　　7.7.9　Insulin. 186
　　　7.7.10　Glucagon. 187
　　　　　　Gastrointestinal Tract Hormones 187
　　　7.7.11　Secretin. 187
　　　7.7.12　Gastrin 187
7.8　　Steroid Hormones, Precursors and Metabolites 188
　　　　　　The Adrenal Cortex. 189
　　　7.8.1　Glucocorticoids. 189
　　　7.8.2　Mineralocorticoids. 195
　　　7.8.3　Sex Hormones 196
7.9　　Bilirubin 200
7.10　Porphyrins and Related Compounds 200
7.11　Carbohydrates 204
　　　7.11.1　Introduction. 204
　　　7.11.2　Biochemistry 205

7.11.3 Clinical Aspects. 207
7.12 Lipids and Lipoproteins 216
7.12.1 Lipoproteins. 217
7.12.2 Blood Lipids. 217
7.12.3 Alcoholic Fatty Liver. 227
7.13 Organic Acids 229
7.13.1 Lactate, Acetoacetate, Beta-Hydroxybutyrate and Pyruvate . 229
7.13.2 Acetate 230
7.13.3 Glucaric Acid 230
7.14 Biologically Active Amines and their Metabolites. 230
7.14.1 Introduction. 230
7.14.2 Serotonin. 230
7.14.3 Catecholamines 232
7.14.4 Condensation Reactions 238
7.14.5 Central Nervous System Amines. 240
7.15 Vitamins 241
7.15.1 Vitamin A 241
7.15.2 Vitamin B_1 242
7.15.3 Vitamin B_2 243
7.15.4 Vitamin B_6 243
7.15.5 Vitamin B_{12} 244
7.15.6 Folic Acid 245
7.15.7 Vitamin C 247
7.15.8 Vitamin D 247
7.15.9 Vitamin E 248
7.15.10 Pantothenic Acid. 248
7.15.11 Niacin 248
7.16 References 248

Appendix. 279

Index 281

Author's Preface

The biochemical disturbances observed in man following long and short term alcohol abuse are complex. The increasing incidence of alcohol abuse and addiction has meant that the clinician and clinical chemist need more than ever to be aware of the range and extent of alterations in biochemical parameters which can occur in people who abuse or have become addicted to alcohol.

Much of the literature on the biochemical disturbances accompanying or resulting from alcohol abuse has been concerned with animal studies. Moreover many of the reports on the subject present conflicting data. The clinician, clinical chemist, or medical student, who wishes to understand or interpret the results of biochemical tests performed on a patient known or suspected of having abused alcohol, is faced with a morass of information and data, much of it being of no direct value in the human situation. This book attempts to outline the salient features of alcohol metabolism and the range of biochemical disturbances which occur in man. The authors acknowledge the important role that animal studies have played in the elucidation of alcohol metabolism, but nevertheless consider that a book restricted soley to human studies would be of considerable value to those workers who are involved in the diagnosis and management of alcohol abuse and addiction.

Birmingham March 1979

L J Kricka
P M S Clark

List of Abbreviations

A	alpha-amino-n-butyric acid
ACTH	adrenocorticotropin or adrenocorticotrophic hormone
ADh	alcohol dehydrogenase
ADH	antidiuretic hormone
AFP	alpha-foetoprotein
ALA	delta-aminolaevulinic acid
AlaT	alanine aminotransferase
AMP	adenosine-5'-phosphate
cAMP	adenosine-3', 5'-cyclic phosphate
AP	alkaline phosphatase
AspT	aspartate aminotransferase
ATP	adenosine 5'-triphosphate
CEA	carcinoembryonic antigen
CK	creatine phosphokinase
CNS	central nervous system
CoA	coenzyme A
CRF	corticotrophin releasing factor
csf	cerebrospinal fluid
DHA	dehydroepiandrosterone
DHAS	dehydroepiandrosterone sulphate
2,3-DPG	2,3-diphosphoglycerate
ECW	extra-cellular water
FFA	free fatty acid
FIGLU	formiminoglutamate
FMN	flavin mononucleotide
FSH	follicle-stimulating hormone
GABA	gamma-aminobutyric acid
GLDH	glutamate dehydrogenase
GGT	gamma-glutamyl-transferase
GH	growth hormone

GIT	gastro-intestinal tract
GSH	glutathione (reduced form)
GSSG	glutathione
HCG	human chorionic gonadotrophin
HDL	high density lipoprotein
5-HIAA	5-hydroxyindole-3-acetic acid
HVA	homovanillic acid
ICD	isocitrate dehydrogenase
ICW	intra-cellular water
IU	international unit(s)
i.v.	intra venous
Km	Michaelis-Menten constant
L	leucine
LCAT	lecithin cholesterol acyltransferase
LDH	lactate dehydrogenase
LDL	low density lipoprotein
LH	luteinising hormone
LHRH	luteinising hormone-releasing hormone
MAO	monoamine oxidase
MCV	mean corpuscular volume
MEOS	mitochondrial ethanol oxidising system
MHPG	3-methoxy-4-hydroxy phenylethylene glycol
MSH	melanocyte-stimulating hormone
NAD	nicotinamide adenine dinucleotide
NADII	nicotinamide adenine dinucleotide (reduced form)
NADP	nicotinamide-adenine dinucleotide phosphate
NADPH	nicotinamide-adenine dinucleotide phosphate (reduced form)
OCT	ornithine carbamoyl transferase
OD	ornithine dehydrogenase
Pa	Pascal
PBG	porphobilinogen
SDH	sorbitol dehydrogenase
SHBG	sex hormone binding globulin
TBW	total body water
TCA	tricarboxylic acid
THF	tetrahydrofolate
TRH	thyrotropin-releasing hormone
TSH	thyroid-stimulating hormone or thyrotropin
UDP	uridine-5′-pyrophosphate
VLDL	very low density lipoprotein
VMA	3-methoxy-4-hydroxy mandelic acid
WBC	white blood cell(s)

CHAPTER 1

Definitions of Alcoholism

1.1 INTRODUCTION†

There are as many definitions of alcoholism as there are types of alcoholics. This has led to some confusion: what one person would call alcoholic, another would not. In an attempt to overcome the problems associated with the term 'alcoholism', workers have used other words to describe the 'alcoholic' e.g.: alcohol-dependent, addicted, problem drinker, etc. This chapter deals with the difficulties of defining alcoholism and outlines the relative advantages and disadvantages of the various definitions.

The main problem in defining the 'alcoholic' is that an alcoholic is a member of a heterogeneous population afflicted with an ailment that is multifactorial in origin. Alcoholism cannot be compartmentalised for several reasons. Firstly, there are many facets of alcoholism: biochemical, psychiatric, moral, sociological and legal. One view might prefer definitions based on observable consequences which result from uncontrolled drinking, such as increasing problems with health, work, and social life, whilst another view might be based on the quantity of alcohol drunk (See Fig. 1.1).

Secondly, there are many patterns of alcoholism. Many people believe that alcoholics are all down-and-outs or Skid Row drinkers. This is not so. Alcohol use and abuse cover a spectrum of drinking. At one extreme of the spectrum there is the teetotaller who never drinks alcohol or the person who drinks socially. Then there are excessive drinkers who have personal and medical problems but who are not necessarily alcoholics. At the other end of the spectrum there are those who are addicted to alcohol and who may also suffer physical, mental and sociological damage (Kessel and Walton, 1965; Forrest, 1975). In defining alcoholism, one is taking a point in this spectrum and saying that up to this point drinking is normal, but beyond it is abnormal. In reality this is impossible, as so many factors will influence one's concept of normal/abnormal drinking. Social and cultural factors influence attitudes to alcohol use

†Ethanol and alcohol are used interchangeably in this book.

and abuse. It is possible to classify cultures in relation to their drinking practices and attitudes. There may be four classes (O'Conner, 1977).

(i) *Abstinent Cultures.* Here the use of alcohol is prohibited. Such cultures, occur in many countries, or among religious groups, for example Christian Scientists, Seventh Day Adventists. Whilst normal drinking is rare, and since there are no norms for drinking, alcoholism is likely.

(ii) *Ambivalent Cultures.* Contradictory attitudes to alcohol exist within the same society. Thus the culture may have no inbuilt controls, and the individual is in a situation of ambivalence which may lead to alcoholism. Such cultures exist in Ireland and the United States.

(iii) *Permissive Cultures.* Favourable attitudes to alcohol exist, but drunkenness and other alcohol-associated deviant behaviour are frowned upon. Spanish and Italian cultures show these characteristics.

(iv) *Over-permissive Cultures.* Here favourable attitudes exist both to drinking and drunkenness, as illustrated by the culture of France. The Anglo-Saxons may represent a culture in transition from a permissive to an over-permissive culture.

Patterns of use of alcohol in different cultures and hence abuse, will vary. In France drinking throughout the day and at meal times is common. Intoxication is at least tolerable and at most humorous and associated with virility. On the other hand Italians, who also drink wine, drink mainly at meal times and regard drunkenness as a disgrace. Thus different patterns of alcohol use exist in these countries and a person designated a problem drinker in one, might not be in another.

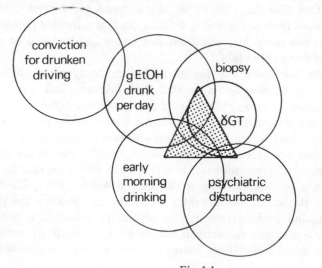

Fig. 1.1
Defining alcoholism: The use of different parameters in defining a multifactorial problem.

Researchers have therefore tried to pinpoint more accurately what is meant by normal drinking and from there to decide what is abnormal. This has been done by considering daily intake of alcohol. The ranges of ethanol intake per day thought to be consistent with 'moderate drinking', and 'heavy drinking' or 'alcoholic drinking' are shown in Tables 1.1 and 1.2. These show what enormous variation exists from country to country, in the amount which is considered to be excessive (Lelbach, 1974).

Whilst attitudes and quantities of alcohol drunk do vary from culture to culture, there is also great variation in concepts of normality within a society. Thus parental and peer group factors influence our attitudes. The task of defining the alcoholic is difficult. It is further complicated by variations in drinking patterns within society and over a period of time in a given individual. These variations have given rise to such terms as 'heavy', 'moderate', 'social', 'spree', 'Skid Row' and 'binge' drinker. It would appear, therefore, difficult if not impossible to define normal and abnormal drinking, and hence to define the alcoholic. In an attempt to overcome these problems, workers in the field have tried to distinguish between alcohol dependence and alcohol related disabilities (WHO, 1977). Such an approach is thought to overcome many of these problems, and together with other definitions of alcoholism is considered in more detail later.

Table 1.1
Range of ethanol intake per day thought to be consistent with 'drinking in moderation'.
(Reproduced by permission from Lelbach 1974 In *Res. Adv. in Alcohol and Drug Problems,* John Wiley & Sons Inc.)

Definition of Drinking Habits	Equivalent to Grams of Ethanol per Day (if daily consumption is assumed)	Country
Alcohol 'users'	(a) <5.8 g	USA
	(b) >5.8 g	
Moderate use	7–18 g	USA
Moderate consumer	8–12 g	Sweden
Regular light drinker	9 g	England
Moderate steady drinker	18 g	
Moderate use	17–21 g	West Germany
Moderate alcohol intake	47–75 g (20% of total calories)	USA
Moderate drinking	Less than 80 g	Chile
Moderate use to Moderate drinking	Less than 80 g	Switzerland
Moderate drinking	Up to 80 g	Chile

Table 1.2
Range of ethanol intake per day found in 'heavy drinkers' or 'alcoholics'.
(Reproduced by permission from Lelbach 1974 In *Res. Adv. in Alcohol and Drug Problems*, John Wiley & Sons Inc.)

Definition of Drinking Habits	Beverage	Equivalent to Grams of Ethanol per Day (if daily consumption is assumed)	Country
'Strong consumer'	Spirits	33 g or more	Norway
Considerable consumption	Beer, wine	40 g	Switzerland
Excessive consumption	Beer, wine; whiskey	>21–45 g	USA
Alcoholics, moderate drinking	–	Not more than 50–60 g	USA
Alcoholic	Beer, wine; whiskey	>50–75 g	USA
Alcoholic	Beer, wine; spirits (for several years)	>80 g	Switzerland
Continuous drinking	Wine	>80 g	Chile
Continuous drinking		Daily up to inebriation	
Alcoholic	Wine	>80 g	Chile
Heavy drinker	Saké (15.5% v/v)	>66–110 g	Japan
Alcoholics, excessive drinking	Beer, wine; spirits	>100 g	Australia
High consumption	Beer or equivalent	72–135 g	Australia
Very high consumption		>135 g	
Alcoholic	Beer, wine	>60–120 g	Austria
Alcoholic	Wine or equivalent	>120 g	West Germany
Alcoholic	Wine or equivalent	>120 g	West Germany
Excessive drinking	Beer, wine; spirits	80–120 g (multiplied by 2 to 3)	Austria
High alcohol consumption	Beer, wine	>120 g	Australia
Alcoholic	Beer, wine; spirits	>120 g (plus once/twice weekly consid. more)	South Germany
Average alcoholic	Beer; wine; spirits	160 g	Sweden
Chronic alcohol abuse	Wine	>160 g	Italy
Chronic excessive	Whiskey or equivalent	>160–188 g	USA
Average chronic alcoholic	Wine; spirits	176 ± 132 g ($\bar{x}$ ± 2s)	Switzerland
Chronic alcoholics	Beer; must, wine; spirits	Average: 180 g	West Germany
Chronic alcoholic	Wine	Average: 180 g	Italy (Alto Adige)
Heavy drinking	Absolute alcohol	160–240 g	Switzerland
Excessive drinking		>240 g	
'Terrain éthylique'	Absolute alcohol	160–240 g	France
Alcoholic	Whiskey	80–376 g	USA
'Active alcoholic'	Whiskey	160–300 g (up to terminal illness)	USA
Heavy drinker	Spirits	Up to 320–400 g	Sweden

1.2 ALCOHOL DEPENDENCE AND ALCOHOL-RELATED DISABILITIES (WHO, 1977)

(i) *'An alcohol related disability* is deemed to exist when there is an impairment in the physical, mental or social functioning of an individual, of such nature that it may be reasonably inferred that alcohol is part of the causal nexus determining that disability'.

Such disabilities are discussed more fully in Chapter 2.

(ii) *'The alcohol dependence syndrome* is manifested by alterations at the behavioural, subjective and psychobiological levels with, as a leading symptom, an impaired control over intake of the drug ethyl alcohol. The alcohol dependence syndrome exists in degrees. Its varied manifestations are influenced by modifying personal and environmental factors so as to give many different presentations'.

'Not all people manifesting alcohol-related disabilities are alcohol-dependent, but they may be at increased risk of developing alcohol dependence'.

An approach to alcoholism which distinguishes between dependency and disability has several advantages. It emphasises that a person might suffer harm due to alcohol without being addicted to the drug whilst also allowing for the numerous factors that will influence the dependence syndrome itself.

This report avoids the problems of defining alcoholism by realising that alcohol abuse is not an all-or-nothing response. There have been several attempts in the past to define alcoholism more closely. In criticising these, the advantages of not using the term alcoholism became apparent.

(i) *World Health Organisation (1952)* defines alcoholics as 'Those excessive drinkers whose dependence on alcohol has attained such a degree that it shows a noticeable mental disturbance or an interference with their bodily and mental health, their interpersonal relations, and their smooth social and economic functioning; or who show the prodromal signs of such development. They therefore require treatment'.

Whilst such a definition is suitably broad and emphasises the various influencing factors in alcoholism, such as interpersonal relations, and social and economic functioning, it has several disadvantages. The definition is long and cumbersome, and it relies on the use of the word 'excessive'. Thus there remains the problem of defining excessive drinking which has been discussed previously. (Seeley, 1959; Edwards, 1967).

(ii) *National Council on Alcoholism/American Medical Society on Alcoholism Committee of Definitions.* 'Alcoholism is a chronic, progressive, and potentially fatal disease. It is characterised by tolerance and physical dependency or pathologic organ changes or both - all the direct or indirect consequences of the alcohol ingested' (Seixas *et al.*, 1976).

Such a definition might be useful in describing extreme forms of alcohol abuse but it fails to point out that alcoholism is just one end of a spectrum, and that problems associated with alcohol may occur before dependency. This definition emphasises the physical aspects of alcoholism without mentioning pyschological, social and economic factors.

(iii) *Jellinek (1960)* in a classic paper described five different types of alcoholic disease. These are called Alpha, Beta, Gamma, Delta and Epsilon Alcoholism.

Alpha Alcoholism. A purely psychological, continual dependence or reliance upon the effect of alcohol to relieve emotional or bodily pain. This is not undisciplined drinking and does not lead to an inability to abstain. Damage caused by this type of drinking is restricted to inter-personal relationships.

Beta Alcoholism. This type of alcoholism leads to the development of alcohol-related pathologies, e.g. cirrhosis, polyneuropathy, gastritis; but there is no physical or psychological dependence upon alcohol.

Gamma Alcoholism. In this type of alcoholism there is an acquired increased tissue tolerance to alcohol, adaptive cell metabolism, withdrawal symptoms and physical dependence, and loss of control (i.e. inability to stop once drinking has started).

Delta Alcoholism. Delta alcoholism has all the features of gamma alcoholism except that, instead of loss of control, there is an inability to abstain from alcohol.

Epsilon Alcoholism. This is an intermittent form of alcoholism characterised by periodic loss of control.

A similar classification *(Episodic Excessive Drinking; Habitual Excessive drinking* and *Alcohol Addiction)* has been drawn up by the American Psychiatric Association (1968).

Whilst the disease concept of alcoholism has many benefits and has removed much of the stigma associated wth alcohol abuse, the classification into types does have disadvantages. Jellinek's work emphasises the many patterns of alcohol drinking that occur, but it does tend to lead to compartmentalization, whereas in fact little is gained by giving such a specific label.

The daily amount of alcohol ingested has also been used as a means of differentiating various drinking patterns, drinking in moderation being equated with an alcohol intake of less than 80 grammes of ethanol[†] per day.

Heavy drinkers and alcoholics would be those persons whose ethanol intake was greater than 176-220 grammes of ethanol per day. There are difficulties with such a definition as the amount of alcohol drunk per day varies with occasion and culture. Individual tolerances vary also.

1.3 CONCLUSIONS

There are many definitions of alcoholism reflecting the difficulties associated with describing a phenomenon in which social, psychological and physical

---

[†]Average ethanol content of alcoholic beverages: beer (4% v/v) 31.8g/1; wine (10% v/v) 79.3g/1; fortified wines (15–20% v/v) 119-158.7 g/1; spirits (38–50 v/v) 301.6-306.9 g/1 (70° proof UK is equivalent to 40% v/v).

factors play varying parts. A broad approach is required and perhaps a useful one is that of the WHO which does not attempt to define either normal or abnormal drinking. The problem is discussed in terms of alcohol related disability and dependence. Keeping this in mind, perhaps the most useful concise definition of alcoholism is that of Davies (1973): 'the intermittent or continual ingestion of alcohol leading to dependency or harm'. This shows that a variety of drinking patterns may be involved and distinguishes between the two effects of alcohol; dependency and harm which may co-exist or occur separately. Whilst this is a useful starting point in the study of alcoholism it should not deter the researcher, particularly the biochemist, from stating the parameters used in the selection of subjects.

1.4 REFERENCES

American Psychiatric Association. (1968) *Diagnostic and statistical manual of Mental Disorders.* 2nd ed. Washington, D.C.

Davies, D. L. (1973) Implications for medical practice of an acceptable concept of alcoholism. *In* alcoholism – A medical profile. Proceedings 1st International Federal Conference on Alcoholism. London. Ed., K., Kessell, Hawker A., and Chalke, M., Edsall., B. London.

Edwards, G. (1967) The meaning and treatment of alcohol dependence. *Hosp. Med.,* 2, 272.

Forrest, G. G. (1975) *In* The Diagnosis and Treatment of Alcoholism. pp. 11-22, pp. 5-10. Charles C. Thomas, Springfield, Illinois.

Jellinek, E. M. (1960) *In* The Disease Concept of Alcoholism. New Haven, Conneticut. College and University Press in association with Hillhouse Press, New Brunswick, N. J.

Kessel, N., and Walton, H. (1965) *In* Alcoholism. Penguin Books.

Lelbach, W. K. (1974) Organic pathology related to volume and pattern of alcohol use. *Res. Adv. Alcohol and Drug Problems,* 1, 93-198.

O'Connor, J. (1977) Social and cultural factors influencing drinking habits. *In* Aspects of Alcoholism. The Alcohol Education Centre, London.

Seeley, J. R. (1959) The W.H.O. definition of alcoholism. *Q. J. Stud. Alcohol,* 20, 352-356.

Seixas, F. A., Blume, S., Cloud, L. A., Lieber, C. S., and Simpson, R. K. (1976) Definitions of Alcoholism. *Ann. Intern. Med.,* 85, 764.

World Health Organization (1952) *Tech. Rep. Ser.,* No. 48.

World Health Organization (1977) Report of a W.H.O. group of investigators on criteria for identifying and clarifying disabilities related to alcohol consumption. W.H.O. Offset publications No. 32.

CHAPTER 2

Incidence and Diseases Associated with Alcohol Abuse

Extensive and prolonged ingestion of alcohol is injurious to health but, despite this, alcohol abuse and addiction are growing and constitute serious problems in many communities. The social and economic damage caused by alcohol in terms of human relationships, damage to life and property, and absenteeism is immense. The economic cost of alcohol abuse and alcoholism in America in 1971 was estimated to be in excess of 25 billion dollars. Lost industrial production and medical costs together accounted for more than half of this total. An indication of the magnitude of the social problems associated with alcohol abuse may be obtained by examining the figures for drunkenness and drunk in charge offences. In England and Wales convictions for drunkenness offences have risen from 157 to 276 per 100,000 during the period 1955-1975, whilst convictions for drinking and driving and drunk in charge offences have risen from 49.4 to 153.6 per 100,000 during the seven year period between 1968 and 1975.

2.1 HISTORICAL ASPECTS

It is likely that alcoholic beverages were known to man as much as 100,000 years ago. Such beverages probably arose from natural fermentation of grapes, grain or honey during storage in pottery jars or rock cavities. Neolithic man some 8,000 years ago certainly made wines as judged from the discovery of packed grape seeds in his rubbish dumps. Some anthropologists have even suggested that early Stone Age agricultural settlements arose from a need to make wine rather than grow food. In ancient Egypt wine was known as far back as the fifth and fourth millenium B.C.

The Bible has numerous references to wine, beginning with Noah:

'Noah was the first tiller of the soil.
He planted a vineyard; and he drank of
the wine, and became drunk, and lay
uncovered in his tent . . .'

Genesis 9:20–1

The role played in society by alcoholic beverages, especially wine, has undergone profound changes since earliest times. Originally wine was a scarce commodity and the privilege of the few. The use of wine was intimately linked with early religion and religious rites. Red wine is reminescent of blood, and cuneiform writing on tablets at Erach in the Persian Gulf mention the use of wine for sacremental purposes. Although wine still fulfills a religious role it is now, like other alcoholic beverages, no longer the privilege of the few, being relatively cheap, plentiful and readily available in most parts of the world.

Drinking and the subsequent problems of intoxication and drunkenness have been a feature of many civilisations. Early Egyptian frescoes and hieroglyphic texts depict and describe scenes of drunkenness. An Egyptian legend tells of the goddess Hathor whom the god Ra sent as a vengeance on rebellious mankind. Hathor slew them without mercy and was only stopped when Ra poured beer over the earth and Hathor drinking it became drunk and 'recognised mankind no longer'. The Greeks also had a wine god, Dionysus, who was honoured in drunken orgies which later gave way to wine festivals called Dionysia. A parallel development was the 'symposia', which was a drinking party. By 400 B.C. social drinking had become an established feature of Greek life. In Western Civilisation alcohol has also been a feature of daily life. Alcoholism and drunkenness were rife in Victorian England, alcohol consumption reaching a peak in the mid-1870's. Alcohol abuse has continued to be a major problem up to modern times and there is no sign of a fall in its prevalence.

2.2 INCIDENCE OF ALCOHOLISM

Despite legislation limiting the sale of alcohol and penalising the alcohol intoxicated person the incidence of alcoholism has risen. In England and Wales the incidence is approximately 1100 per 100,000 adults, males being particularly affected. This is however not as serious as the incidence in America, approximately 4400 per 100,000 and the incidence in France 5000-7000 per 100,000.

There are several sources of information available for the estimation of the prevalence of alcoholism, and all suffer from one disadvantage or another. Yet the accurate determination of incidence is essential in order to assess, for example, the efficiency of treatment. The following methods have been used:

Surveys and interviews. These are usually small and may exclude the homeless or those in institutions. It has been suggested that such surveys reveal only 20-70% of national consumption.

Alcohol Consumption Statistics. Government figures of total consumption of alcoholic beverages show an increase in recent years and may parallel the increase in alcoholism. Total consumption of alcoholic beverages in the United Kingdom has shown a dramatic increase during the period 1955-1975 (Figs. 2.1, 2.2, and 2.3.) Consumption of beer has increased by 47%, spirits by 156% and wine by a staggering 314%. Such figures may, however, exclude imports and home brewing.

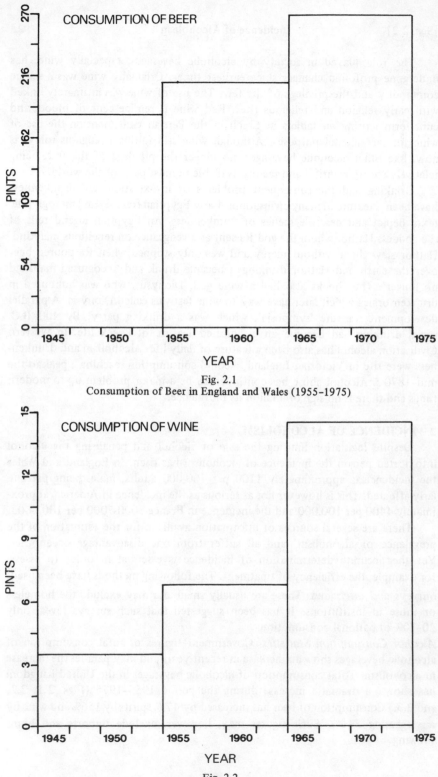

Fig. 2.1
Consumption of Beer in England and Wales (1955–1975)

Fig. 2.2
Consumption of Wine in England and Wales (1955–1975)

CONSUMPTION OF SPIRITS

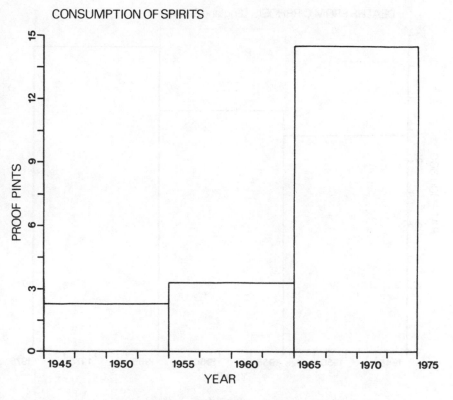

Fig. 2.3
Consumption of Spirits in England and Wales (1955–1975)

Law enforcement. Arrests, reports and convictions for alcohol-related offences such as a drunken driving, breach of the peace and being drunk and disorderly may indicate the extent of alcoholism in a community. However, such figures reflect current law and the degree to which such law is enforced may vary considerably.

Clinical records. These tend to be inaccurate in that only a minority of alcoholics (11–25%) are in contact with official agencies. This method may grossly under-estimate the prevalence of alcoholism.

Liver cirrhosis mortality rates. Such a figure indicates retrospectively the incidence of alcoholism (statistics for deaths in England and Wales due to alcohol cirrhosis are shown in Fig. 2.4). The relationship between liver disease and alcoholism may vary from country to country and with time. It should also be realised that only a minority of alcoholics (approximately 12%) develop liver cirrhosis.

DEATHS FROM CIRRHOSIS (England & Wales)

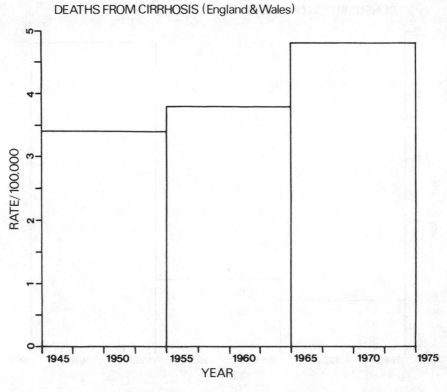

Fig. 2.4
Deaths from Cirrhosis in England and Wales (1955–1975)

It can therefore be seen that it is difficult to obtain accurate figures of the incidence of alcoholism. An increasing awareness of the problems and changes in criteria for diagnosis may in part contribute to the reported increase in alcoholism over the past few years. It seems likely, though, that there has been a real increase in alcoholism and alcohol-related problems, particularly among women and children.

2.3 DISEASES ASSOCIATED WITH ALCOHOLISM
Alcohol abuse is associated with a wide variety of psychiatric and physical illnesses. Amongst the more commonly encountered conditions are acute alcohol intoxication, psychoses, delirium tremens, malnourishment, malabsorption, liver disease and sexual dysfunction. In some cases it is difficult to ascertain the exact relationship between disease and alcohol abuse, for example psychiatric illness may predispose to alcoholism and *vice versa*.

The death rate amongst alcoholics is higher than in the general population. This is particularly marked in the younger groups, especially amongst females (Table 2.1).

Table 2.1
Overall Mortality in Alcoholics in England and Wales (1953-1974)

Age Group	Males	Females
	(ratio of observed to expected deaths[†])	
15-39	11.5	17.4
40-59	3.3	4.9
60 and over	1.2	1.9

†Death rate in alcoholics compared with expected number of deaths if alcoholics had the same death rate as the respective male and female population of England and Wales

In the older age groups the death rate approaches that of the general population. One problem with such statistical data is that it may under-estimate deaths due to alcoholism. Under-reporting of deaths due to alcoholism occurs because of the stigma associated with alcoholism, unawareness of previous alcoholism in the deceased, or uncertainty of the relationship of alcoholism to the cause of death.

Depressive or manic-depressive psychosis is the psychiatric illness most closely linked with alcoholism. In 1975 more than 7% of admissions to psychiatric hospitals in England and Wales were due to alcoholism or alcoholic psychosis. Suicide and self-inflicted injuries are more prevalent in alcoholics than in the general population by a factor of approximately 20. Disease of the digestive system (e.g. liver disease, pancreatitis, and gastritis) are amongst the most commonly encountered diseases in alcoholics. Table 2.2 presents ratios of observed to expected deaths due to various causes amongst alcoholics. In some cases alcohol abuse has been shown to be the prime causative factor, whereas other diseases encountered in alcoholics may be secondary to alcohol abuse, e.g. due to malnutrition.

The influence of the extent and duration of alcohol abuse as a causative factor of a disease is best exemplified by the incidence of liver dysfunction in heavy drinkers and alcoholics (Table 2.3). In those people consuming less than 160 g ethanol per day an increase in the duration of drinking from 3.5 to 21 years leads to three-fold increase in the number of cases of liver dysfunction. Consumption of more than 160 g of alcohol per day, however, causes a massive rise in the incidence of liver dysfunction, from 11% to 73% for those persons whose average duration of drinking was 3.5 years and approximately 21 years, respectively.

Table 2.2

Mortality by Cause Amongst Alcoholics in England and Wales (1953-1974)

	Males	*Females*
	(ratio of observed to	
Cause	expected deaths)	
Infective and Parasitic Diseases	5.05	2.86
Neoplasms	1.17	1.75
Mental Disorders	27.08	28.57
Disease of the Circulatory System	1.30	1.53
Diseases of the Respiratory System	2.70	4.61
Diseases of the Digestive System	6.78	7.18
(Liver, gall bladder and pancreatic disease	15.08	19.18)
Accidents, Poisoning and Violence	14.13	17.81
Other causes	1.54	2.12

Table 2.3

Influence of Extent and Duration of Alcohol Abuse on Liver Dysfunction
Adapted from Lelbach (1974)

		BELOW 160g ethanol/day		ABOVE 160g ethanol/day	
Group	Duration years	Number of cases	% of cases with Liver Dysfunction	Number of cases	% of cases with Liver Dysfunction
1	3.5 ± 1.3	74	6	55	11
2	7.8 ± 1.4	76	16	79	37
3	12.8 ± 1.5	30	17	64	40
4	21.1 ± 5.4	6	17	33	73

In comparison with liver disease and diseases of the digestive system the increased mortality in alcoholics due to other diseases is not very great. An increased incidence of neoplasms especially carcinoma of the larynx, pharynx and oesophagus, does occur in alcoholics but this may be due to the fact that many alcoholics are also smokers. Likewise alcoholism carries only a moderately increased risk of circulatory system disease. Alcohol is known to be a cardiotoxin but thiamine deficiency (beri beri heart) and other components of alcoholic beverages, e.g. cobalt (cobalt cardiomyopathy), can also cause heart disease.

The diseases encountered in alcoholics may complicate the results of biochemical tests on alcoholics and can also complicate tests for alcoholism. These problems are dealt with in greater detail in Chapters 5 and 6.

2.4 SUMMARY

The incidence of alcoholism has continued to rise over the last decade, with deleterious social and economic consequences. In comparison with other drugs alcohol is relatively inexpensive and has gained a considerable degree of social acceptability. Perhaps the most alarming and far-reaching aspect of the incidence of alcohol abuse is the finding that a younger and younger age group is experimenting with and abusing alcohol. If this trend is continued it can only lead to an increase in the number of people requiring treatment for alcoholism and alcohol related pathologies.

2.5 REFERENCES

Adelson, A., and White, G. (1976) Alcoholism and mortality. *Population Trends,* **6,** 7-13.

Advisory Committee on Alcoholism (1978) *In* The Pattern and Range of Services for Problem Drinkers. H.M.S.O., London.

Donnan, S., and Haskey, J. (1977) Alcoholism and cirrhosis of the liver. *Populations Trends,* **7,** 18-24.

Finnish Foundation for Alcohol Studies and WHO Regional Office Europe (1977) *In* International Statistics on Alcoholic Beverages, Akateeminen Kirjakauppa, Helsinki.

Hawker, A. (1978) *In* Adolescents and Alcohol. B. Edsall & Co. Ltd., London.

Kessel, N., and Walton, H. (1965) *In* Alcoholism. Penguin Books.

Lelbach, W. K. (1974) Organic pathology related to volume and pattern of alcohol use. *Res. Adv. Alcohol Drub Probs.,* **1,** 93-198.

Lieber, C. S. (*ed.*) (1977) *In* Metabolic Aspects of Alcoholism. MTP Press Ltd., Lancaster.

Kissin, B., and Begleiter, H. (1974) *In* The Biology of Alcoholism. Vol. 3. Plenum Press.

Mowat, N. A. G., and Brunt, P. W. (1976) Alcohol and the gastrointestinal tract. *Res. Adv. Gastroenterol,* **3,** 150-177.

United States Department of Health, Education and Welfare (1974) *In* Alcohol and Health. U.S. Government Printing Office, Washington D.C.

Wilkins, R. H. (1974) *In* The Hidden Alcoholic in General Practice. Elek Science, London.

CHAPTER 3

Absorption, Excretion and Metabolism of Ethanol

3.1 INTRODUCTION

Ethanol is a polar substance which is completely miscible with water. The small size and weak charge of the molecule enable it to diffuse easily through cell membranes, transfer occurring by a process of simple passive diffusion.

Metabolism of ethanol occurs principally in the liver where the zinc-containing metallo-enzyme alcohol dehydrogenase (ADh), located in the cytosol of the hepatocyte, oxidises ethanol to acetaldehyde. Ethanol may also be oxidised to acetaldehyde by a microsomal ethanol oxidising system (MEOS) and possibly by the enzyme catalase located in peroxisomes. Acetaldehyde produced by oxidation of ethanol is further oxidised to acetate by a cytoplasmic aldehyde dehydrogenase. About 75% of ethanol taken up by the liver is released as acetate into the circulation (Lundquist *et al.*, 1962). Acetate is then oxidised to carbon dioxide *via* the citric acid cycle (Krebs or tricarboxylic acid cycle). Alternatively acetyl CoA, an activated form of acetate and a key intermediary metabolite can undergo reaction to form fatty acids, ketone bodies, amino acids, and steroids (Fig. 3.1).

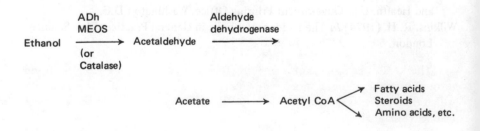

Fig.3.1 — Metabolism of ethanol

Numerous books, reviews, and articles have presented detailed accounts of both human and animal studies of ethanol absorption and metabolism.[†] This chapter, however, is restricted to human studies.

3.2 ABSORPTION OF ETHANOL

Ethanol is readily absorbed unchanged from the gastrointestinal tract from where it diffuses rapidly and uniformly throughout the body water (Fig. 3.2). Absorption occurs along the whole length of the gastrointestinal tract, but mainly from the duodenum and jejunum and to a lesser extent from the stomach and large intestine (Kalant, 1971). Ethanol can also be absorbed when administered *per rectum* (Mardones, 1963). In contrast, the absorption of ethanol from the mouth is minimal. A further route of ethanol absorption into the blood is by inhalation of vapour and by passage across the pulmonary epithelium (Gibson, 1975). At levels of 103–140 p.p.m. approximately 14% of inspired ethanol is retained (Nomiyama and Nomiyama, 1974a, 1974b). Ethanol may also be absorbed into the blood by any parenteral route, e.g., intra-peritoneal, intrathecal, or subarachnoid injection.

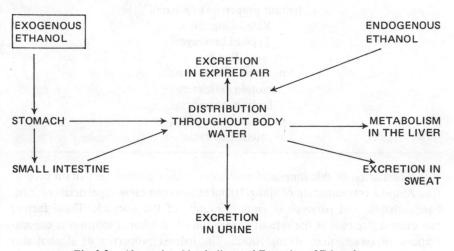

Fig. 3.2 – Absorption, Metabolism and Excretion of Ethanol

The keratin layer of skin is impermeable to ethanol, and hence absorption through intact skin does not occur. Similarly, the urinary bladder is impermeable which thus prevents reabsorption of any ethanol contained in urine stored in the bladder (Kalant, 1971).

[†]Books, reviews, and articles which have appeared since 1965 dealing with the metabolism and absorption of ethanol are identified by asterisks* in the list of references at the end of this chapter.

3.3 FACTORS INFLUENCING ETHANOL ABSORPTION

The absorption of ethanol is influenced by a large number of factors (National Centre etc., 1968; Kalant, 1971) and these are listed in Table 3.1.

Since ethanol is absorbed by a process of simple diffusion, the higher the concentration of ethanol the greater the resulting concentration gradient and the more rapid the absorption—for example the mean amount of ethanol absorbed from a test meal introduced into the stomach *via* a gastric tube increases as the concentration of ethanol in the test meal increases. At concentrations of 7.9 and 55.8 mg/ml the mean amount of ethanol absorbed from the test meals was approximately 850 and 5500 mg, respectively (Cooke and Birchall, 1969). In addition, any factor which serves to maintain the concentration gradient, such as rapid removal of ethanol from the site of absorption by an efficient blood flow, will also promote absorption.

Table 3.1
Factors Affecting Ethanol Absorption

Concentration of ethanol
Blood flow at site of absorption
Irritant properties of ethanol
Rate of ingestion
Type of beverage
Food
Emptying of the stomach
Protein deficiency
Body temperature
Physical exercise
Menstrual cycle

A limitation of this simplistic mechanism is that ethanol has irritant properties. Above a concentration of 30mg/100ml ethanol can cause superficial erosions, haemorrhages, and paralysis of smooth muscle of the stomach. These factors can cause a decrease in the rate of absorption of an ethanol solution at concentrations of greater than 30 mg/100ml. The irritant properties of alcohol also limit absorption by inhalation, the maximum tolerable concentration in inspired air being 20 mg per litre of air (Kalant, 1971). The rate of ingestion of ethanol also affects absorption. Peak blood alcohol levels develop more slowly if a beverage is ingested rapidly (Payne *et al.*, 1966; Moskowitz and Burns, 1976). However, peak blood ethanol levels are higher if a given dose of alcohol is ingested as a single dose rather than in a small doses. This is presumably because the ethanol concentration gradient is higher in the former case than in the later.

Absorption of ethanol is retarded by the chemicals other than ethanol (congeners) in alcoholic beverages (see Chapter 4). The ethanol in distilled spirits is absorbed much more rapidly than the ethanol contained in wines and beers, even when the beverages are diluted to the same alcohol concentration. Substances in alcoholic beverages responsible for the retardation of absorption and the mechanism by which the retardation occurs have not been identified. The presence of food in the stomach delays gastric emptying and thus reduces the rate and efficiency of absorption of ethanol. The longer the time interval between eating and drinking the less the retardation of absorption. Ingestion of food either accompanied or preceded by a dose of ethanol has been shown to decrease peak ethanol concentrations and increase the time taken to reach peak concentrations compared to ingestion on an empty stomach (Lin *et al.*, 1976; Wilkinson *et al.*, 1977).

A larger amount of food has a greater effect on the absorption of ethanol than a little food, and the type of food is also important. Welling and co-workers (1977) have shown that at low doses of ethanol (0.2ml of 99% ethanol/kg body weight), when there are no problems of delayed stomach emptying or decreased absorption due to gastric irritation, food has a dramatic effect on serum ethanol levels. Inhibition of ethanol absorption by foods in order of increasing effectiveness was high protein, high fat, and foods with a high carbohydrate content.

Foods with a high carbohydrate content inhibited ethanol absorption compared to the fasted state to such an extent that in three of the six subjects tested extremely low levels of ethanol were recorded (Fig. 3.3). The mechanism of the inhibition of ethanol absorption by food is not known.

Rapid emptying of the stomach, e.g. in the 'dumping syndrome', promotes ethanol absorption. Similarly in patients who have undergone gastrectomy, absorption of ethanol is very rapid since the absence of the stomach allows the ethanol to reach the highly absorptive jejunum and duodenum more quickly.

Various other factors affect the rate of alcohol absorption by altering either gastrointestinal mobility or the circulation. Absorption is increased in protein deficiency states, following insulin induced hypoglycaemia, ingestion of cholinergic drugs, at elevated body temperatures or following previous ingestion of water. The last factor acts presumably by emptying the stomach of mucus and residual food.

Decreased absorption occurs with decreasing body temperature, following mental or physical exercise, and under the action of anti-cholinergic and sympathomimetic drugs. The decreased rate of absorption following physical exercise is possibly due to changes in the splanchnic circulation from the gastrointestinal tract (Krebs *et al.*, 1969).

There are several complicating factors in the study of ethanol absorption. Great intra-individual variation in the percentage dose of ethanol absorbed has been found (Wagner and Patel, 1972) and variations in hormonal status, e.g. stage of the menstrual cycle, have also been shown to affect ethanol absorption (Jones and Jones, 1975).

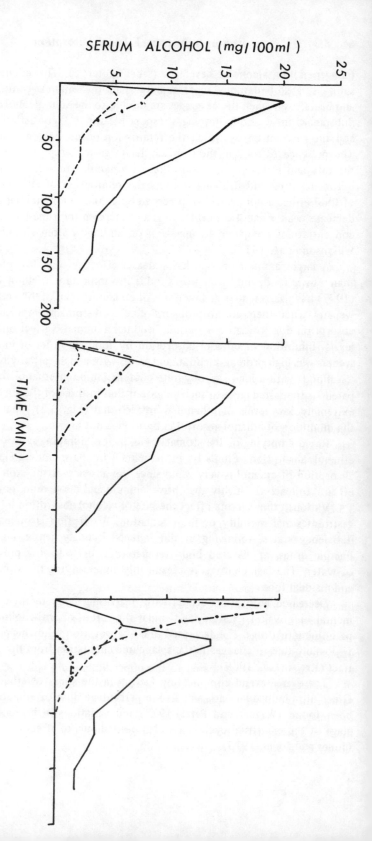

SERUM ALCOHOL (mg/100ml)

TIME (MIN)

Fig.3.3 – Individual serum levels of alcohol after a dose of 0.2 mls 95% alcohol per kg to fasted (——) and nonfasted subjects following high carbohydrate (·······), high fat (– – – –), and high protein (–·–·–·–), meals. Reproduced by permission from Welling et al., *Journal of Clinical Pharmacology* (1977).

3.4 ENDOGENOUS ETHANOL

Exogenous ethanol in body fluids may be supplemented by trace amounts synthesised endogenously (Lester, 1961; Anonymous, 1963; Harger and Forney 1963, 1967; Jansson and Larsson, 1969). Endogenous ethanol is thought to arise both from bacterial fermentation in the gut and from the action of alcohol dehydrogenase on acetaldehyde derived from pyruvate.

$$\text{Pyruvate} \xrightarrow{\text{Pyruvate kinase}} \text{Acetaldehyde} \xrightarrow[\text{Dehydrogenase}]{\text{Alcohol}} \text{Endogenous ethanol}$$

Experiments in rats (Krebs and Perkins, 1970) have demonstrated the presence of ethanol in the gastro-intestinal tract and in portal blood. Levels of endogenous ethanol were diminished but not abolished in animals treated with antibiotics, indicating that some endogenous ethanol is produced by a process other than fermentation in the gut. It is probable that the physiological role of hepatic alcohol dehydrogenase is to detoxify endogenous ethanol carried from the intestine in portal blood. Blood levels of endogenous ethanol in man are very low ranging up to 1.5 mg/1 of blood (Walker and Curry, 1966; Lin et al., 1976). Gas-liquid chromatography–mass spectrometry studies have confirmed the presence of ethanol in breath in the range 0.05-0.36 ppm (mean 0.13 ppm).

Endogenous ethanol intoxication ('Meiteisho') has been reported in a patient who had undergone gastrojejunostomy. The ethanol was considered to have arisen from the action of *Candida albicans* on intestinal contents in dilated jejunal segments (Yamashita et al., 1974).

3.5 DISTRIBUTION OF ETHANOL IN BODY FLUIDS

The rate of equilibration of ethanol with tissue depends on a series of factors such as the blood flow, permeability, and the mass of the tissue. Penetration of ethanol by diffusion is slow, and a rich blood supply speeds up the process. Thus, organs such as the brain, lungs, kidneys and liver reach equilibrium rapidly, whilst skeletal muscle, which has a poorer blood supply, reaches equilibrium with ethanol slowly (Wallgren and Barry, 1970). The mass of tissue is also an important factor. Ethanol concentrations in the cubital vein of the elbow are significantly higher than in blood samples taken from a suitable vein on the opposite foot during the first hour after drinking. This is due to the greater mass of the lower as compared to the upper limb and a consequent slower rate of equilibration (MaCallum and Scroggie, 1960). Whilst the rate of equilibration varies, the equilibrium concentration of ethanol in tissues depends only on the relative water content. This has been demonstrated by analysis of body fluids and tissue from both cadavers and live subjects. Ethanol content follows closely the absolute water content of the fluid or tissue (Table 3.2).

Table 3.2
Concentration of Ethanol in Various Body Fluids and Tissues.
Adapted by courtesy from Kalant, *Biology of Alcoholism Vol. 1,*
Plenum Press (1971)

Tissue or body fluid	Ethanol concentration relative to that in blood	Absolute water content %
Blood	1	80.5
Serum	0.91–1.17	–
Plasma	0.91–1.18	–
Urine	1.33	–
Saliva	1.21	–
Bile	1.10	98
Cerebrospinal fluid	1.27	99
Brain	0.74	76
Kidney	0.92	77
Liver	0.64	70
Muscle	0.84	74
Myocardium	0.83	77
Spleen	0.88	77
Testis	0.97	86

The distribution of ethanol in various body fluids, e.g., blood, urine, breath (Payne *et al.*, 1966; Alobaidi *et al.*, 1976) cerebrospinal fluid, maternal milk, vitreous humour (Felby and Olsen, 1969), sweat (Brusilow and Gordes, 1966; Pawan and Grice, 1968) ascitic fluid (Danopoulos, *et al.*, 1954), and cord blood (Chapman and Williams, 1951), has been studied.

A typical course of ethanol concentrations in arterial and venous blood, breath and urine with time is shown in Figure 3.4. The difference between the arterial and venous blood alcohol levels is due to a combination of the high solubility of alcohol in blood and tissue and the relatively poor blood flow to muscle. During the initial phase alcohol diffuses rapidly into the tissues from arterial blood and, when absorption is complete, arterial concentrations fall and alcohol diffuses from tissues into the capillaries and into venous blood. Levels in peripheral venous blood then remain higher than those in arterial blood because of lower rates of metabolism and excretion. Blood ethanol levels estimated from breath levels underestimate arterial concentrations although there is usually an initial period of high readings due to alcohol retained in the mouth. Peak urine levels of ethanol are usually reached in 30–190 minutes after drinking, depending on whether the ethanol was taken in a single or a series of doses.

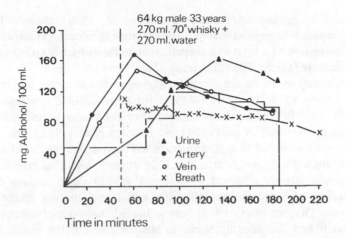

Fig. 3.4 – The changing relationship with time between the alcohol concentration in arterial and venous blood, breath and urine in a 33-year old man. The dotted perpendicular line indicates the point when drinking ceased. The urine: blood ratio of 1.32 has been used to convert the alcohol concentrations in urine to blood. As the urine figures represent the mean values of the altering concentrations during secretion the conversion to blood has been plotted as the mean value against time and is represented by the shaded areas. The peak blood concentrations were reached soon after the end of drinking: the urine peak was not reached until over an hour later, after which good agreement with blood was obtained.
Reproduced by permission from Payne *et al.*, *British Medical Journal* (1966).

3.6 EXCRETION OF ETHANOL

Small amounts of ethanol are excreted unchanged in urine, expired air, and sweat (Brusilow and Gordes, 1966). Usually less than 2% of a dose of ethanol is excreted *via* these routes, although at elevated temperatures and at high blood alcohol levels (200 mg/100 ml), combined pulmonary excretion and excretion in sweat and urine may exceed this value.

Excretion of ethanol in expired air at a blood level of 100mg/100ml amounts to 238mg/h assuming a resting ventilation rate of 8 l/minute and an ethanol in blood: expired air ratio of 2100:1. In subjects exposed to ethanol vapour the fall in the concentration of ethanol in expired air after cessation of exposure was very rapid. The ratio of respiratory elimination to retained ethanol (approximately 5:1) indicated that considerable quantities of inspired ethanol were re-excreted in expired air (Nomiyama and Nomiyama, 1974b).

Urinary excretion of ethanol is a passive process and ethanol clearances of between 0.9–12.7ml/minute have been reported (Blackmore and Mason, 1968).

3.7 HEPATIC METABOLISM OF ETHANOL

The liver is the principal site of ethanol metabolism. Hepatic vein catheterisation studies have shown that approximately 75% of a dose of ethanol is eliminated by hepatic metabolism (Winkler *et al.*, 1969). Maximal hepatic metabolic capacity is approximately 2 mmol ethanol/minute (Tygstrup *et al.*, 1974), as compared to a total extrahepatic metabolism which is estimated to be 0.4 mmol/minute (Larsen, 1959; Lindeneg *et al.*, 1964).

The enzymology of human alcohol metabolism has been the subject of an extensive review article by Li (1976) and for more detailed coverage of the enzymes involved in hepatic alcohol metabolism the reader is referred to this and articles by Wartburg *et al.* (1974) and Branden *et al.* (1975). The average metabolic rate for alcohol in a 70 kg person has been determined to be approximately 100mg/kg/body weight/hour or 170g ethanol/day. This rate has been derived using a formula proposed by Widmark (1932) which assumes a linear rate of decline of blood alcohol after the initial equilibration period. More recent studies (Wagner *et al.*, 1976) have indicated that ethanol disappearance from blood is best described by Michaelis-Menten kinetics. The metabolic rate for ethanol based on calculations assuming Michaelis-Menten kinetics is 120–150 mg/kg/h (200–240 g/day). Chronic ethanol ingestion amongst other factors can, however, greatly increase the metabolic elimination of ethanol (see section 3.8). Various early studies of ethanol elimination capacity in humans have been reviewed by Lelbach (1974).

3.7.1 Alcohol Dehydrogenase

Human alcohol dehydrogenase (ADh) (alcohol: NAD^+ oxidoreductase, EC 1.1.1.1) is a dimer with a zinc content of 2–2.5 atoms per molecule. Each sub unit may also contain an additional two zinc atoms *in vivo* (Branden *et al.*, 1975). Chromatographic and electrophoretic analysis has shown that the enzyme exists as a complex mixture of isoenzymes. Considerable variation in the pattern of isoenzymes occurs both during development and between individuals (Smith *et al.*, 1971). The variations arise due to the synthesis of different polypeptide sub-units α, β, and γ from three different gene loci. Two common alleles occur at the locus coding for γ sub-units giving rise to structurally distinct forms of the γ sub-unit, γ^1 and γ^2 (Wartburg *et al.*, 1974).

Atypical alcohol dehydrogenase isoenzymes also exist (Wartburg *et al.*, 1965, Li *et al.*, 1977). The activities of these isoenzymes are 3–6 times greater than normal ADh and the pH optima lie around 7.5–8.8, whereas the pH optima for the normal isoenzymes are around 10.8–11.5. The Michaelis-Menten constant (Km) for ethanol of atypical ADh is approximately three times that of normal ADh (Km 1100×10^{-6}M). Population studies have demonstrated the presence of an atypical ADh in European, North and South American, Greek and Japanese populations (Edwards and Evans, 1967; Wartburg and Schurch 1968; Ugarte *et al.*, 1970; Wartburg *et al.*, 1974). Frequencies of 4%, 20%, 43%, and 90% have been found for atypical ADh in English, Swiss, Chilean, and Japanese populations, severally.

The ADh activity of a whole liver containing the atypical enzyme is approximately 12,000 I.U. compared to an activity of 2700 I.U. for a normal liver. Various studies on the rate of ethanol metabolism in individuals with the atypical enzyme have shown both normal and increased rates of metabolism. The latter, however, do not correspond to the 3-6 fold increase in *in vitro* activity of the atypical enzyme. This is because reoxidation of reduced nicotinamide adenine dinucleotide (NADH) is the rate limiting step in alcohol metabolism. Evidence in support of this comes from studies of children with Type I glycogen storage disease (Glucose-6-phosphatase deficiency) who have a metabolic rate of ethanol oxidation of 460 compared to 100mg/kg/h in normal individuals. This is due to an efficient re-oxidation of NADH by the excessive amounts of pyruvate present in this disease (Lowe and Mosovich, 1965; Sadeghi-Nejad *et al.*, 1975). ADh activity is located primarily in the liver but activities have also been demonstrated in other organs (Table 3.3). Both the normal and atypical enzyme exhibit broad but differing substrate specificities converting a range of alcohols to the corresponding aldehydes and *vice versa* (Wartburg *et al.*, 1964, 1965; Blair and Vallee, 1966). Substrates studied apart from ethanol include methanol, ethylene glycol, 1,2-and 1,3-propane diol, 2-methoxy-and 2-ethoxyethanol, *iso*-propanol, cyclohexanol, *n*-butanol, phenol, *n*-octanol, formaldehyde, and glyoxylic acid, ethanol being the most readily oxidised substrate. ADh will also oxidise certain 3-β-hydroxysteroids, however, compared to ethanol they are poor substrates (Pietruszko *et al.*, 1972).

Table 3.3
Alcohol dehydrogenase Activity in International Units per 100g of Fresh Tissue in Various Human Organs

Organ	Activity (mean and/or range)
Liver	200 (44–470)
Stomach	9.7 (1.7-19)
Intestine	0-7.1
Lung	2.2-11.1
Kidney	1.2-2.4
Spleen	0-0.9
Omentum	0-1.9
Prostate	0-1.1
Appendix	
Colon	
Sigma	
Rectum	trace
Gall and Urinary bladder	
Testes	
Adrenal	
Brain	

3.7.2 Microsomal Ethanol Oxidising System

In addition to alcohol dehydrogenase, ethanol may be oxidised by a NADPH-dependent microsomal ethanol oxidising system (MEOS) (Lieber and DeCarli, 1970). Several workers (Mezey and Tobon, 1971; Kostelnik and Iber, 1973) have shown that the activity of MEOS is increased in alcoholic patients as compared to controls and that the increased activity persists for 2-3 weeks after withdrawal. Introduction of MEOS activity is associated with a proliferation of the hepatic smooth endoplasmic reticulum which is part of the microsomal fraction. Other microsomal drug metabolising enzymes are stimulated by ethanol, and this explains the resistance of sober alcoholics to drugs such as pentobarbital and meprobamate (Kater *et al.*, 1969a, 1969b; Carulli *et al.*, 1971; Misra *et al.*, 1971). Hepatic hydroxylation of pentobarbital and benzpyrene is stimulated by ethanol (Rubin and Lieber, 1968), and the finding that serum bilirubin levels are lower in children of mothers given intravenous ethanol during labour suggests that ethanol may also stimulate enzymes involved in the conjugation of bilirubin (Waltman *et al.*, 1969).

3.7.3 Catalase

The enzyme catalase, in conjunction with an hydrogen peroxide generating system such as xanthine oxidase, could oxidise ethanol to acetaldehyde. Although the hepatocyte contains catalase, located mainly in peroxisomes, this enzyme does not play a major role in the metabolism of ethanol (Lieber, 1977).

3.8 FACTORS INFLUENCING ELIMINATION AND METABOLISM OF ETHANOL

Many factors have been shown to alter the rate of metabolism and elimination of ethanol and some of these are listed in Table 3.4.

Table 3.4

Factors Influencing Elimination and Metabolism of Ethanol.

Adapted by courtesy from Wartburg, *Biology of Alcoholism. Vol. 1,*
Plenum Press (1971).

Maturity of the liver
Liver damage
Drugs
Food
Menstrual cycle
Time of day
Ageing
Race

An immature liver and associated immature ADh activity can greatly reduce the metabolism of ethanol (Seppela *et al.*, 1971; Gartner and Ryden, 1972). In a study in which intravenous ethanol was given to low birth-weight infants, elimination of alcohol was found to be only about 50-65% of the adult value (Wagner *et al.*, 1970). Pikkarainen and Raiha (1967) have determined the ADh activity in foetal livers from legal abortions and shown that ADh activity is only 3-4% of the adult value which is reached at about five years of age. The ADh activity at term is approximately 20% of the adult value.

A diminution in overall hepatic function due to liver damage may also cause a reduction in ethanol metabolism. Significantly reduced hepatic ADh activities have been found in alcoholics with cirrhosis or steatosis (Figuerao and Klotz, 1962, Ugarte *et al.*, 1967). Reduced clearances of ethanol have also been found in alcoholics with jaundice (Kater *et al.*, 1969a) although in a group of alcoholics with either acute hepatitis or fatty infiltration no significant alteration in metabolism was detected (Wilkinson *et al.*, 1969). As well as decreased and normal rates of ethanol metabolism, increased rates have been observed in alcoholics with liver disease. Ugarte and co-workers (1977) have reported that the rates of ethanol metabolism in chronic alcoholics with biopsy-proven steatosis (rate: 207±20mg ethanol/kg body weight/h) or steatosis, necrosis and fibrosis (256±20.5) were significantly higher than in alcoholics with a normal liver (154±17) or with mild fibrosis (174±11.0). The reason for this enhancement in metabolism in the diseased liver has not been ascertained.

Drugs can affect the rate of metabolism of ethanol by inducing MEOS activity, altering hepatic blood flow, or by increasing the rate of reoxidation of NADH (Mezey, 1976).

Induction of the mitochondrial ethanol oxidising system by ethanol leads to increased rates of metabolism (Iber, 1971; Vesell *et al.*, 1971; Ugarte *et al.*, 1972). For example, the latter group of workers have studied a group of recently drinking alcoholics free of overt liver disease and found that the clearance of ethanol was nearly twice that in normal subjects, (49.4±9.5 as compared to 24.7±10.2 mg ethanol/100ml blood/h).

In a heavy drinker accustomed to large quantities of ethanol, an absolute limit to ethanol elimination is 360g/day and blood ethanol levels have reached 200-300 mg/100ml (Bonnischen *et al.*, 1968).

Barbiturates, by inducing the mitochondrial drug metabolising system, can also increase ethanol metabolism (Mezey and Robles, 1974). Oral contraceptive therapy may also affect ethanol metabolism. Bode (1974) has reported that significant increases in the rate of ethanol elimination have been detected in four users of oral contraceptives.

Drugs may also inhibit ethanol metabolism by inhibiting ADh (Maling, 1970). Ingestion of chloral hydrate half an hour before taking a dose of ethanol caused peak blood ethanol levels to be higher and reached earlier than without pre-medication (Sellers *et al.*, 1972). This is due to competitive inhibition of ADh by trichloracetaldehyde (Fig. 3.5) which reduces metabolism of ethanol to acetaldehyde by ADh.

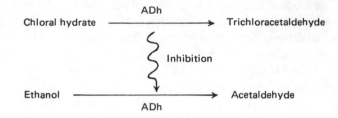

Fig. 3.5 – Competitive inhibition of Alcohol Dehydrogenase by Trichloracetaldehyde

The effects of various substances on ethanol metabolism have been investigated in a search to discover a substance which would accelerate metabolism and thus provide a rapid means of reducing blood alcohol levels and reversing the effects of ethanol.

Conflicting results on the effect of tri-iodothyronine (T_3) on ethanol metabolism have appeared. Both significant increases (Goldberg et al., 1960) and no increase in metabolism following T_3 treatment (Kalant et al., 1962) have been reported. Elimination of ethanol is said to be raised in patients with thyrotoxicosis (Ugarte and Ituriaga, 1976). Likewise contrary reports on the efficiency of fructose in accelerating ethanol metabolism have appeared. The rate of ethanol metabolism is dependent upon the rate of reoxidation of the ADh :NADH complex in the liver. A substrate such as fructose could by reoxidising this complex, make the ADh : NAD complex available for ethanol metabolism. Usually regeneration of NAD from NADH formed during ethanol metabolism takes place via shuttle mechanisms which indirectly transport the hydrogen into mitochondria where it is oxidised in the respiratory chain. The shuttle mechanisms are necessary because of the impermeability of the mitochondrion to NADH. The metabolism of fructose is outlined in Fig. 3.6.

The normal metabolism of fructose is via fructose-1-phosphate and glyceraldehyde, the latter being converted to glycerate and then metabolised in the Embden Meyerhof pathway to pyruvate. When ethanol and fructose are given together the metabolism of fructose is shunted to the production of sorbitol and glycerol via NADH requiring pathways due to the unavailability of NAD. However, the overall effect is to regenerate NAD for ethanol metabolism. Studies in human volunteers (Tygstrup et al., 1965) have shown that when given ethanol plus fructose as compared to ethanol alone—

(i)   sorbitol and glycerol are found in the liver and are detectable in hepatic veins,

(ii) hepatic output of lactate and pyruvate decreases whilst output of glucose
increases and

(iii) a two fold increase in the oxidation of ethanol to acetate occurs.

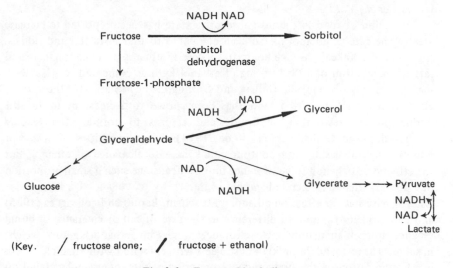

(Key. / fructose alone; / fructose + ethanol)

Fig. 3.6 — Fructose Metabolism

Blood sorbitol levels increase 2–3 fold in patients given ethanol plus fructose
compared with fructose alone. Fructose does not affect acetaldehyde levels but
does partially prevent the ethanol-mediated elevation of lactate/pyruvate and
β-hydroxybutyrate/acetoacetate ratios in blood (Rawat, 1977). These findings
support the view that in the presence of ethanol the metabolism of fructose
is shunted from NAD to NADH requiring pathways, and thus effective reoxidation
of NADH to NAD takes place making NAD available for ethanol oxidation.
Various reports on the effect of both oral and intravenous fructose have indicated the magnitude of the effect on ethanol metabolism to be somewhere
between a quantitatively modest to a 50% increase (Lundquist and Wolthers,
1956; Merry and Marks, 1967; Pawan, 1968b, Patel et al., 1969; Lowenstein
et al., 1970a, 1970b; Brown et al., 1972; Soterakis and Iber, 1975). In a recent
prospective double blind trial with glucose as the control, intravenous fructose
was shown to have no effect on the rate of ethanol metabolism. Indeed, the
significant elevations in the serum urate and lactate in patients receiving fructose
were deemed a potential risk (Levy et al., 1977; see also Iber, 1977).

Other sugars, such a glucose and galactose, have no significant effect on the
rate of ethanol metabolism. Because vitamins are involved in the pathways by
which NADH is reoxidised to NAD, it has been suggested that vitamins may
indirectly increase ethanol metabolism by increasing the reoxidation of NADH
to NAD. However, administration of vitamin supplements does not increase
the rate of ethanol metabolism (Pawan, 1968b).

Post-ethanol treatment with L-dopa, aminophylline, and/or ephedrine has been shown to reduce significantly some of the deleterious effects of ethanol. However, no significant changes in the rate of ethanol elimination were detected (Alkana *et al.*, 1977).

Ingestion of food in the post-absorptive state has been reported to increase greatly the rate of ethanol metabolism compared to that in fasting individuals. Ingestion of 1000 calories one hour after a dose of ethanol produced an increased rate of metabolism of 178±11.9 mg of ethanol/kg/h as compared to 81.5±3.55 mg/kg/h in fasting subjects (Millar and Stirling, 1966). Similarly, the rate of elimination of ethanol from blood has been shown to decrease by up to 50% during protein restriction or fasting and returns to normal after feeding (Creutzfeldt and Graham, 1971; Bode, 1974). Large quantities of water or diuretics by increasing urine output could increase clearance of ethanol, but the effect is anticipated to be of minor importance, since such a small proportion of a dose of ethanol is excreted *via* that route.

Exercise has no effect on ethanol metabolism. Barnes and colleagues (1965) and Pawan (1968) found no difference in the rate of fall or clearance of blood ethanol: in their first study, mean clearances were 75mg ethanol/kg body weight in subjects at rest, and 76mg/kg/h in subjects who exercised with ethanol.

Complications in the study and interpretation of rates of ethanol metabolism arise from factors such as time of day of testing, phase of the menstrual cycle, age, race, and genetic characteristics. Even repeated ethanol clearance tests on a single subject under standardised conditions employing an identical dose of ethanol can give a wide range of results (Wagner & Patel, 1972).

The chronopharmacokinetics of ethanol metabolism has been the subject of a number of recent studies. These have demonstrated that the rate of metabolism is dependent upon the time of day and follows a 16h cycle (Fig. 3.7) (Sturtevant *et al.*, 1975, 1976). Jones (1974) has also found a rhythmicity in rate of elimination of ethanol, elimination being greater in the afternoon than in the evening.

The phase of the menstrual cycle has also been shown to affect ethanol metabolism. Blood ethanol elimination rate was found to be increased in the second part of the cycle (Bode, 1974).

Apart from the problems associated with immature hepatic ADh activity in neonates, the age of a subject does not affect rate of ethanol elimination. Although differences in peak ethanol levels have been detected in old, as compared to young, age groups, this may be accounted for by a decrease in extra-cellular fluid volume and total body water with ageing (Vestal *et al.*, 1977).

Racial variations have been discovered in the rate at which ethanol is metabolised, although the studies to date have been fragmentary and preliminary in nature (Gilbert and Schaefer, 1977). Dietrich and Collins (1977) have recently reviewed the pharmacogenetics of ethanol metabolism in both animals and man. The rate of metabolism of ethanol by Canadian Indians and Eskimos is reported to be significantly less than thay by Caucasians--a finding which has been challenged (Fenna *et al.*, 1971, Lieber, 1972; Bennion and Li, 1976). Evidence from other studies of the relationship between alcoholism and serum complement (C_3), blood groups A, S and D, and other serological markers has indicated that that there may possibly be a genetic influence on the variability in the metabolism of ethanol (Hill *et al.*, 1975). Further evidence for genetic control of the variation in rate of ethanol metabolism has come from the studies of Vesell and colleagues (1971). In a study of 14 pairs of twins, inter-pair differences in rate of ethanol metabolism were greater in fraternal than in identical twins. A considerable range (0.11-0.24mg ethanol/ml of blood/h) in rates was observed, thus supporting the claims of an earlier study that different individuals have characteristic 'burning rates' for ethanol (Shumate *et al.*, 1967).

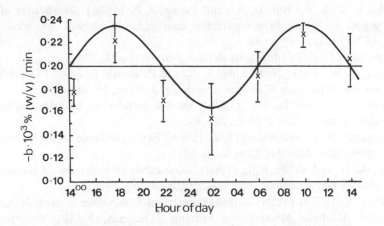

Fig. 3.7 – Variation of rate of ethanol metabolism (estimated slope (β) of ethanol disappearance curve) with the time of day in a repeat dose 30 hour experiment. The rate of metabolism follows a 16 hour cycle.
Reproduced by permission from Sturtevant *et al.*, *Archives of Pharmacology* (1976).

3.9 SUMMARY

Ethanol is absorbed by a process of passive diffusion, absorption occurring principally from the duodenum and jejunum. Increased gastric emptying and any factor which serves to maximise or maintain the concentration gradient at the site of absorption will facilitate the absorption of ethanol. Factors which have been shown to influence absorption include the concentration of ethanol in the beverage, and the type of beverage, the blood flow at site of absorption, the irritant properties of ethanol, the rate of ingestion, food, emptying of the stomach, protein deficiency, the body temperature, physical exercise, and phase of the menstrual cycle.

Following absorption, some ethanol is excreted in urine and in expired air, but most is metabolised in the liver. Alcohol dehydrogenase and the mitro-chondrial ethanol oxidising system are the principal enzymes of ethanol oxidation. The rate of oxidation is approximately 120–150 mg/kg/h but hepatic enzyme induction by drugs, especially ethanol, may double this rate of oxidation. Other factors which influence ethanol metabolism include the maturity and patency of the liver, food, phase of the menstrual cycle, time of day, age and ethnic origin.

3.10 REFERENCES

Alkana, R. L., Parker, E. S., Cohen, H. B., Birch, H., and Noble, E. P. (1977) Reversal of ethanol intoxication in humans: An assessment of the efficacy of L-dopa, aminophylline and ephedrine. *Psychopharmacol.*, **55**, 203-212.

Alobaidi, T. A. A., Hill, D. W., and Payne, J. P. (1976) Significance of variations in blood: breath partition coefficient of alcohol. *Br. Med. J.*, **2** 1479-1481.

Anonymous (1963) Endogenous alcohol. *Nutr. Rev.*, **21**, 324-326.

Barnes, E. W., Cook, N. J., King, A. J., and Passmore, R. (1965) Observations on the metabolism of alcohol in man. *Br. J. Nutr.*, **19**, 485-489.

Bennion, L. J., and Li, T-K. (1976) Alcohol metabolism in American Indians and whites. *N. Eng. J. Med.*, **294**, 9-13.

Blackmore, D. J., and Mason, J. K. (1968) Renal clearance of urea, creatinine and alcohol. *Med. Sci. Law*, **8**, 50-53.

Blair, A. H. and Vallee, B. L. (1966) Some catalytic properties of human liver alcohol dehydrogenase. *Biochemistry*, **5**, 2026-2034.

Bode, J. C. (1974) Factors influencing ethanol metabolism in man. *In* Alcohol and Aldehyde Metabolizing Systems (Thurman, R. G., Yonetani, T., Williamson, J. R., Chance, B. *eds.*) pp 457-468, Academic Press, New York.

Bonnischen, R., Dimberg, R., Maehley, A. (1968) Die Alkohol verbrennung bei Alkoholikern und bei ubrigen Versuchspersonen. *Blutalkohol*, **5**, 301.

Branden, C-I., Jornvall, H. E., and Furugren, B. (1975) Alcohol dehydrogenases *In* The Enzymes (Boyer P. D. *ed.*) Vol 11, pp. 103-190., Academic Press, New York.

Brown S. S., Forrest, J. A. H., and Roscoe, P. (1972) A controlled trial of fructose in the treatment of acute alcohol intoxication. *Lancet*, **ii**, 898-900.

*Browne-Mayers, A. N., Seelye, E. E., Stokes, P. E., and Seixas, F. (1971) Alcoholism. *Prog. Neurol. Psychiatry*, **26**, 473-490.

*Browne-Mayers, A. N., Seelye, E. E., Seixas, F., and Stokes, P. (1973) Alcoholism and drug abuse. *Progr. Neurol. Psychiatry*, **28**, 449-467.

Brusilow, S. W., and Gordes, E. H. (1966) The permeability of the sweat gland to non-electrolytes. *Am. J. Dis. Child.*, **112**, 328-333.

Carulli, N., Manenti, F., Gallo, M., and Salvioli, G. F. (1971) Alcohol-drugs interaction in man. Alcohol and tolbutamide. *Europ. J. Clin. Invest.*, **1**, 421-424.

Chapman, E. R., and Williams, P. T. (1951) Intravenous alcohol as an obstetrical analgesia. *Am. J. Obstet. Gynecol.*, **61**, 676-679.

Cooke, A. R., and Birchall, A (1969) Absorption of ethanol from the stomach. *Gastroenterology*, **57**, 269-272.

Creutzfeld, W., and Graham, G. R. (1971) Hemmung des Athanolabbaues durch Proteinmangel beim Menschen. *Dtsch. Med. Wochschr.*, **96**, 1576-1577.

Danopoulos, E., Maratos, E., and Legolhetopoulos, J. (1954) Studies on the alcohol's metabolism in patients with atrophic liver cirrhosis. *Acta Med. Scand.*, **148**, 485-492.

Deitrich, R. A., and Collins, A. C. (1977) Pharmacogenetics of alcoholism *In* Alcohol and Opiates (Blum, K. *ed.*) pp 109-139, Academic Press, New York.

Edwards, J. A., and Evans, P. D. A. (1967) Ethanol metabolism in subjects possessing typical and atypical liver alcohol dehydrogenase. *Clin. Pharmacol. Ther.*, **8**, 824-829.

Felby, S., and Olsen, J. (1969) Comparative studies of postmortem ethyl alcohol in vitreous humour, blood and muscle. *J. Forensic Sci.*, **14**, 93-101.

Fenna, D., Mix, L., Schaefer, O., and Gilbert, J. A. L. (1971) Ethanol metabolism in various racial groups. *Can. Med. Assoc. J.*, **105**, 472-475.

Figueroa, R. B., and Klotz, A. P. (1962) Alterations of liver alcohol dehydrogenase and other hepatic enzymes in alcoholic cirrhosis. *Gastroenterology*, **43**, 10-12.

Gartner. U., and Ryden, G. (1972) The elimination of alcohol in the premature infant. *Acta Paediatr. Scand.*, **61**, 720-721.

Gibson, A. G. (1975) Alcohol can be absorbed through the respiratory tract. (A case report). *Med. Sci. Law,* **15**, 64.

Gilbert, J. A. L., and Schaefer, O. (1977) Metabolism of ethanol in different racial groups. *Can. Med. Assoc. J.*, **116**, 476.

Goldberg, M., Hehir, R., and Hurowitz, M. (1960). Intravenous tri-iodothyronine in acute alcoholic intoxication. *N. Eng. J. Med.*, **263**, 1336-1339.

Harger, R. N. and Forney, R. B. (1963) Aliphatic alcohols. *Prog. Chem. Toxicol.*, **1**, 53-134.

Harger, R. N., and Forney, R. B. (1967) Aliphatic Alcohols. *Prog. Chem. Toxicol.*, **3**, 1-61.

Hill, S. Y., Goodwin, D. W., Cadoret, R., Osterland, C. K., and Doner, S. M. (1975) Association and linkage between alcoholism and eleven serological markers. *J. Stud. Alcohol,* **36**, 981-992.

*Hoensch, H. (1972) The effects of alcohol on the liver. *Digestion,* **6**, 114-123.

Iber, F. L., (1971) Increased drug metabolism in alcoholics. *In* Biological Aspects of Alcohol (Roach, M. K., McIsaac, W. M., and Creaven, P. J. *eds.*) pp. 94-105. University of Texas Press, Austin.

Iber, F. L. (1977) The effect of fructose on alcohol metabolism. *Arch. Intern. Med.*, **137**, 1121.

*Israel, Y. (1970) Cellular effects of alcohol. *Q. J. Stud. Alcohol,* **31**, 293-316.

Jansson, B. O. and Larson, B. T. (1969) Analysis of organic compounds in human breath by gas chromatography–mass spectrometry. *J. Lab. Clin. Med.*, 74, 961–966.

Jones, B. M. (1974) Circadian variation in the effects of alcohol on cognitive performance. *Q. J. Stud. Alcohol*, 35, 1212–1219.

Jones, B. M., and Jones, M. K. (1975) Effects of a moderate dose of alcohol on female social drinkers at different times in the menstrual cycle. *Chronobiologia*, **Supp.** 1, 34 (Abstr).

Kalant, H. (1971) Absorption, diffusion, distribution and elimination of ethanol: Effects on biological membranes. *In* The Biology of Alcoholism (Kissin, B., and Begleiter, H., *eds.*) Vol. 1. pp 1–62. Plenum Press, New York.

Kalant, H., Sereny, G., and Charlebois, R. (1962) Evaluation of tri-iodothyronine in the treatment of acute alcoholic intoxication. *N. Engl. J. Med.*, 267, 1–6.

Kater, R. M. H., Carulli, N., and Iber, F. L. (1969a) Differences in the rate of ethanol metabolism in recently drinking alcoholic and non-alcoholic subjects. *Am. J. Clin. Nutr.*, 22, 1608–1617.

Kater, R. F., Tobon, F., and Iber, F. L. (1969b) Increased rate of tolbutamide metabolism in alcoholic patients. *J. Am. Med. Assoc.*, 207, 363–365.

Kater, R., Roggin, Tobon, F., Zieve, P., and Iber, F. L. (1969c) Increased rate of clearance of drugs from the circulation of alcoholics. *Am. J. Med. Sci.*, 258, 35–39.

Kostelnik, M. E., and Iber, F. L. (1973) Correlation of alcohol and tolbutamide blood clearance rates with microsomal alcohol-metabolizing enzyme activity. *Am. J. Clin. Nutr.*, 26, 161–164.

Krebs, H. A., and Perkins, J. R. (1970) The physiological role of liver alcohol dehydrogenase. *Biochem. J.*, 118, 635–644.

Krebs, H. A., Cunningham, D. J. C., Stubbs, M., and Jenkins, D. J. A. (1969) Effect of ethanol on postexercise lactacidemia. *Isr. J. Med. Sci.*, 5, 959–962.

Larsen, J. A. (1959) Extrahepatic metabolism of ethanol in man. *Nature (Lond).*, 184, 1236.

Lelbach, W. K. (1974) Organic pathology related to volume and pattern of alcohol use. *Res. Adv. Alcohol Drug Probl.*, 1, 93–198.

Lester, D. (1961) Endogenous ethanol: A review. *Q. J. Stud. Alcohol.*, 22, 554–574.

Levy, R. Elo, T., and Hanenson, I. B. (1977). Intravenous fructose treatment of acute alcohol intoxication. *Arch. Intern. Med.*, 137, 1175–1177.

Li, T-K. (1976) Enzymology of human alcohol metabolism. *Adv. Enzymol. Relat. Areas Mol. Biol.*, 45, 427–433.

Li, T-K., Bosron, W. F., Dafeldecker, W. P., Lange, L. G., and Vallee, B. L. (1977) Isolation of II–alcohol dehydrogenase of human liver: Is it a determinant of alcoholism? *Proc. Natl. Acad. Sci.*, 74, 4378–4381.

*Lieber, C. S., (1966) Alcohol and the liver. *Prog. Liver Dis.*, 2, 134–154.

*Lieber, C. S., (1966) Hepatic and metabolic effects of alcohol. *Gastroenterology*, **50**, 119-133.

*Lieber, C. S., (1967) Metabolic derangement induced by alcohol. *Annu. Rev. Med.*, **18**, 35-54.

Lieber, C. S., (1972) Metabolism of ethanol and alcoholism. Racial and acquired factors. *Ann. Intern. Med.*, **76**, 326-327.

*Lieber, C. S. (1973) Liver adaptation in alcoholism. *N. Eng. J. Med.*, **288**, 356-362.

*Lieber, C. S. (1973) Hepatic and metabolic effects of alcohol (1966 to 1973). *Gastroenterology*, **65**, 821-846.

*Lieber, C. S. (1975) Alcohol and malnutrition in the pathogenesis of liver disease. *J. Am. Med. Assoc.*, **233**, 1077-1082.

*Lieber, C. S. (1977) Metabolism of ethanol. *In* Metabolic Aspects of Alcoholism (Lieber, C. S., *ed.*) pp. 1-29, MTP Press Limited, Lancaster.

Lieber, C. S., and DeCarli, L. M. (1970) Hepatic microsomal ethanol-oxidizing system. *J. Biol. Chem.*, **245**, 2505-2512.

Lin, Y., Weidler, D. J., Garg, D. C., and Wagner, J. C. (1976) Effects of solid food on blood levels of alcohol in man. *Res. Commun. Pathol. Pharmacol.*, **13**, 713-722.

Lindeneg, O., Mellemgaard, K., Fabricius, J., and Lundquist, F. (1964) Myocardial utilisation of acetate, lactate and free fatty acids after ingestion of ethanol. *Clin. Sci. (Oxf.)*, **27**, 427-435.

Lowe, C. U. , and Mosovich, L. L. (1965) The paradoxical effect of alcohol on carbohdrate metabolism in four patients with liver glycogen disease. *Pediatrics*, **35**, 1005-1008.

Lowenstein, L. M., Simone, R. C., Boulter, P., and Nathan, P. (1970a) Éffect of fructose on blood ethanol levels. *Fed. Proc.*, **29**, 632 (Abstr.)

Lowenstein, L. M., Simone, R., Boulter, P., and Nathan P. (1970b) Effect of fructose on alcohol concentrations in the blood of man. *J. Am. Med. Assoc.*, **213**, 1899-1901.

Lundquist, F., and Wolthers, H. (1958) The influence of fructose on the kinetics of alcohol elimination in man. *Act. Pharmacol. Toxicol.*, **14**, 290-294.

Lundquist, F., Tygstrup, N., Winkler, K., Mellemgaard, K., and Munck-Petersen, S. (1962) Ethanol metabolism and production of free acetate in human liver. *J. Clin. Invest.*, **41**, 955-961.

MaCallum, N. E. W. and Scroggie, J. G. (1960) Some aspects of alcohol in body fluids. Part III. Study of alcohol in blood in different parts of the body. *Med. J. Aust.*, **II**, 1031-1032.

*McKinley, A. R., and Moorhead, H. H. (1967) Alcoholism. *Progr. Neurol. Psychiatry*, **22**, 459-468.

Maling, H. M. (1970) Toxicology of a single dose of ethyl alcohol. *In* International Encyclopedia of Pharmacology and Therapeutics, section 20, Volume II (Tremolieres, J., *ed.*) pp. 227-299, Pergamon Press, Oxford.

Mardones, J. (1963) The alcohols. *In* Physiological Pharmacology (Root, W. S. and Hofman, F. G., *eds.*) Vol. I, pp. 99-183, Academic Press, New York.

*Mendelson, J. H. (1970) Biologic concomitants of alcoholism. *N. Eng. J. Med.,* **283**, 24-32.

Merry, J., and Marks, V. (1967) Effect on performance of reducing blood-alcohol with oral fructose. *Lancet,* **ii**, 1328-1330.

Mezey, E. (1976) Ethanol metabolism and ethanol-drug interactions. *Biochem. Pharmacol.,* **25**, 869-875.

Mezey, E., and Tobon, F. (1971) Rates of ethanol clearance and activities of the ethanol-oxidizing enzymes in chronic alcoholic patients. *Gastroenterology,* **61**, 707-715.

Mezey, E., and Robles, E. A. (1974) Effects of phenobarbital administration on rates of ethanol clearance and on ethanol-oxidizing enzymes in man. *Gastroenterology,* **66**, 248-253.

Millar, D. S., and Stirling, J. L. (1966) The effect of a meal on the rate of ethanol metabolism in man. *Proc. Nutr. Soc.,* **25**, xl.

Misra, P. S., Lefevre, A., Ishii, H., Rubin, E., and Lieber, C. S. (1971) Increase of ethanol, meprobamate, and pentobarbital metabolism after chronic ethanol treatment in man and in rats. *Am. J. Med.,* **51**, 346-351.

Moskowitz, H., and Burns, M. (1976) Effects of rate of drinking on human performance. *J. Stud. Alcohol,* **37**, 598-605.

Mowat, N. A. G., and Brunt, P. W. (1976) Alcohol and the gastrointestinal tract. *Rec. Adv. Gastroenterol.,* **3**, 150-177.

National Centre for Prevention and Control of Alcoholism (1968). Alcohol and Alcoholism Public Health Service Publication No. 1640. U.S. Government Printing Office, Washington D.C.

Nomiyama, K., and Nomiyama, H. (1974a) Respiratory retention, uptake and excretion of organic solvents in man. *Int. Arch. Arbeitsmed.,* **32**, 75-83.

Nomiyama, K., and Nomiyama, H., (1974b) Respiratory elimination of organic solvents in man. *Int. Arch. Arbeitsmed.,* **32**, 85-91.

*Nordmann, R., and Nordmann, J. (1971) Effects of alcohol on hepatic metabolism. *Rev. Eur. Etud. Clin. Biol.,* **16**, 965-969.

Patel, A. R., Paton, A. M., Rowan, T., Lawson, D. H., and Linton, A. R. (1969) Clinical studies on the effect of laevulose on the rate of metabolism of ethyl alcohol. *Scott. Med. J.,* **14**, 268-271.

Pauly, J. E., Scheving, L. E., Sturtevant, F. M., and Sturtevant, R. P. (1975) Evidence for circadian variation in the metabolism of ethanol in man. *Proc. X. Int. Cong. Anat. Tokyo,* 522.

Pawan, G. L. S. (1968a) Physical exercise and alcohol metabolism in man. *Nature (Lond.),* **218**, 966-967.

Pawan, G. L. S. (1968b) The effect of vitamin supplements and various sugars on the rate of metabolism of ethanol in man. *Biochem. J.,* **107**, 25P-26P.

Pawan, G. L. S. and Grice, K. (1968) Distribution of alcohol in urine and sweat after drinking. *Lancet,* **ii,** 1016.

Payne, J. P., Hill, D. W., and King, N. W. (1966) Observations on the distribution of alcohol in blood, breath, and urine. *Br. Med. J.,* **1,** 196-202.

Pietruszko, R., Theorell, H., and de Zalenski, C. (1972) Heterogeneity of alcohol dehydrogenase from human liver. *Arch. Biochem. Biophys.,* **153,** 279-293.

Pikkarainen, P. H., and Raiha, N. C. R. (1967) Development of alcohol dehydrogenase activity in the human liver. *Pediatr. Res.* **1,** 165-168.

*Porta, E. A., Koch, O. R., and Hartroft, W. S. (1970) Recent advances in molecular pathology. A review of the effects of alcohol on the liver. *Exp. Mol. Pathol.,* **12,** 104-132.

Rawat, A. K. (1977) Effects of fructose and other substances on ethanol and acetaldehyde metabolism in man. *Res. Commun. Chem. Pathol. Pharmacol.,* **16,** 281-290.

Rubin, E., and Lieber, C. S. (1968) Hepatic microsomal enzymes in man and rat. Induction and inhibition by ethanol. *Science (Wash. D. C.),* **162,** 690-691.

Sadeghi-Nejad, A., Hochman, H., Senior, B. (1975) Studies in Type 1 glycogenosis. The paradoxical effect of ethanol on lactate. *J. Pediatr.,* **86,** 37-42.

Sedman, A. J., Wilkinson, P. K., Sakamar, E., Weidler, D. J., and Wagner, J. G. (1976). Food effects on absorption and metabolism of alcohol. *J. Stud. Alcohol,* **37,** 1197-1214.

Sellers, E. M., Lang, M., Koch-Weser, J., Le Blanc, E., and Kalant, H. (1972) Interaction of chloral hydrate and ethanol in man. *Clin. Pharmacol. Ther.,* **13,** 37-49.

Seppela, M., Raiha, N. C. R., and Tamminan, V. (1971) Ethanol elimination in a mother and her premature twins. *Lancet,* **ii,** 1188-1189.

Shumate, R. P., Crowther, R. F., Zarafshan, M. (1967) A study of the metabolism rates of alcohol in the human body. *J. Forensic Med.,* **14,** 83-100.

Smith, M., Hopkinson, D. A., and Harris, H. (1971) Developmental changes and polymorphism in human alcohol dehydrogenase. *Ann. Hum. Genet.,* **34,** 251-271.

Soterakis, J., and Iber, F. L. (1975) Increased rate of alcohol removal from blood with oral fructose and sucrose. *Am. J. Clin. Nutr.,* **28,** 254-257.

Sturtevant, F. M., Sturtevant R. P., Scheving, R. P., and Pauly, J. E. (1975) Chronopharmokinetics of ethanol in man. *Pharmacologist,* **17,** 194 (Abstr.).

Sturtevant, F. M., Sturtevant, R. P., Scheving, L. E., and Pauly, J. E. (1976) Chronopharmokinetics of Ethanol. II. Circadian rhythm in rate of blood level decline in a single subject. *Naunyn-Schmiedeberg's Arch. Pharmacol.,* **293,** 203-208.

Thieden, H. I. D. (1975) Ethanol metabolism in the liver. *Acta Pharmacol. Toxicol.,* **36, Suppl. 1,** 1-51.

Tygstrup, N., Winkler, K., and Lundquist, F. (1965) The mechanism of the fructose effect on the ethanol metabolism in human liver. *J. Clin. Invest.*, **44**, 817-830.

Tygstrup, N., Ranek, L., Ramscoe, K., and Keiding, S. (1974) The effect of submaximal ethanol elimination on hepatic redox levels in man. *In* Alcohol and Aldehyde Metabolizing systems (Thurman, R. G., Yonetani, T., Williamson, J. R., and Chance, B., *eds.*) pp. 469-481, Academic Press, New York.

*Ugarte, G., and Iturriaga, H. (1976) Metabolic pathways of alcohol in the liver. *Front. Gastrointest. Res.*, **2**, 150-193.

Ugarte, G., Pino, M. E., and Insunza, I. (1967) Hepatic alcohol dehydrogenase in alcoholic addicts with and without hepatic damage. *Am. J. Dig. Dis.*, **12**, 589-592.

Ugarte, G., Pino, M. E., Altschiller, H., and Pereda, T. (1970) Atypical alcohol dehydrogenase in Chilean alcohol addicts with and without hepatic damage. *Q. J. Stud. Alcohol*, **31**, 571-577.

Ugarte, G., Pereda, T., Pino, M. E., and Iturriaga, H. (1972) Influence of alcohol intake, length of abstinence and meprobamate on the rate of ethanol metabolism in man. *Q. J. Stud. Alcohol*, **33**, 698-705.

Ugarte, G., Iturriaga, H., and Pereda, T., (1977) Possible relationship between the rate of ethanol metabolism and the severity of hepatic damage in chronic alcoholics. *Dig. Dis.*, **22**, 406-410.

Vesell, E. S., Page, J. G., and Passananti, G. T. (1971) Genetic and environmental factors affecting ethanol metabolism in man. *Clin. Pharmacol. Ther.*, **12**, 192-201.

Vestal, R. E., McGuire, E. A., Tobin, J. D., Andres, R. , Norris, A. H., and Mezey, E. (1977) Aging and ethanol metabolism. *Clin. Pharmacol. Ther.*, **21**, 343-354.

Wagner, J. G., and Patel, J. A. (1972) Variations in absorption and elimination rates of ethyl alcohol in a single subject. *Res. Commun. Chem. Pathol. Pharmacol*, **4**, 61-76.

Wagner, L., Wagner, G., and Guerrero, J. (1970) Effect of alcohol on premature newborn infants. *Am. J. Obstet. Gynecol.*, **108**, 308-315.

Wagner, J. G., Wilkinson, P. K., Sedman, A. J., Kay, D. R., and Weider, D. J. (1976) Elimination of alcohol from human blood. *J. Pharm. Sci.*, **65**, 152-154.

Walker, G. W., and Curry, A. S. (1966) 'Endogenous' alcohol in body fluids, *Nature, (Lond).* **210**, 1368.

Wallgren, H., and Barry, H. (1970) *In* Actions of Alcohol, Vol 1, pp. 17-73, Elsevier Pub. Co., New York.

Waltman, R., Bonura, F., Nigrin, G., and Pipat, C. (1969) Ethanol and neonatal bilirubin levels. *Lancet, ii*, 108.

Wartburg, J. P. von (1971) The metabolism of alcohol in normals and alcoholics: Enzymes. *In* The Biology of Alcoholism (Kissin, B., and Begleiter, H. *eds.*) Vol 1, pp. 63–102, Plenum Press, New York.

Wartburg, J. P. von and Schurch, P. M. (1968) Atypical human liver alcohol dehydrogenase. *Ann. N. Y. Acad. Sci.*, **151**, 936–946.

Wartburg, J. P. von, Bethune, J. L., and Vallee, B. L. (1964) Human-liver alcohol dehydrogenase: Kinetic and physicochemical properties. *Biochemistry*, **3**, 1775–1782.

Wartburg, J. P. von, Papenberg, J., and Aebi, H. (1965) An atypical human alcohol dehydrogenase. *Clin. J. Biochem.*, **43**, 889–898.

Wartburg, J. P. von, Berger, D., Buhlmann, Ch., Dubied, A., and Ris, M. M. (1974) Heterogeneity of pyridine nucleotide dependent alcohol and aldehyde metabolizing enzymes. *In* Alcohol and Aldehyde Metabolizing Systems (Thurman, R. G., Yonetani, T., Williamson, J. R. and Chance, B. *eds.*) pp. 33–44, Academic Press, New York.

Welling, P. G., Lyons, L. L., Eliot, R., and Amidon, G. L. (1977) Pharmokinetics of alcohol following single low doses to fasted and non-fasted subjects. *J. Clin. Pharmacol.*, **17**, 199–206.

Widmark, E. (1932) Die Theoretischen Grundlagen und die praktische Verwendbarkeit gerichtlich-medizinischen Alkololbestimmung, Urban and Schwarzenberg, Berlin.

Wilkinson, P., O'Day, D. M., and Rankin, J. G. (1969) Alcohol degradation and bromsulphthalein metabolism in acute alcoholic liver disease. *Gut*, **10**, 241–244.

Wilkinson, P. K., Sedman, A. J., Sakmar, E., Lin, Y-L., and Wagner, J. G. (1977) Fasting and non-fasting blood ethanol concentrations following repeated oral administration of ethanol to one adult. *J. Pharmacokinet. Biopharm.*, **5**, 41–52.

Winkler, K., Lundquist, F., and Tygstrup, N. (1969) The hepatic metabolism of ethanol in patients with cirrhosis of the liver. *Scand. J. Clin. Lab. Invest.*, **23**, 59–69.

Yamashita, Y., Inoue, N., Shirabe, T., Ohnishi, A., and Kuroiwa, Y. (1974). A case of malabsorption syndrome 'Meiteisho' (endogenous ethanol intoxication) and polyneuropathy. *Clin. Neurol. (Tokyo)*, **14**, 17–23.

Ylikahri, R. H., Leino, T., Huttunen, M. O., Pösö, A. R., Eriksson, C. J. P., and Nikkilä, E. A. (1976) Effects of fructose and glucose on ethanol-induced metabolic changes and on the intensity of alcohol intoxication and hangover. *Europ. J. Clin. Invest.*, **6**, 93–102.

CHAPTER 4

Congeners in Alcoholic Beverages

4.1 INTRODUCTION

4.1.1 Definitions

Alcoholic beverages contain numerous chemicals other than ethanol and these are called congeners. The word, which strictly means 'of the same kind', has also been defined as 'all alcohols other than ethyl alcohol' (Leake & Silverman, 1971). The congener content of the different alcoholic beverages varies, although they include mainly the aliphatic and aromatic primary alcohols other than ethanol, aldehydes and esters. Khan (1969) in a tabulation lists approximately 400 compounds which have been identified in alcoholic beverages, whilst Leake and Silverman (1966, 1971) have described in detail the chemical composition of the five basic kinds of alcoholic beverages: beers, table wines, dessert or cocktail wines, liqueurs or cordials, and distilled spirits. Carroll (1970) has also described the congener content of many alcoholic beverages. Table 4.1 lists a few of the common congeners and their concentrations in various alcoholic beverages.

The term fusel oil is frequently used as a synonym for congener. It is however more correctly defined as the oily residue left on the surface of any beverage after all the ethanol has been removed. The main ingredients of the fusel oils are 3-methyl-1-butanol and 2-methyl-1-butanol. These compounds in particular have a bad taste and usually efforts are made to remove them from alcoholic beverages. Despite this, significant amounts of iso-amyl alcohol and trace amounts of other compounds remain in alcoholic beverages (Webb et al., 1952; Carroll, 1970).

Considerable interest has centred on the possible relationship between the presence of congeners in beverages and alcohol addiction and related pathologies.

Some of the congeners have toxic or irritant properties, whilst others exert a pharmacological action. Congeners may also act as competitive substrates with ethanol or acetaldehyde for alcohol dehydrogenase and aldehyde dehydrogenase respectively. Whilst the importance of individual congeners in the development of addiction or pathological changes is equivocal, there is a school of thought which attributes the deleterious effects of alcoholic beverages to congeners.

Table 4.1
Congener content of alcoholic beverages (g per 100 litres at 50% alcohol.)
Adapted from Carroll, 1970.

	vodka	gin	whisky	cognac
acetaldehyde	0.44	0.33	1.71	7.14
ethyl formate	0.50	0.40	1.11	3.93
ethyl acetate	0	0.06	14.70	53.58
methanol	0.49	2.33	2.82	14.76
n-propanol	0	0.06	2.19	16.67
i-butanol	1.35	1.17	5.56	39.60
i-amyl alcohol	0.52	0	18.45	116.60
Total	3.30	4.35	46.54	252.28

4.1.2 Origins
Congeners may either originate from the raw materials of beverages, e.g. methyl anthranilate from grapes, or they may result from the fermentation process, bacterial contamination or accumulate in the ageing process (Murphree, 1971). In distilled spirits some of them are removed in the distillation process (Grab, 1961).

4.1.3 Analysis
The analysis of congeners in alcoholic beverages began in an attempt to identify the compounds giving flavour to beverages and for the purposes of quality control in the brewing industry. Earlier analytical techniques were tedious and included fractional distillation, titrimetry and column chromatography, as well as functional group analysis (Soumalainen & Nykänen, 1968). With the advent of gas chromatography the identification and quantitation of many more congeners in beverages has been possible.

4.1.4 Metabolism
There is little information of the metabolic fate of congeners in man. Studies on experimental animals show that of the primary alcohols, methanol is metabolised to formaldehyde and formate, whilst the higher primary alcohols are probably oxidised to the corresponding aldehyde and fatty acid. Human studies also support this as a mode of methanol metabolism, see Section 4.3.2,

(Haggard *et al.*, 1945). These compounds may contribute to the pharmacological and toxic actions of alcoholic beverages and will be considered in more detail elsewhere.

Secondary alcohols are oxidised only as far as the corresponding ketone, whilst tertiary alcohols which cannot be oxidised biochemically are slowly excreted.

Diols, such as ethylene and propylene glycol, are not normally found in alcoholic beverages. Both of these glycols are highly toxic: for instance, the former is oxidised in part to oxalic acid which damages renal tubules. Compounds with more than two hydroxy groups have reduced toxicity. Aliphatic esters are probably hydrolysed; the most prevalent are ethyl esters giving rise to ethanol. Aromatic esters are only hydrolysed with difficulty, if at all. The aldehydes, with the exception of acetaldehyde, are present in only small amounts and are oxidised to fatty acids. The metabolic fate of the congeners is outlined in Fig. 4.1.

$$R-CH_2OH \longrightarrow R-CHO \longrightarrow R-COOH$$

$$R^1.R^{11}.CHOH \longrightarrow R^1.R^{11}.C = O \longrightarrow\!\!\times\!\!\longrightarrow$$

$$R^1.R^{11}.R^{111}.COH \longrightarrow\!\!\times\!\!\longrightarrow$$

$$R^1.CO.OR^{11} \longrightarrow R^1.CO.OH + HOR^{11}$$

R = alkyl group

Fig. 4.1 – Metabolism of some congeners in man.

Haggard *et al.*, (1973) gave ethanol to a human volunteer, either as highly purified or as commercial spirit, and found that with the higher congener mixture there was a significant decrease in the oxidation of ethanol. This work, supported by studies in experimental animals (Gaillard & Derache, 1964 and 1965), suggests that a competitive inhibition of common metabolic pathways might lead to an accumulation of congeners in blood after prolonged or heavy drinking (Lelbach, 1974).

4.1.5 Blood and Urine levels

In a search for congeners in the blood of alcoholics, Majchrowitz and Mendelson (1970a,b) found blood acetaldehyde concentrations to be twice as high in those who drank bourbon whiskey than in those who consumed pure grain ethanol. This may be due to the presence of acetaldehyde both as a congener and as a metabolite of ethanol. In contrast, methanol levels in blood were shown to be only slightly higher in bourbon drinkers than in grain alcohol drinkers and it was suggested that the methanol came from endogenous sources (Majchrowicz and Mendelson, 1970c). This work is discussed more fully in Section 4.3.

In recent years the technique of gas–chromatography/mass–spectrometry has been used to separate and identify many of the compounds found in urine. Some of these compounds are also congeners, see Table 4.2, (Suomalainen & Nykänen, 1968; Khan, 1969; Carroll, 1970).

Table 4.2
Some compounds identified in urine that are also congeners.

Compounds identified in urine	Reference
4-hydroxybenzoic acid	Mrochek *et al.,* (1971)
citric acid, tartaric acid, *p*-hydroxybenzoic acid	Horning and Horning (1971)
lactic acid, succinic acid, citric acid	Thompson and Markey (1975)
l-propanol limonene acetic acid benzaldehyde	Zlatkis and Liebach (1971)
benzene benzaldehyde	Matsumato *et al.,* (1973)

The origin of these compounds in urine is not known because drinking histories were not given. It is, however, possible that these compounds are not derived from alcoholic beverages and are normal urine constituents, so that the toxicity of congeners may not be relevant.

4.1.6 Pharmacology and Toxicity

Richardson (1869) was the first to show that the pharmacological action of the primary alcohols increases in proportion to the number of carbon atoms. He proposed that these substances were responsible for such toxic effects of alcoholic beverages as hangover. Since then there have been numerous studies on the toxicity of congeners in various experimental animals and *in vitro* systems. Macht (1921) reviews much of the earlier work showing that the higher alcohols have great pharmacological action, although studies of different beverages have been less clear. Such studies have measured, for instance, the effect of different alcoholic beverages on the sleeping time of mice (Blum *et al.*, 1970), enzymatic activity and histological appearance of rat liver (Kiessling and Pilstom, 1968). The study of congener toxicity in humans has been less extensive. Many congeners are known to be toxic if inhaled or swallowed in the pure form, and most are irritants causing damage to the gastrointestinal tract, respiratory system, kidney, heart or liver. To illustrate their toxicity, Table 4.3 lists the threshold limit values (TLV) for some congeners. These values are accepted by the American Governmental Hygienists (Muir, 1971) and they 'represent conditions under which it is believed that nearly all workers may be repeatedly exposed day after day without adverse effect'.

Table 4.3
Threshold limit values and some properties of selected congeners.

Congener	Ethyl acetate	Acetaldehyde	i-Butyl alcohol
TLV ppm of air at 25°C 760 mm Hg	400	200	100
Toxic effects	Irritant Kidney, liver damage	Headaches Drowsiness Irritation GIT Anaemia Delirium Hallucinations Loss of intelligence	Irritant
	Propanol	*Methanol*	
	200	200	
	Irritant Narcotic	Dizziness Stupor Cramps Irritation Central nervous-system damage Kidney damage Liver damage Heart damage	

From 'Hazards in the Chemical Laboratory'
ed. G. D. Muir, Royal Institute of Chemistry 1971

Gosselin *et al.*, (1976) classify and list the probable oral lethal dose of many compounds which are congeners as follows:

Classification	Probable Oral Lethal Dose
6 Super toxic	< 5 mg/kg
5 Extremely	5–50 mg/kg
4 Very	50–500 mg/kg
3 Moderately	0.5–5 g/kg
2 Slightly	5–15 g/kg
1 Practically non-toxic	> 15 g/kg

Compound	Classification
Benzoic acid	3
Benzene	4
Amyl alcohol	3
Benzyl alcohol	3
n-Butyl alcohol	3
Ethanol	2
3-Methyl-1-butanol (*i*-amyl)	4
2-Propanol (*i*-propyl)	2
Methanol	3
1-Propanol	3
Acetaldehyde	3
Carbamates	3–1

Little is known however about the toxicity of these compounds as congeners in alcoholic beverages.

Barlow *et al.*, (1936) showed that whiskey had a greater effect on gastrointestinal mobility than pure alcohol. A study of cardiovascular effects in men found changes in heart rate, pulse and blood pressure, though the exact relation to congener content was not made clear (Starr *et al.*, 1970). Enhanced catecholamine release caused by the congeners was the suggested mechanism. The effect of congeners on the incidence of nystagmus has been studied using vodka, bourbon whiskey, and a 'super bourbon' with high congener content (Murphree *et al.*, 1966; Murphree *et al.*, 1967). No difference was found in blood ethanol concentration or incidence of nystagmus produced by the bourbon and vodka. However the synthetic 'super bourbon' produced a much greater incidence of nystagmus, which persisted after the blood ethanol had fallen to nothing. It should be realised that the 'super bourbon' represents an extremely high concentration of congeners. Other workers (Murphree, 1969; Murphree *et al.*, 1970) have investigated the effect of different beverages on the electro-encephalogram (EEG) of humans. Qualitative changes were found in those who had consumed beverages with a high congener content.

4.1.7 Pathology

There is little evidence to suggest that congeners play an important role in the development of organic lesions in humans. Most clinical evidence suggests that the source of ethanol is of no importance in the occurrence of diseases complicating alcoholism (Lelbach, 1974). In the development of liver disease the choice of beverage is not important. Lelbach (1968) compared two groups of alcoholics, one drinking beer and the other only spirits. The two groups were matched for age and sex but no differences were found in the degree of hepatic dysfunction of the two groups. Schmidt and Bronetto (1962) showed a significant relationship between cirrhosis mortality and consumption of cheap, native wines, but not of beer or spirits. This may be due to the fact that wines are a cheap source of ethanol (Doctor, 1967; Rubington, 1968). Some congeners have been linked with specific pathologies. In a study of oesophageal cancer in central Africa, the high incidence of the cancer was attributed to the presence of nitrosoamines in the local alcoholic beverages (McGlashan, 1969). More recent studies, however, were unable to detect nitrosoamines in spirits from Africa (Gough, 1977).

Similarly polycyclic aromatic hydrocarbons, which have been found in whiskies, have been implicated in oesophageal carcinogenesis (Richardson, 1869). High contents of lead, iron and cobalt in alcoholic beverages have been shown to cause specific organ lesions but these may not be considered as congeners. There is some evidence that congeners might play a part in the overall intoxicating effect of alcoholic beverages (Lelbach, 1974). Much of the early work supported this, but experiments were badly designed and the data ambiguous (Murphree, 1971).

Similarly, experiments designed to test the effects of congeners on 'hangover' suffer also from this criticism. Chapman (1970) found more frequent and severe 'hangover' in subjects given bourbon than in those given vodka, though Nathan et al., (1970) showed that hangover was essentially dependent on the amount of ethanol ingested. The role of congeners in the addictive process is unclear but, in view of their greater depressant and acute toxic activities, investigation into this might be useful.

4.1.8 Behaviour

Studies of the effect of different alcoholic beverages on behaviour have suggested that congeners may affect behaviour, but the results are inconclusive.

Katkin et al., (1970) found increased risk-taking in subjects given doses of high congener beverages as compared with those given doses of low congener beverages. Other studies have reported conflicting results from their studies of the effect of congeners on reaction time and perceptual motor performance (Katkin and Hayes, 1967; Wilson et al., 1970).

Finally the most extreme view supporting the clinical importance of congeners is that of Gyorgy (1961), who denies that ethanol is in any way implicated in the pathogenesis of alcoholic cirrhosis.

4.2 THE HIGHER ALCOHOLS

The higher alcohols are found as congeners in alcoholic beverages. Although the toxicity of the pure compounds in animals has been widely studied, much remains to be learnt about their importance as congeners and about their metabolism and toxicology in man (Derache, 1970).

4.2.1 Absorption and Metabolism

We know little about the absorption or metabolism of the higher alcohols, although some of the alcohols have been shown to be absorbed through the oral mucosa in dogs (Siegel et al., 1976).

Animal experiments (Haggard et al., 1945) suggest that the higher primary alcohols are probably oxidised to the corresponding aldehydes and fatty acids, and the secondary alcohols to the corresponding ketones. The fate of the tertiary alcohols is uncertain.

Gaillard and Derache (1965) studied the relative rates of disappearance of the different alcohols in rats. They showed that methanol, i-propanol and t-butanol reach higher blood levels than ethanol and remain in the blood for longer. Conversely n-butanol, i-butanol, n-propanol and i-amyl alcohols are much weaker than ethanol and disappear very rapidly from the blood. Methanol, ethanol and i-propanol were found in urine, whereas no amyl or i-amyl alcohols were found. In vitro experiments with horse material (Winer, 1958) indicate that higher alcohols are probably oxidised by ADh and some at a greater rate than ethanol.

Wartburg et al., (1965) studied human ADh and found that it was capable of metabolising the higher alcohols to a certain extent. This is discussed further in Chapter 3.

It has been suggested that those alcohols, occurring in higher concentrations in blood than ethanol, may accumulate as a result of competition with ethanol for ADh (Greenberg, 1970).

Iso-propanol, when ingested, is metabolised to acetone (15%) which is excreted for 3–6 days (Arena, 1970). When the intake is small only acetone can be found in the urine, and when it is large both acetone and i-propanol have been found (Stolman and Steward, 1960; Anon, 1977).

4.2.2 Metabolic Effects

The metabolic effects of the higher alcohols have not been extensively investigated, so it is difficult to assess their clinical importance. Studies in animals have indicated that some alcohols such as i-propanol, may affect acid-base status, glucose homeostasis and lipid metabolism. Iso-propanol may also affect acid-base status in man (Derache 1970).

4.2.3 Toxicity and Pharmacology

The toxicity of the higher alcohols is well documented, but the exact nature of the effect depends on the experimental animal, the route of administration, and the measure of toxicity employed. Many methods, including lethal dose (Haggard *et al.*, 1945) cell culture (Mai *et al.*, 1965) and 'state of ebriety' of animals (Wallgren, 1960) have been used as a measure of toxicity. It has been found as a general rule that the acute toxicity of the alcohols in animals increases with the number of carbons and decreases with isomerism according to Richardson's Law (Richardson, 1869; Macht, 1921; Wallgren, 1960) (See Table 4.4).

Table 4.4
The acute lethal doses of some congeners. (Adapted from and with the permission of Macht (1921) J. Pharmacol. Exp. Ther., The Williams and Wilkins Co., Baltimore).

Alcohol	Acute lethal dose per kilo weight (ml)
Methyl	118
Ethyl	100
Propyl	40
Butyl	6
Amyl	15
Iso propyl	5
Iso butyl	18
Iso amyl	26
Benzyl	60

In discussing the toxicities of the alcohols, a distinction should be made between acute or intermediate effects, and the secondary effects due to metabolites (Macht, 1921).

Similarly, the pharmacological effects, i.e. the narcotic effects, of the higher alcohols seem to increase with increase in the number of carbon atoms, and to decrease with isomerism (Wesse, 1928). However this relationship may only reflect differences in the ability of the different alcohols to reach the central nervous system from the blood. For example in the monkey the blood brain barrier is not very permeable to alcohols (Raichle *et al.*, 1976), and hence other measures of narcotic activity have been sought.

It has been shown that a strong concentration of ethanol blocks the transmission of the frog nerve impulse through membrane depolarisation (Gallego, 1948), and this has been used as a test of narcotic activity. The effect of ethanol on potentiating the effect of acetylcholine on frog muscle and the secretion of hydrochloric acid by isolated rat stomach have also been used (Nelemens, 1962; Sachdev *et al.*, 1963; Sait-Blanquat and Derache, 1966). Inhibition of the oxidative process, in the rat brain, has been found to increase with the number of carbons and concentration, *n*-pentanol being the most active (Beer and Quastel 1958a). These authors and Lindenbohm and Wallgren (1962) suggest that the alcohols bring about a narcotic effect at the cell membrane level. Further evidence from Nisenbaum *et al.* (1976) indicates that propanol and benzyl alcohol affect the stability of cell membranes—*n*-butanol, butane-2, 3-diol and octanol were found to have similar effects (De Bruijne and Steveninck, 1977).

4.3 METHANOL

Despite its low concentration in alcoholic beverages, methanol is an important congener because of its great toxicity.

4.3.1 Absorption and Metabolism

After absorption, which can occur through the alimentary mucosa, skin and pulmonary alveolae, methanol is widely distributed in the body tissues. It is found in the cerebrospinal fluid, breath, urine, blood and gastric juices. As little as 3% is excreted unchanged (Koivusalo, 1970).

Methanol is oxidised to formaldehyde and then to formic acid. The latter may then be excreted or further metabolised to carbon dioxide and water. In man 5% of the dose may be excreted as formic acid with maximal blood and urinary levels of this acid at 2-3 days after ingestion. Blood and urine concentrations of formic acid are directly related to the amount of methanol consumed (Roe, 1946; Lund, 1948; Cooper and Kini, 1962; Koivusalo, 1970; Closs and Solberg, 1970) though it has not been isolated in other studies of methanol poisoning (Cooper and Kini, 1962, Koivusalo, 1970).

Studies on methanol metabolism in experimental animals, reviewed by Koivusalo (1970) and Cornish (1975), have shown that both ADh and the catalase system metabolise ethanol. The relative importance of each enzyme system depends on the animal studied. *In vitro* experiments have implicated the MEOS in the oxidation of methanol, though its significance in man is not known. It would appear that in man ADh is the principal enzyme involved in the oxidation of methanol to formaldehyde (Cooper and Kini, 1962; Koivusalo,

1970; Cornish, 1975), formaldehyde dehydrogenase oxidising it to formate and then catalase to carbon dioxide and water (Cooper and Kini, 1962). The latter two steps are not confirmed in man. Alternative pathways of metabolism through aldehyde dehydrogenase, alcohol dehydrogenase, xanthine oxidase, aldehyde oxidase or glyceraldehyde-3-phosphate dehydrogenase have been suggested from animal experiments (Koivusalo, 1970).

Mani *et al.*, (1970) showed that human ADh oxidises methanol at approximately 1/10 of the rate of ethanol. Kinetic studies have indicated that there are similarities of human ADh to horse and yeast ADh: however human liver ADh has the lowest Km value for methanol, and so is the best catalyst for this reaction (Wartburg *et al.*, 1965; Blair and Vallee, 1966).

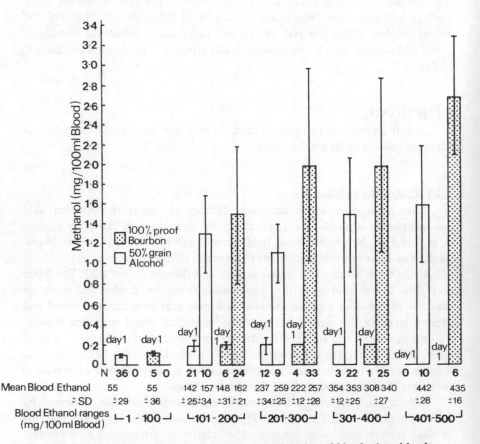

Fig. 4.2 – Blood methanol concentration as a function of blood ethanol levels in bourbon and grain alcohol drinkers following cessation of drinking. The values are means ± standard deviation. (Reproduced by permission from Majchrowicz and Mendelson (1970) from Recent Advances in Studies of Alcoholism, National Institute of Health/National Institute of Mental Health, U.S.A.)

The common biochemical pathway of oxidation of ethanol and methanol may account for the clinical observations that the administration of ethanol may ameliorate the toxic sequelae of methanol poisoning (Roe, 1943, Zatman 1946; Smith, 1961; Majchrowicz and Mendelson, 1970a,c).

4.3.2 Blood Levels

Blood levels of methanol in acute methanol poisoning have been reviewed by Koivusalo (1970). There is evidence that methanol may also be found in man endogenously (Western and Ozburn, 1949; Erikson and Kulkarni, 1963). Some of this methanol may originate from pectin-rich foods which contain ester-bound methanol or from the activity of the intestinal flora (Koivusalo, 1970), but endogenous methanol may arise metabolically. Axelrod and Daly (1965) identified an enzyme system which metabolised S-adenosylmethionine to methanol and to S-adenosylhomocysteine in the pituitary. Tyce (1977) found that demethylation of catecholamine metabolites in human erythrocytes led to the formation of methanol. Although trace amount of methanol may be innocuos, accumulation in the alcoholic from congeners may be important. Majchrowicz and Mendelson (1970a) (see Figs 2 & 3) found an increase in blood methanol levels from 0.2 mg/100 ml to 2.7 mg/100 ml in drinking alcoholics. They suggest that part of this is endogenous and part derives from the alcoholic beverage. Blood methanol levels decreased at a rate of 0.29 mg/100 ml/h but only

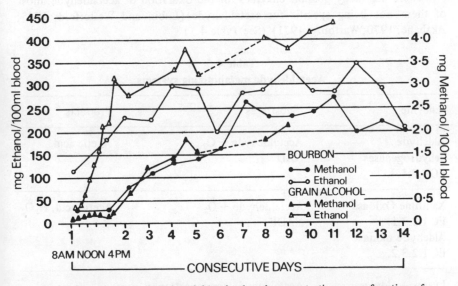

Fig. 4.3 – Blood methanol and blood ethanol concentrations as a function of time in bourbon and grain alcohol drinkers. (Reproduced by permission from Majchrowicz and Mendelson (1970) from Recent Advances in Studies of Alcoholism, National Institute of Health/National Institute of Mental Health, U.S.A.)

after blood ethanol levels decreased to 70–20 mg/100 ml. Blood methanol disappearance lagged behind the linear disappearance of ethanol by approximately 6–8h. Methanol probably accumulated in the blood as a result of competitive inhibition of ADh by ethanol. Endogenously-formed methanol or its metabolites may contribute to the severity of intoxication and withdrawal.

4.4 ACETALDEHYDE

Acetaldehyde has a dual role in alcohol consumption, because it is found both as a constituent of many alcoholic beverages and also as a metabolite of ethanol. This is important, because it is 10–30 times more toxic than ethanol (Akabane, 1970; Truitt and Walsh, 1971). Many of its effects have been studied (see for instance Finnish Foundation, 1975).

4.4.1 Metabolism

Acetaldehyde is metabolised rapidly (Lieber, 1968): mainly it is thought to acetate and then to acetyl CoA (Lunquist *et al.*, 1962; Wartburg, 1971). Animal studies have indicated that oxidation of acetaldehyde occurs mainly in the mitochondria, though at high concentrations oxidation may occur in the cytosol, whereupon the reduced equivalents are transported to the mitochondria by the malate-aspartate cycle (Parilla *et al.*, 1974; Peterson *et al.*, 1977).

There are many possible enzymes for the oxidation of acetaldehyde, most of them not being specific for acetaldehyde (Lubin and Westerfold, 1945; Akabane, 1970; Wartburg, 1971). (See Table 4.5).

Table 4.5
Acetaldehyde metabolizing systems.

Enzyme	Substrates	Products
Aldehyde dehydrogenases EC 1.2.1.3.	Acetaldehyde + O_2 NAD	Acetic acid
Xanthine Oxidase EC 1.2.3.1. Aldehyde oxidase EC 1.2.3.2.	Acetaldehyde + O_2 NADP	Acetic acid, H_2O_2
Lyases − aldolases	Acetaldehyde condensation reactions e.g. Acetaldehyde + Pyruvate → Acetoin	

Thus there are many pathways for acetaldehyde metabolism. The relative importance of each pathway may vary with species, tissue, diet and many other factors (Wartburg, 1971). However, it is likely that in man aldehyde dehydrogenase is the most important acetaldehyde metabolizing enzyme.

Human acetaldehyde dehydrogenase (E.C.1.2.3.1.) has two actions, namely (1) the conversion of acetaldehyde to acetate, and (2) the hydroxylation of non-aldehydic heterocyclic compounds. It is a flavoprotein, similar to xanthine oxidase, oxidised by NAD^+ with a pH optimum of 9-10. It is not stimulated by coenzyme A and its action is irreversible. The human enzyme can be fractionated into several components by chromatography and electrophoresis. Their significance is not known (Johns, 1967; Kraemer and Deitrich, 1968; Blair and Bodley, 1969).

4.4.2 Blood Acetaldehyde Levels

Much of the earlier work on blood acetaldehyde levels, (reviewed by Truitt and Walsh (1977)), was carried out on experimental animals, and on humans after ingestion of disulfiram and after acute ingestion of ethanol. These results show a wide range of blood acetaldehyde levels, partially due to analytical variability. (Table 4.6).

Table 4.6

Blood acetaldehyde levels in humans (μg/ml).

CH_3 CHO after alcohol	Drug pretreatment	CH_3 CHO after alcohol and drug
16.06	—	—
1.05	disulfiram	5.64–8.0
6.9–9.6	,,	15.4–48.4
—	,,	~5.0–9.0
3.61	,,	10.0
—	glucose	1.9–6.6
5.9–17.0	disulfiram	6.4–25.1
30	—	—
0.3	—	—
1.0	—	—
13.75	—	—
2.5	disulfiram	5.2
0.1–0.56	—	—
7–14	—	—

(Sources: Stotz, 1943; Akabane, 1970; Truitt and Walsh, 1971)

It is perhaps more interesting to consider blood acetaldehyde levels following chronic alcohol administration. It had been postulated that an induction of ADh might take place due to repeated drinking and that this would lead to an increased generation of acetaldehyde (Truitt and Walsh, 1971). However, increased levels of ADh have not been found in alcoholics (Chapter 3).

Freund and O'Hollaren (1965) found a plateau of acetaldehyde concentration in human alveolar air following ethanol administration. The relationship to ethanol metabolism was, however, not defined. These researchers reported higher levels in alcoholics, particularly those suffering from brain damage. It was therefore proposed that acetaldehyde might be implicated in brain damage.

Majchrowicz and Mendelson (1970 a,b) recorded blood acetaldehyde levels ranging from 0.04–0.15 mg/100 ml in chronic alcoholism after a period of acute intoxication, (see Fig. 4.4). The levels depended on the source of alcohol, but no dose or dose-time relationships were found between blood ethanol and blood acetaldehyde concentrations. High congener drinks gave rise to higher blood acetaldehyde levels than was the case in low congener beverages. This may be due either to the presence of acetaldehyde as a congener, or to competitive inhibition of aldehyde dehydrogenase by aldehydes derived from other alcohols present in the beverages.

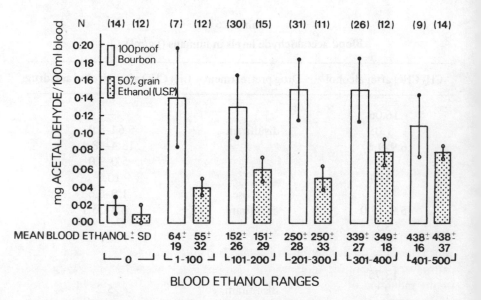

Fig. 4.4 – Blood acetaldehyde concentration as a function of blood ethanol levels in bourbon and grain alcohol drinkers following cessation of drinking. The values are mean ± standard deviation. (Reproduced by permission from Majchrowicz and Mendelson (1970) from Recent Advances in Studies of Alcoholism, National Institute of Health/National Institute of Mental Health, U.S.A.)

The authors concluded that acetaldehyde does not play a significant role in the process of tolerance and physical dependence on alcohol. These processes show dose and dose-time relationships to blood ethanol levels (Isabell *et al.*, 1955). Since such dose-response relationships with blood acetaldehyde levels were not found, they concluded that ethanol and not acetaldehyde is the main addictive agent in alcoholism.

Korsten *et al.* (1975) found a relationship between blood acetaldehyde and ethanol in humans after i.v. administration of ethanol yielding concentrations high enough to saturate intra-hepatic ethanol oxidising systems, ADh, MEOS and catalase. This study showed that acetaldehyde levels remained fairly constant despite variation in the blood alcohol levels. However, the acetaldehyde plateau ends abruptly when ethanol concentrations reach 110 mg/100 ml, a concentration corresponding to MEOS saturation (Fig. 4.5).

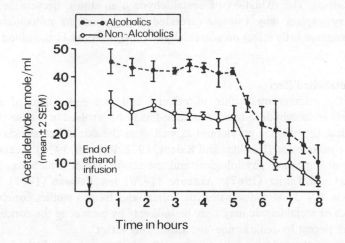

Fig. 4.5 – Comparison of blood acetaldehyde levels of alcoholic and non-alcoholic subjects following i.v. alcohol infusion. (Reprinted by permission from the New England Journal of Medicine, **292**, 386, 1975).

The plateau of acetaldehyde was higher in alcoholics than non-alcoholics. This observed fall in blood acetaldehyde concentration at blood ethanol levels which are fully saturating for ADh suggests the *in vivo* operation of a non-ADh pathway of alcohol metabolism. The high plateau of acetaldehyde may be due to the induction of the MEOS or due to mitrochondrial changes in the liver (Lieber *et al.*, 1975). Whether or not ethanol consumption alters the activity of acetaldehyde dehydrogenase is unproven; because both increases, and no changes, in this enzyme have been found in experimental animals (Lieber *et al.*, 1975). It is also possible that acetaldehyde oxidation is limited by the availability of NAD.

In contrast Truitt (1971) using GC methods found no statistically significant difference in blood acetaldehyde levels between alcoholics and non-alcoholics.

In summary where higher blood acetaldehyde levels have been found in alcoholics the following mechanisms have been proposed:

(a) Increased generation of acetaldehyde from ethanol due to the increased activity of ADh or MEOS.

(b) The presence of acetaldehyde in beverages.

(c) Inhibition of aldehyde dehydrogenase by aldehydes generated from higher alcohols present in beverages.

(d) Mitochondrial changes.

Fructose, glucose, sucrose and alanine were found not to increase the clearance of acetaldehyde after administration of alcohol to alcoholics (Rawat, 1977). Castro and Malkus (1977) suggest that acetaldehyde metabolism, unlike ethanol metabolism, is less sensitive to shifts in the redox state of the NAD couples. The oxidation of acetaldehyde is an almost irreversible process. This may explain why fructose-mediated changes on the mitochondria and cytoplasm have little effect on acetaldehyde concentrations in the blood.

4.4.3 Metabolic Effects

As the primary metabolite of ethanol and as a constituent of alcoholic beverages, acetaldehyde, a toxic compound, may be involved in the development of physical dependence on alcohol as well as in the side effect associated with ethanol consumption (Hawkins and Kalant, 1972; Rahwan, 1974). Acetaldehyde has several important physiological and metabolic effects, which are discussed by Truitt and Duritz (1967), Akabane (1970) and Rahwan (1975). Dietrich and Erwin (1975) in a discussion of animal and human studies conclude that the effect of acetaldehyde may only be indirect—by increasing the concentration of a more potent biogenic amine-'the amplifying effect'.

Many of the studies carried out on the toxicity of acetaldehyde were on animals, and these are described in the reviews listed above. A few of the human studies are described in the following pages:

(1) OXIDATIVE PHOSPHORYLATION AND COENZYME A ACTIVITY

Animal experiments indicate that acetaldehyde depresses oxidative phosphorylation. This may occur, it is suggested, through a coupling of a metabolite of pyruvate leading to increased acetoin levels (Rehak and Truitt, 1958). An impairment of the NADH-ubiquinone oxidoreductase complex may also be involved (Cederbaum et al., 1974; Cederbaum et al., 1976). The reduction in oxidative phosphorylation due to acetaldehyde has been confirmed by Beer and Quastel (1958b) who also found that this inhibition was reversed by NAD. However Truitt and Duritz (1967) conclude that this is not the cause of ethanol brain depression. The inebriating action of ethanol appears too quickly after alcohol ingestion and with little or no acetaldehyde measurable. This effect, however, may become more important in chronic drinking.

Acetaldehyde has also been shown in animal experiments to depress coenzyme A activity in brain and liver. This may be due to the blocking of the active site (Ammon et al., 1969; Ammon et al., 1971).

(2) BIOGENIC AMINE METABOLISM

Acetaldehyde may play a role in biogenic amine metabolism. In alcoholics there is an alteration in both serotonin and norepinephrine metabolism leading to an increase in the reductive pathway and a decrease in the oxidative pathway. This increase in the reductive pathway may be due to an increase in hepatic NADH, due to the oxidation of ethanol. Another possible mechanism, relevant to the discussion of congeners, is the competitive inhibition of aldehyde dehydrogenase, an enzyme involved in amine metabolism, by acetaldehyde.

(3) RELEASE OF CATECHOLAMINES

Alcohol has been shown to produce stress-like increases in urinary excretion of catecholamines in animals and man, as reviewed by Truitt and Walsh (1971). Animal experiments both in vitro and in vivo indicate that this might be due to acetaldehyde (Walsh and Truitt, 1968; Greenberg and Cohen, 1973; Rahwan et al., 1974; Schneider, 1971, 1974a; O'Neill and Rahwan, 1975; Lahti, 1975). This effect has been implicated in the development of alcoholic cardiomyopathy (Jones and Beer, 1967 and 1968). Evidence for central effects of acetaldehyde in animals is not conclusive (Truitt and Walsh, 1971).

(4) TETRAHYDROISOQUINOLINES

Acetaldehyde condenses with catecholamines to form unstable Schiff bases which cyclise to form tetrahydroisoquinolines (Whaley and Govindachari, 1951). Such compounds have been found in biological tissue in vitro, in vivo in laboratory animals (Truitt and Duritz, 1967; Cohen and Collins, 1970; Davis and Walsh, 1970a,b,c; Truitt and Walsh, 1971; Davis, 1973; Rahwan et al., 1974; Rahwan, 1975; Lahti, 1975) and in humans (Sandler et al., 1973) following the administration of ethanol and/or dopa. These compounds are structurally related to naturally-occurring psychoactive plant products and may play a role in ethanol dependence. Acetaldehyde-derived tetrahydroisoquinoline derivatives have been shown to act as false neurotransmitters and also to alter adrenergic function, and hence to cause side effects (Cohen, 1973).

Many compounds capable of complexing with acetaldehyde may interfere with the synthesis of these compounds and hence they may protect against acetaldehyde toxicity.

(5) TETRAHYDRO-β-CARBOLINES

Acetaldehyde condenses with indoleamines to form tetrahdro-β-carbolines *in vivo* following administration of ethanol or acetaldehyde to laboratory animals (McIsaac, 1961; Dajani and Saheb, 1973). These compounds are structurally related to the hallucinogenic agent 10-methoxylharmalan, which could arise through aberrant metabolism of serotonin in the presence of acetaldehyde. Thus these compounds may play a role in ethanol dependence (Rahwan, 1975). Mainly because it has not been possible to repeat experiments and to isolate these compounds their role in alcohol addiction remains open to criticism. Seevers (1970) however based his criticism on the dissimilarity between physical dependence and withdrawal from morphine as compared with alcohol. There is moreover a lack of concordance between tolerance and dependence of these compounds. Davis and Walsh (1970a,b,c) suggest that these anomalies are due to the diffuse action of morphine and the localised action of acetaldehyde.

4.4.4 Organ Effects

MUSCLE

Liver damage in alcoholics can be related to metabolism of ethanol at that site. However, muscle does not metabolise ethanol to a large extent and yet a myopathy has been described in alcoholics (Geller and Rubin, 1977). It has been suggested, therefore, that this is due to the action of a metabolite of ethanol such as acetaldehyde.

Ethanol and acetaldehyde alter the activity of healthy human muscle ATPase, probably through altering the binding of calcium to muscle proteins (Puszkin and Rubin, 1976).

A similar decrease in muscle ATPase has been noted in chronic alcoholics (Rubin *et al.*, 1976). They concluded that the damage may not be due directly to acetaldehyde as these changes were found 12–24 h after alcohol consumption.

Much remains to be learnt of the possible role of acetaldehyde in alcoholic myopathy.

BRAIN

The direct effects of acetaldehyde on the human brain are incompletely understood. Much work has been carried out on animals, reviewed by Truitt and Walsh (1971). These studies suggest that acetaldehyde might play a role in central nervous system (CNS) depression. Truitt and Walsh (1971) suggest that it may be the relative blood levels of acetaldehyde and ethanol which are important. For example acetaldehyde levels are high relative to ethanol during alcohol withdrawal, a time during which hallucinations are common in alcoholics. Thus they suggest that acetaldehyde may effect the CNS. However it is possible that these effects are indirect and are due to the release of catecholamines stimulated by acetaldehyde. There are further complications in that recent studies suggest that there is a blood-brain barrier to acetaldehyde, at least in mice (Tabakoff *et al.*, 1976).

ERYTHROCYTES

Several erythrocyte abnormalities are found in chronic alcoholics—altered cell morphology, increased osmotic fragility and decreased erythrocyte filterability.

Gaines *et al.*, (1977) have shown using human erythrocyte ghosts that acetaldehyde binds to erythrocyte membrane proteins, spectin and actin, giving rise to morphological changes. There is also evidence that acetaldehyde binds to haemoglobins. It is suggested that these changes could lead to the erythrocyte abnormalities found in alcoholics.

CARDIOVASCULAR SYSTEM

Variation in patient characteristics makes the assessment of the aetiological agents in alcoholic heart disease difficult (Bing and Tillmanns, 1977). Acetaldehyde has been implicated in its pathology. It has been suggested that the changes found in the cardiovascular system in alcoholics may arise from the myocardial and adrenal release of catecholamines due to acetaldehyde (James and Bear, 1967).

Asmussen, *et al.*, (1948) found that the administration of acetaldehyde to humans to a level of 0.2-0.7 mg/100 ml led to an increase in heart rate, ventilation and dead space. At the same time a decrease in alveolar carbon dioxide was found. Similar symptoms are found in patients on Antabuse[†], which gives rise to high blood acetaldehyde levels.

There is also evidence from experimental animals that acetaldehyde might inhibit the synthesis of cardiac proteins (Schrieber *et al.*, 1972; Schreiber *et al.*, 1974).

Acetaldehyde is also found in cigarette smoke (Newsome, 1965), and elevated blood acetaldehyde concentrations during chronic alcohol consumption combined with heavy cigarette smoking could play a role in cardiovascular disease (Egle, 1972).

4.4.5 Miscellaneous Effects

PORPHYRINS

The porphyrinogenic action of alcohol may not be due to ethanol itself but may be due to changes in liver redox state or ethanol metabolites (Held, 1977).

†Antabuse is a Registered Trade Mark

DISULFIRAM (ANTABUSE)

Acetaldehyde is believed to give rise to the toxic manifestations of the disulfiram-ethanol reaction (Akabane, 1970; Truitt and Walsh, 1971).

TERATOLOGY

It has been suggested that acetaldehyde could be responsible for some of the effects seen in the foetal alcohol syndrome. However animal studies have shown that acetaldehyde does not cross the placenta in appreciable amounts and may, in fact, be metabolized by the placenta (Randall, 1977).

Studies of ethanol and acetaldehyde levels in the milk and peripheral blood of lactating women after ethanol administration have shown (Kesäniemi, 1974) that ethanol but not acetaldehyde is found in the milk of drinking women. The amount of ethanol which a suckling could recieve during maternal ethanol metabolism is low and unlikely to cause harmful effects when maternal use of alcohol is temporary.

4.5 REFERENCES

Akabane, J. (1970) Aldehydes and related compounds. *In* International Encyclopedia Pharmacology and Therapeutics Section 20 (Tremolieres, J. *ed.*) Vol 2, pp. 523-560, Pergamon Press, Oxford.

Ammon, H. P. T. (1971) *Biological Aspects of Alcoholism* (Roach, M. K., McIsaac, W. M., and Creaven, P. J. *eds.*) University of Texas Press, Austin.

Ammon, H. P. T., Estler, C. J., and Heim, F. (1969) Inactivation of coenzyme A by ethanol, I, Acetaldehyde as mediator of the inactivation of coenzyme A following the administration of ethanol *in vivo. Biochem. Pharmacol.*, 18, 29-33.

Anon. (1977) *The Extra Pharmacopoeia* (Martindale II) pp. 42-43, Plenum Press.

Arena, J. M. (1970) *Poisoning*, p.165, Charles C. Thomas, Springfield Illinois.

Asmussen, E., Hald, J., and Larsen, V. (1948) The pharmacological action of acetaldehyde on the human organism. *Acta Pharmacol. Toxicol.*, 4, 311-320.

Axelrod, J., and Daly, J. (1965) Pituitary gland: Enzymic formation of methanol from S-adenosylmethione. *Science*, 150, 892-893.

Barlow, O. W., Beams, A. J., and Goldblatt, H. (1936) Studies on the pharmacology of ethyl alcohol. *J. Pharmacol. Exp. Ther.*, 56, 117-146.

Beer, C. T., and Quastel, J. H. (1958a) The effects of aliphatic alcohols on the respiration of rat brain cortex slices and rat brain mitochondria. *Can. J. Biochem. Physiol.*, 36, 543-556.

Beer, C. T., and Quastel, J. H. (1958b) The effects of aliphatic aldehydes on the respiration rate of rat brain cortex slices and rat brain mitochondria. *Can. J. Biochem. Physiol.*, 36, 531-541.

Bing, R. J., and Tillmans, H. (1977) The effect of alcohol on the heart, *In* Metabolic Aspects of Alcoholism (Lieber, C. S. *ed.*) pp. 117-134, MTP Press Ltd., Lancaster.

Blair, A. H., and Bodley, F. R. (1969) Human liver aldehyde dehydrogenase: partial purification and properties. *Can. J. Biochem.*, **47**, 265-272.

Blair, A. H., and Vallee, B. L. (1966) Some catalytic properties of human liver alcohol dehydrogenase. *Biochemistry*, **5**, 2026-2034.

Blum, K., Ryback, R. S., and Geller, I. (1970) Effects of vodka and bourbon on sleeping time in mice. *Q. J. Stud. Alcohol*, **Suppl. 5**, 62-66.

Carroll, R. B. (1970) Analysis of alcoholic beverages by gas-liquid chromatography. *Q. J. Stud. Alcohol*, **Suppl. 5**, 6-25.

Cederbaum, A. I., Lieber, C. S., and Rubin, E. (1974) The effect of acetaldehyde on mitochondrial function. *Arch. Biochem. Biophys.*, **161**, 26-29.

Cederbaum, A. I., Lieber, C. S., and Rubin, E. (1976) Effect of chronic ethanol consumption and acetaldehyde on partial reactions of oxidative phosphorylation and CO_2 production from citric acid cycle intermediates. *Arch. Biochem. Biophys.*, **176**, 525-538.

Chapman, L. E. (1970) The experimental induction of hangover. *Q. J. Stud. Alcohol*, **Suppl. 5**, 67-86.

Closs, K., and Solberg, C. O. (1970) Methanol poisoning. *J. Am. Med. Assoc.*, **211**, 497-499.

Cohen, G. (1973) A role for tetrahydroisoquinoline alkaloids as false adrenergic neurotransmitters in alcoholism. *Adv. Exp. Med. Biol.*, **35**, 33-44.

Cohen, G., and Collins, M. (1970) Alkaloids from catecholamines in adrenal tissues: possible role in alcoholism. *Science*, **167**, 1749-1751.

Cooper, J. R., and Kini, M. M. (1962) Biochemical aspects of methanol poisoning. *Biochem. Pharmacology*, **11**, 405-416.

Cornish, H. C. (1975) Solvents and Vapours in Toxicology: The basic science of poisons (Casarett, L. J., and Doull, J. *eds.*) pp. 503-526, Macmillan Publishing Co., New York.

Dajani, R. M., and Saheb, S. E. (1973) A further insight into the metabolism of certain β-carbolines. *Ann. N. Y. Acad. Sci.*, **215**, 120-123.

Davis, V. E. (1973) Neuroamine-derived alkaloids: A possible common denominator in alcoholism and related drug dependancies. *Ann. N. Y. Acad. Sci.*, **215**, 111-115.

Davis, V. E., and Walsh, M. J. (1970a) Alcohols, amines and alkaloids: a possible biochemical basis for alcohol addiction. *Science*, **167**, 1005-1007.

Davis, V. E., and Walsh, M. J. (1970b) Alcohol addiction and tetrahydropapaveroline. *Science*, **169**, 1105-1106.

Davis, V. E., and Walsh, M. J. (1970c) Ans. Morphine and ethanol physical dependance and a critique of a Hypothesis. *Science*, **170**, 1114-1115.

DeBruijne, A. W., and Van Steveninck, J. (1977) The influence of anesthetics on glycerol and K^+ translocation across the membrane of red blood cells. *Biochem. Pharmacol.*, **26**, 779-781.

Deitrich, R. A., and Erwin, V. G. (1975) Involvement of biogenic amine metabolism in ethanol addiction. *Fed. Proc.*, **34**, 1962-1968.

Derache, R. (1970) Toxicology, pharmacology, and metabolism of higher alcohols. *In* International Encyclopedia of Pharmacology and Therapeutics, Section 20 (Tremolieres, J. *ed.*) Vol 2, pp. 507-522, Pergamon Press.

Doctor, R. F. (1967) Drinking practices of skid row alcoholics. *Q. J. Stud. Alcohol*, **28**, 700-708.

Egle, J. L. (1972) Effects of inhaled acetaldehyde and propionaldehyde on blood pressure and heart rate. *Toxicol. Appl. Pharmacol.*, **23**, 131-135.

Eriksen, S. P., and Kulkarni, A. B. (1963) Methanol in normal human breath. *Science*, **141**, 639-640.

Finnish Foundation for Alcohol Studies (1978) The role of acetaldehyde in the actions of ethanol. (Lindros, H. O., and Eriksson, C. J. P. *eds.*) Vol 23, Helsinki.

Factor, S. M. (1976) Intramyocardial small vessel disease in chronic alcoholism. *Am. Heart J.*, **92**, 561-575.

Freund, G., and O'Hollaren, P. (1965) Acetaldehyde concentrations in alveolar air following a standard dose of ethanol in man. *J. Lipid Res.*, **6**, 471-477.

Gaillard, D., and Derache, R. (1964) Vitesse de la métabolisation de différents alcools chez le rat. *C. R. Seances Soc. Biol. (Paris)*, **158**, 1605-1608.

Gaillard, D., and Derache, R. (1965) Métabolisation de différents alccols présents dans les boissons alcooliques chez le rat. *Trav. Soc. Pharm. Montpellier*, **25**, 51-62.

Gaines, K. C., and Salhany, J. M., Tuma, D. J., and Sorrell, M. F. (1977) Reaction of acetaldehyde with human erythrocyte membrane proteins. *FEBS Letts.*, **75**, 115-119.

Gallego, A. (1948) On the effect of ethyl alcohol upon frog nerve. *J. Cellular Comp. Physiol.*, **31**, 97-106.

Geller, S. A., and Rubin, E. (1977) The effect of alcohol on striated and smooth muscle. *In* Metabolic Aspects of Alcoholism (Lieber, C. S. *ed.*) pp. 187-213, MTP Press Ltd., Lancaster.

Gosselin, R. E., Hodge, H. C., Smith, R. P., and Gleason, M. N. (1976) *Clinical Toxicology of Commercial Products*, Williams and Wilkins Co, Baltimore.

Gough, T. A. (1977) A search for volatile nitrosamines in East African Spirit. *Gut*, **18**, 301-302.

Grab, W. (1961) Pharmakologische Problems bei Wein und Spirituosen. *Arzneium Forsch.*, **11**, 73-80.

Greenberg, L. A. (1970) The appearance of some congeners of alcoholic beverages and their metabolites in blood. *Q. J. Stud. Alcohol*, **Suppl. 5**, 439-445.

Greenberg, R. S., and Cohen, G. C. (1973) Tetrahydroisoquinoline alkaloids. Stimulated secretion from the adrenal medulla. *J. Pharmacol. Exp. Ther.*, **184**, 119-128.

György, P. (1961) Discussion of Klatskin, G., Experimental studies on the role of alcohol in the pathogenesis of cirrhosis. *Am. J. Clin Nutr.*, **9**, 439-445.

Haggard, H. W., Greenberg, L. A., and Cohen, L. H. (1943) The influence of the congeners of distilled spirits upon the physiological action of alcohol. *Q. J. Stud. Alcohol*, **4**, 3-56.

Haggard, H. W., Miller, D. P., and Greenberg, L. A. (1945) The amyl alcohols and their metabolic fates and comparative toxicities. *J. Ind. Hyg. Toxicol.*, **27**, 1-14.

Halushka, P. V., and Hoffman, P. C. (1970) Alcohol addiction and tetrahydropapaveroline. *Science*, **169**, 1104-1105.

Hawkins, R. D., and Kalant, H. (1972) The metabolism of ethanol and its metabolic effects. *Pharmacol. Rev.*, **24**, 67-157.

Held, H. (1977) Effect of alcohol on the heme and porphyrin synthesis interaction with phenobarbital and pyrazole. *Digestion*, **15**, 136-146.

Horning, E. C., and Horning, M. G. (1971) Metabolic profiles: Gas-phase methods for analysis of metabolites. *Clin. Chem.*, **17**, 802-809.

Isabell, H., Fraser, H. F., Wickler, F. A., Belleville, M. A., and Eisemen, A. J. (1955) An experimental study of the aetiology of rum fits and delirium tremens. *Q. J. Stud. Alcohol*, **16**, 1-33.

James, T. N., and Bear, E. S. (1977) Effects of ethanol and acetaldehyde on the heart. *Am. Heart J.*, **74**, 243-255.

James, T. N., and Bear, E. S. (1968) Cardiac effects of some simple aliphatic aldehydes. *J. Pharmacol. Exp. Ther.*, **163**, 300-308.

Johns, D. G. (1967) Human liver aldehyde oxidase: Differential inhibition of oxidation of charged and uncharged substrates. *J. Clin. Invest*, **46**, 1492-1505.

Kahn, J. H. (1969) Compounds identified in whiskey, wine and beer: A tabulation. *J. Assoc. Off. Anal. Chem.*, **52**, 1166-1178.

Katkin, E. S., and Hayes, W. N. (1967) Differential effects upon reaction time and perceptual motor performance of alcoholic beverages differing in congener content. *Amer. Psychol. Assoc.*, Washington.

Katkin, E. S., Hayes, W. N., Teger, A. I., and Pruitt, G. (1970) Effects of alcoholic beverages differing in congener content on psychomotor tasks and on risk taking. *Q. J. Stud. Alcohol*, **Suppl. 5**, 101-104.

Kesäniemi, Y. A. (1974) Ethanol and acetaldehyde in the milk and peripheral blood of lactating women after ethanol administration. *J. Obs. Gynecol. Brit. Common.*, **81**, 84-86.

Kiessling, K. H., and Pilström, L. (1968) Effect of ethanol on rat liver. V Morphological and functional changes after prolonged consumption of various beverages. *Q. J. Stud. Alcohol*, **29**, 819-827.

Koivusalo, M. (1970) Methanol. *In* International Encyclopedia Pharmacology and Therapeutics Section 20 (Tremolieres, J. *ed.*) Vol 2, pp. 465-505, Pergamon Press, Oxford.

Korsten, M. A., Matsuzaki, S., Feinman, L., and Leiber, C. S. (1975) High blood acetaldehyde levels after ethanol administration. *N. Engl. J. Med.*, **292**, 386-389.

Kraemer, P. J., and Deitrich, R. A. (1968) Isolation and characterization of human liver aldehyde dehydrogenase. *J. Biol. Chem.*, **243**, 6402-6408.

Lahti, R. A. (1975) Alcohol aldehydes and biogenic amines. *Adv. Exp. Med. Biol.*, **56**, 239-253.

Leake, C. D., and Silverman, M. (1966) *Alcoholic Beverages in Clinical Medicine.* pp. 14-47 World Publishing Co., Cleveland.

Leake, C. D., and Silverman, M. (1971) The chemistry of alcoholic beverages. *In* The Biology of Alcoholism (Kissin, B., and Begleiter, H. *eds.*) Vol 1, pp. 575-612, Plenum Press, New York.

Lelbach, W. K. (1968) Liver damage from different alcoholic drinks. *Gen. Med. Mon.*, **13**, 31-39.

Lelbach, W. K. (1974) Organic pathology related to volume and pattern of drug use. *Research Advances in Alcohol and Drug Problems,* Vol 1, (Gibbins, R. J., Israel, Y., Kalant, H., Bopham, R. E., Schmidt, W., Smart, R. G. *eds.*) pp. 93-198, Wiley.

Lieber, C. S. (1967) Metabolic derrangement induced by alcohol. *Annu. Rev. Med.*, **18**, 35-54.

Lieber, C. S. (1968) Metabolic effects produced by alcohol in the liver and other tissues. *Adv. Int. Med.*, **14**, 151-199.

Lieber, C. S., DeCarli, L. M., Feinman, L. Hasumara, Y., Korsten, M., Matsuzaki, S., and Teschke, R. Effect of chronic alcohol consumption on ethanol and acetaldehyde metabolism. *Adv. Exp. Med. Biol.*, **59**, 185-227.

Lindenbohm, R., and Wallgren, H. (1962) Changes in respiration in rat brain cortex slices induced by some aliphatic alcohols. *Acta Pharmacol. Toxicol.*, **19**, 53-58.

Lubin, M., and Westerfold, W. W. (1945) The metabolism of acetaldehyde. *J. Biol. Chem.*, **161**, 503-512.

Lundquist, F., Tygstrup, N., Winkler, K., Mellemgaard, K., and Munck-Petersen, S. (1962) Ethanol metabolism and production of free acetate in the human liver. *J. Clin. Invest.*, **41**, 955-961.

Lund, A. (1948) Excretion of metabolism and formic acid in man after methanol consumption. *Acta Pharmacol. Toxicol.*, **4**, 205-212.

McGlashan, N. D. (1969) Oesophageal cancer and alcoholic spirits in central Africa. *Gut*, **10**, 643-650.

McIsaac, W. M. (19610 Formation of 1-methyl-6-methoxy-1, 2, 3, 4,-tetrahydro-2-carboline under physiological conditions. *Biochim. Biophys. Act,* **52**, 607-609.

Macht, D. I. (1921) A toxicological study of some alcohols with especial reference to isomers. *J. Pharmacol. Exp. Ther.*, **16**, 1-10.

Mai, R., Sassine, A., Lindenberg, A. B., Boucomont, L. (1965) Toxicité différentielle des alcools à l'égard des tissus en culture sur milieux semisynthetiques. *Monographie INSERM*, No. **32**, 153-162.

Majchrowicz, E., and Mendelson, J. H. (1970a) Blood levels of acetaldehyde and methanol during chronic ingestion and withdrawal. *In* Recent Advances in Studies of Alcoholism. (Mello, N. K. and Mendelson, J. H. *eds.*) pp. 200-216, NIM, NIMH, Government Printing Office, Washington DC.

Majchrowicz, E., and Mendelson, J. H. (1970b) Blood concentrations of acetaldehyde and ethanol in chronic alcoholics. *Science*, **168**, 1100-1102.

Majchrowicz, E., and Mendelson, J. H. (1970c) High blood ethanol levels appear to produce blood methanol build-up. *J. Am. Med. Assoc.*, **212**, 1454.

Mani, J. C., Pietruszko, R., and Theorell, H. (1970) Methanol activity of alcohol dehydrogenase from human liver, horse liver and yeast. *Arch. Biochem. Biophys.*, **140**, 52-59.

Matsumoto, K. E., Partridge, D. H., Robinson, A. B., and Pauling, I. (1973) The identification of volatile compounds in human urine. *J. Chromatogr.*, **85**, 31-34.

Muir, C. D. (*ed.*) (1971) *Hazards in the Chemical Laboratory*, RIC.

Murphree, H. B. (1969) Effects of alcoholic beverages containing large and small amounts of congeners, *Biochemical and Clinical Effects of Alcohol Metabolism* (Sardesai, V. M. *ed.*) pp. 259-265, Charles C. Thomas, Springfield, Ills.

Murphree, H. B. (1971) The importance of congeners in the effects of alcoholic beverages. *In* Biological Basis of Alcoholism. (Israel, Y. and Mardones, J. *eds.*) pp. 209-324, Wiley Interscience.

Murphree, H. B., Price, L. M., and Greenberg, L. A. (1966) Effect of congeners in alcoholic beverages on the incidence of nystagmus. *Q. J. Stud. Alcohol*, **27**, 201-213.

Murphree, H. B., Greenberg, L. A., and Carroll, R. B. (1967) Neuropharmacological effects of substances other than ethanol in alcoholic beverages. *Fed. Proc.*, **26**, 1568-1473.

Murphree, H. B., Schulz, R. E., and Jusko, A. G. (1970) Effects of high congener intake by human subjects on the EEG. *Q. J. Stud. Alcohol*, **Suppl. 5**, 50-61.

Mrocheck, J. E., Butts, W. C., Rainey, W. T., and Burtis, C. A. (1971) Separation and identification of urinary constituents by use of multiple-analytical techniques. *Clin. Chem.*, **17**, 72-77.

Nakan, J., and Kessinger, J. M. (1972) Cardiovascular effects of ethanol, its congeners and synthetic bourbon in dogs. *Eur. J. Pharmacol.*, **17**, 195-201.

Nathan, P. E., Zare, N. E., Ferneau, E. W. Jr., and Lowenstein, L. M. (1970) Effect of congener differences in alcoholic beverages on the behaviour of alcoholics. *Q. J. Stud. Alcohol*, **Suppl. 5**, 87-100.

Nelemans, F. A. (1962) The influence of various substances on the acetyl choline contracture on the frog's isolated abdominal muscle. *Acta. Physiol. Pharmacol. Nearle*, 11, 76–82.

Newsome, J. R., Norman, V., and Keith, C. H. (1965) Vapour phase analysis of cigarette smoke. *Tobacco Sci.*, 9, 102–110.

Nisenbaum, G. D., Okun, I. M., Adzerikha, R. D., Lyskova, T. I., Narishevichus, E. V., Aksentsev, S. L., and Knev, S. V. (1976) Structural rearrangements of membranes induced by anesthetics. *Biofizika*, 21, 271–275.

O'Neill, P. J., and Rahwan, R. G. (1975) Experimental evidence for calcium-independant catecholamine secretion from the bovine adrenal medulla. *J. Pharmacol. Exp. Ther.*, 193, 513–522.

Parrilla, R., Ohkawa, K., Lindros, K. O., Zimmerman, U. J. P., Kobay-Ashi, K., and Williamson, J. R. (1974) Functional compartmentation of acetaldehyde oxidation in rat liver. *J. Biochem.*, 249, 4926–4933.

Peterson, D. R., Collins A. C., and Deitrich, R. A. (1977) Role of liver cytosolic aldehyde dehydrogenase isozymes in control of blood acetaldehyde concentrations. *J. Pharmacol. Exp. Ther.*, 201, 471–481.

Puszkin, S., and Rubin, E. (1976) Effects of ADP, ethanol and acetaldehyde on the relaxing complex of human muscle and its absorption by polysytrene particles. *Arch. Biochem. Biophys.*, 177, 574–584.

Rahwan, R. G. (1974) Speculations on the biochemical pharmacology of ethanol. *Life Sci.*, 15, 617–633.

Rahwan, R. G. (1975) Toxic effects of ethanol: possible role of acetaldehyde tetrahydroisoquinolines and tetrahydro-beta-carbolines. *Toxicol. Appl. Pharmacol.*, 34, 3–27.

Rahwan, R. G., O'Neill, P. J., and Miller, D. D. (1974) Differential secretion of catecholamines and tetrahydroisoquinolines from the bovine adrenal medulla. *Life Sci.*, 14, 1927–1938.

Raichle, M. E., Eichlung, J. O., Straatmann, M. G., Welch, M. J., Larson, K. B., and Ter-Pogossian, M. M. (1976) Blood-brain barrier permeability of ^{11}C-labelled alcohols and ^{15}O-labelled water. *Am. J. Physiol.*, 230, 543–522.

Randall, C. L. (1977) Teratogenic effects. *In utero* ethanol exposure. *In* Alcohol and Opiates: Biochemical and Behavioral Mechanisms (Blum, K. *ed.*) pp. 91–107, Academic Press, New York.

Rawat, A. K. (1977) Effects of fructose and other substances on ethanol and acetaldehyde in man. *Res. Commun. Chem. Pathol. Pharmacol.*, 16, 281–290.

Rehak, M. J., and Truitt, E. B. (1958) Anesthesia LVIII. Biochemical effects of acetaldehyde and other aldehydes on oxidative phosphorylation. *Q. J. Stud. Alcohol*, 19, 399–405.

Richardson, B. W. (1869) Physiological Research on alcohols. *Med. Times Gaz.*, 2, 703–706.

Rφe, O. (1943) Clinical investigations of methyl alcohol poisoning with special reference to pathogenesis and treatment of amblyopia. *Acta Med. Scand.*, **113**, 558-608.

Rφe, O. (1946) Methanol poisoning and its clinical course, pathogenesis and treatment. *Acta Med. Scand.*, **126, Suppl. 182**, 1-253.

Rubin, E., Katz, A. M., Lieber, C. S., Stein, E. P., and Puszkin, S. (1976) Muscle damage produced by chronic alcohol consumption. *Am. J. Pathol.*, **83**, 499-512.

Rubington, E. (1968) The bottle gang. *Q. J. Stud. Alcohol*, **29A**, 943-955.

Sachdev, K. S., Panjwani, M. H., and Joseph, A. D. (1963) Potentiation of the response to acetylcholine on the frog's rectus abdominus by ethyl alcohol. *Arch. Intern. Pharmacodyn.*, **145**, 36-43.

Saint-Blaquat, G., de and Derache, R. (1966) Effet de l'éthanol sur la sécretion gastrique *in vitro* chez le rat. *Biochem. Pharmacol.*, **15**, 1895-1898.

Sandler, M., Carter, S. B., Hunter, K. A., and Stern, G. M. (1973) Tetrahydro-isoquinolines. alkaloids: *In vivo* metabolites of L-Dopa in men. *Nature (Lond).*, **241**, 439-443.

Schmidt, W., and Bronetto, J. (1962) Death from liver cirrhosis and specific alcoholic beverage consumption: an ecological survey. *Am. J. Publ. Health.*, **52**, 1473-1482.

Schneider, F. H. (1971) Acetaldehyde-Induced catecholamine secretion from the cow adrenal medulla. *J. Pharmacol. Exp. Ther.*, **177**, 109-118.

Schneider, F. H. (1974) Effects of length of exposure to and concentrations of acetaldehyde on the release of catecholamines. *Biochem. Pharmacol.*, **23**, 223-229.

Schrieber, S. S., Briden, K., Oratz, M., and Rothschild, M. A. (1972) Ethanol, acetaldehyde and myocardial protein synthesis. *J. Clin. Invest.*, **51**, 2820-2826.

Schreiber, S. S., Oratz, M., Rothschild, M. A., Roff, F., and Evans, C. (1974) Alcoholic cardiomyopathy. II Inhibition of cardiac microsomal protein synthesis by acetaldehyde. *J. Mol. Cell Cardiol.*, **6**, 207-213.

Seevers, M. H. (1970) Morphrine and ethanol physical dependence: A critique of a hypothesis. *Science*, **170**, 1113-1114.

Siegel, I. A., Izutsu, K. T., and Burkhart, J. (1976) Transfer of alcohols and urea across the oral mucosa measured using streaming potentials and radio-isotopes. *J. Pharm. Sci.*, **65**, 129-131.

Smith, M. E. (1961) Interrelations in ethanol and methanol metabolism. *J. Pharmacol. Exp. Ther.*, **134**, 233-237.

Soumalainen, H., and Nykänen, L. (1968) Methods applied in studies on the aroma, composition of alcoholic beverages. *Wallterstein Lab. Commun.*, **31**, 5-15.

Starr, M. B., Murphree, H. B., and Schulz, R. E. (1970) Prolonged cardiovascular effects of alcoholic beverages. *Fed. Proc. Fed. Am. Soc. Exp. Biol.*, **29**, 274.

Stolman, A., and Stewart, C. P. (*eds.*) (1960) *Toxicology*, Vol 1, pp. 51, Academic Press, New York.

Stotz, E. (1943) A colorimetric determination of acetaldehyde in blood. *J. Biol. Chem.*, **148**, 585-591.

Tabakoff, B., Anderson, R. A., and Ritzman, R. F. (1976) Brain acetaldehyde after ethanol administration. *Biochem. Pharmacol.*, **25**, 1305-1309.

Thompson, J. A., and Markey, S. P. (1975) Quantitative metabolic profiling of urinary organic acids by gas chromatography-mass spectrometry. Comparison of isolation methods. *Anal. Chem.*, **47**, 1313-1321.

Truitt, E. B. (1971) Blood acetaldehyde levels after alcohol consumption by alcoholic and non-alcoholic subjects. *In* Biological Aspects of Alcoholism (Roach, M. K., McIsaac W. M., and Creaven, P. J. eds.) pp. 212-232, University of Texas Press, Austin.

Truitt, E. B., and Duritz, G. (1967) The role of acetaldehyde in the actions of ethanol. *In* Biochemical Factors in Alcoholism (Maickel, R. P. *ed.*) pp. 61-69, Pergamon Press, Oxford.

Truitt, E. B., and Walsh, M. J. (1971) The role of acetaldehyde in the actions of ethanol. *In* The Biology of Alcoholism (Kissin, B., and Begleiter, H. *eds.*) Vol 1, pp. 161-195, Plenum Press, London.

Tyce, G. M. (1977) Demethylation of O-methyl metabolites of catecholamines in erythrocytes and a methanol-forming reaction. *Res. Commun. Chem. Pathol. Pharmacol.*, **16**, 669-685.

Wallgren, H. (1960) Relative intoxicating effects on rats of ethyl, propyl, and butyl alcohols. *Acta Pharmacol. Toxicol.*, **16**, 217-222.

Walsh, M. J., and Truitt, E. B. (1968) Release of 7-H^3-norepinephrine in plasma and urine by acetaldehyde and ethanol in cats and rabbits. *Fed. Proc.*, **27**, 601.

Wartburg, J. P. von (1971) The metabolism of alcohol in normals and alcoholics: Enzymes. *In* The Biology of Alcoholism (Kissin, B. and Begleiter, H. *eds.*) Vol 1, pp. 63-102, Plenum Press, London.

Wartburg, J. P. von, Papenburg, J., and Aebi, H. (1965) An atypical human alcohol dehydrogenase. *Can. J. Biochem.*, **43**, 889-898.

Webb, A. D., Kepner, R. E., and Ikeda, R. M. (1952) Composition of a typical grape brandy fusel oil. *Anal. Chem.*, **24**, 675-683.

Weese, H. (1928) Vergleichende Untersuchungen uber die Wirksamseit und Giftigkeit der Dampfe niederes aliphatischen Alcohols. *Arch. Exp. Pathol. Pharmacol.*, **135**, 118-130.

Western, O. C., and Ozburn, E. E. (1949) Methanol and formaldehyde in normal body tissue and fluids. *U. S. Naval Med. Bull.*, **49**, 574-575.

Whaley, W. M., and Govindachari, T. R. (1950) The Pictet-Spengler synthesis of tetrahydroisoquinolines and related compounds. *Org. React.*, **6**, 151-206.

Wilson, A. S., Barboriak, J. J., and Kass, W. A. (1970) Effects of alcoholic beverages and congeners on psychomotor skills in old and young subjects. *Q. J. Stud. Alcohol,* **Suppl, 5,** 115-129.

Winer, A. D. (1958) Substrate specificity of horse liver alcohol dehydrogenase. *Acta Chem. Scand.,* **12,** 1695-1696.

Zatman, L. J. (1946) The effect of ethanol on the metabolism of methanol in man. *Biochem. J.,* **40,** lxviii-lxvix.

Zlatkis, A., and Liebich, H. M. (1971) Profile of volatile metabolites in human urine. *Clin. Chem.,* **17,** 592-594.

CHAPTER 5

Biochemical Effects of Alcohol Abuse

5.1 INTRODUCTION

Alcohol abuse produces a wide range of biochemical disturbances and organic lesions in man. The biochemical disturbances may vary greatly in their direction and magnitude. In some subjects ethanol may cause a minor elevation of a particular substance in blood, whereas in others the opposite effect may be seen. Many of the biochemical changes accompanying alcohol abuse may be understood in terms of the hepatic metabolism of ethanol and the consequent alteration in the the redox state of the liver (*vide infra*).

In order to understand the variation in the biochemical disturbances which may be seen in people who imbibe ethanol, many other factors must be considered and these include:

Extent and duration of ethanol intake and previous experience of ethanol
Time of testing
Type of alcoholic beverage and congeners
Solubility and solvent effect of ethanol
Nutritional status
Endocrine effects of ethanol
Stress due to intoxication
Disease
Genetic factors
Analytical interferences

The interaction of the above factors (Figure 5.1), although incompletely understood, no doubt contribute to the range and variability of biochemical sequelae associated with abuse of ethanol (see Chapter 7). We shall examine the influence of each of these factors on the biochemical changes accompanying ethanol abuse in Sections 5.2 to 5.11.

Enzymatic oxidation of ethanol in the liver results in the production of acetaldehyde and acetate, and in the generation of the reduced cofactor NADH. Many of the biochemical consequences of alcohol abuse have been explained on the basis of these changes.

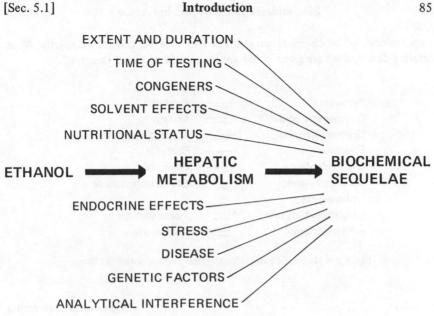

Fig. 5.1 – Factors influencing biochemical sequelae of ethanol metabolism and abuse.

Acetaldehyde derived from ethanol may cause a release in catecholamines, a shift in their metabolism from a reductive to an oxidative pathway (see Chapter 7 Section 14), and an inactivation of acetyl CoA (Truitt *et al.,* 1971). The fate of acetate, or its activated form acetyl CoA, is oxidation to carbon dioxide, steroid or fatty acid synthesis, ketone production or any of the other metabolic transformations available to these intermediary metabolites (Wartburg, 1971). The altered redox state of the liver due to the accumulation of the reduced cofactor NADH in the cytosol has a profound effect on many metabolic transformations *vide infra.*

Re-oxidation of excess NADH takes place in the mitochondrion, but as the mitochondrion is virtually impermeable to NADH, shuttle mechanisms operate to transfer the reduced cofactor into the mitochondrion where it is oxidised in the respiratory chain. Several shuttle mechanisms have been proposed including the malate/aspartate, alpha-glycerophosphate, and fatty acid shuttles. However, the oxidation capacity of the flavo-protein-cytochrome system is limited and there is therefore an increase in the NADH/NAD ratio of the cytosol. This change in the redox state of the liver during the oxidation of ethanol influences the equilibrium of all NAD-dependent reactions. Some examples are given in Figure 5.2. In many cases, the increases in the reduced metabolite will only be found in the hepatocyte, and not in the peripheral blood. However the shift in the lactate/pyruvate ratio of the liver is so large that it is also observable in the peripheral blood. The influence of ethanol metabolism on a number of biochemical parameters will now be considered briefly. More detailed descriptions are given in the appropriate sections of Chapter 7.

Pyruvate	⇌	Lactate
Oxaloacetic acid	⇌	Malate
Glyceraldehyde	⇌	1,3-Diphosphoglycerate
Fructose	⇌	Sorbitol
Glyceraldehyde	⇌	Glycerol
Dihydroxyaceto-phosphate	⇌	Glycerophosphate
β-Hydroxybutyrate	⇌	Acetoacetate
α-Ketoglutarate	⇌	Glutamate

Fig. 5.2 – Metabolic pairs reflecting the redox state of the liver.

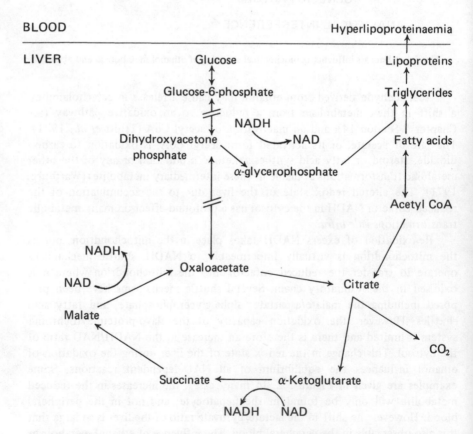

Fig. 5.3 – Effects of ethanol metabolism and altered NADH/NAD ratio on lipid metabolism.

Lipids

Ethanol displaces fat as a metabolic fuel due to the effect of the altered hepatic redox state on various steps in the tricarboxylic acid (TCA) cycle (Figure 5.3). Decreased conversion of malate to oxaloacetate and alpha-ketoglutarate to succinate inhibits metabolism of fat by the TCA cycle and leads to a build up of free fatty acids in the liver. Excess NADH may also promote fatty acid synthesis, thus augmenting the build up of fatty acids (Lieber and De Carli, 1977). Excess fat is exported from the liver in the form of lipoproteins leading to a hyperlipoproteinaemia (hyperlipaemia).

The altered redox state of the liver also increases alpha-glycerophosphate production which in turn leads to an increase in triglyceride production and this augments the hyperlipaemia.

Glucose

In subjects who are drinking and not eating and who also have depleted glycogen stores, ethanol may precipitate hypoglycaemia by inhibition of gluconeogenesis. The main substrates for gluconeogenesis are amino acids derived from hepatic breakdown of proteins (Figure 5.4).

Alterations in the redox state of the liver due to ethanol metabolism reduce pyruvate levels, a precursor of glucose, and also interfere with the TCA cycle, thus inhibiting the utilisation of amino acids such as aspartate, glutamate and proline.

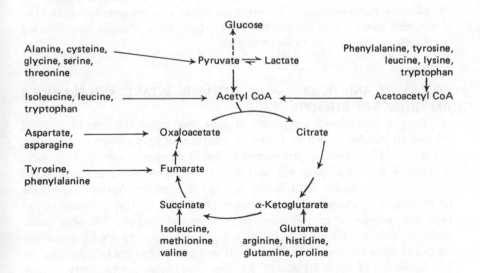

Fig. 5.4 – The catabolism of amino acids.

Ketones

Apart from increased secretion of lipoproteins, another way of disposing of excess free fatty acids (formed in the liver as a consequence of ethanol metabolism) is to convert them to ketones. Free fatty acids are metabolised to acetyl CoA and when in excess this undergoes a series of condensation, reduction and decarboxylation reactions to produce the ketones, acetoacetate, β-hydroxybutyrate and acetone. Excessive production of these substances leads to ketosis.

Lactate

The altered redox state of the liver affects the pyruvate/lactate interconversion resulting in an increase in lactate production. This, together with decreased utilisation of lactate produced peripherally, leads to elevated blood lactate levels and a lactic acidosis.

Urate

Lactate competes with urate for renal excretion in the distal tubule. A consequence of increased lactate levels is an inhibition of urate excretion and hence hyperuricaemia.

Biogenic amines and steroids

A shift in the metabolism of biogenic amines and steroids from oxidative to reductive pathways occurs following prolonged ethanol metabolism and the consequent alteration in the hepatic redox state. These changes are discussed more fully in Chapter 7 Sections 14 and 8.

5.2 EXTENT AND DURATION OF ETHANOL INTAKE AND PREVIOUS EXPERIENCE OF ETHANOL

Dose of ethanol and the period of time over which the dose or doses of ethanol are imbibed have been shown to influence the nature of ethanol-induced alterations of biochemical parameters. Acute as compared with chronic doses of ethanol can have quite different effects on blood and urinary levels of enzymes, lipids, organic acids, hormones, and electrolytes. Previous experience of ethanol, (i.e. abstinent, social drinker, alcoholic), is also a factor in the type and magnitude of the observed biochemical changes following either acute or chronic ethanol intake. Table 5.1 summarises the results of various studies of acute and chronic intake in both healthy subjects and in alcoholics.

Inspection of Table 5.1 reveals the diverse and often contradictory changes which may be seen in acute versus chronic intake by either healthy subjects or alcoholics.

Table 5.1

Effects of acute and chronic doses of ethanol in healthy subjects and in alcoholics.

A. ACUTE STUDIES
Healthy subjects

Biochemical parameter	Effect	dose of ethanol		No. of Subjects	Reference
AspT	N	85g		12	Bang et al., 1958
AspT	N	0.6–0.7g/kg		12	Childs et al., 1963
AlaT	N	1.7g/kg		8	Goldberg and Watts, 1965
ICD	E				
OCT	E				
OCT	E	200–300g		10	Brohult and Reichard, 1965
GLDH, SDH, blood ammonia	N	70g			Müting, 1971
AspT, AlaT, LDH	N	28g		22	Galambos et al., 1963
Cortisol	E	45–60g		15	Jenkins and Connolly, 1968
Triglycerides, insulin	E	1.5g/kg		24	Taskinen and Nikkila, 1977

D; depressed levels, E; elevated levels, N; normal levels.

Table 5.1 (*Continued*)
B. CHRONIC STUDIES
Healthy subjects

Biochemical parameter	Effect	dose of ethanol (duration)	clinical details	No. of Subjects	Reference
Uric acid, lactate, pyruvate, zinc, cholesterol, triglycerides, phospholipids urinary zinc	N	47–75g/day (12 days)			Carey *et al.*, 1971
	E				
LDH, AspT, AlaT, CK	N	400g (3 days)	Carbohydrate poor diet	6	Hed *et al.*, 1972
LDH₂	E				
CK	E	225/day (28 days)		3	Song and Rubin 1972
Cortisol	E	4g/kg (4 days)			Mendelson and Stein, 1966
AspT, uric acid	E	68–170g/day (6–14 days)		5	Rubin and Lieber, 1968
AspT, CK	D	0.75/kg (3 days)		9	Freer and Statland, 1977a
AlaT, GGT, AP	E				
GGT	E	0.75g/kg (2 days)		8	Freer and Statland, 1977b
GGT, AlaT, AspT, bilirubin	N	0.9g/kg		4	Belfrage *et al.*, 1973
triglycerides, α-lipoproteins	E	(5 weeks)			

D; depressed levels, E; elevated levels, N; normal levels.

Table 5.1 (*Continued*)
A. Alcoholics

Biochemical parameter	Effect	dose of ethanol	clinical details	No. of Subjects	Reference
AspT	E	100–135g	chronic alcoholics	35	Bang et al., 1958
AspT, AlaT, AP	N	113g	hospitalised alcoholic	104	Abbot et al., 1963
GLDH, SDH, blood ammonia	E	70g	alcohol induced fatty infiltration	12	Müting, 1971
Asp, AlaT, OD, LDH	N	28g	active hepatocellular injury	42	Galambos et al., 1963
glucose intolerance		200–215g	alcoholic	2	Phillips and Safrit, 1971

D, depressed levels, E; elevated levels, N; normal levels.

Table 5.1 *(Continued)*
B. Alcoholics

Biochemical parameter	Effect	dose of ethanol (duration)	clinical details	No. of Subjects	Reference
cortisol	E	4g/kg (4 days)	alcoholics	4	Mendelson and Stein, 1966
AspT	N	141–300g/day (8–21 days)	alcoholics with alcoholic fatty liver	5	Lieber et al., 1965
AspT, AlaT, CK	E	>160g/day (5 days)	alcoholics without cirrhosis normal diet	12	Dimberg et al., 1967
AspT, AlaT, CK	N		carbohydrate poor diet		
Folate, Mg, K	D	205g/day (22 days)	alcoholic without liver injury	3	Hines and Cowan, 1970
Iron	E				

D; depressed levels, E; elevated levels, N; normal levels.

5.3 TIME OF TESTING

The time of testing is an important consideration in the direction and magnitude of a biochemical change following alcohol abuse. Four different factors may be identified:

(a) Inherent rhythmic changes of biochemical parameters and different body times.
(b) Time dependency of rate of ethanol metabolism.
(c) Direct effect of ethanol on rhythmic pattern of change of biochemical parameters.
(d) Time-dependent response of biochemical parameters following ethanol ingestion and metabolism.

(a) Many substances of biological interest exhibit rhythmic changes having either ultradian (<20h period), circadian (20-28h) or infradian (>28h) rhythms. Figure 5.5 illustrates the timing of some variables in blood and urine. As yet the extent of changes of substances in blood and in urine along the particular cycles has not been reliably quantified. Studies of urea and amino acids in blood have revealed that the extent of change during a 24h cycle may be as much as 20% and 30% of the average values, respectively. Ultra-, circa- or infradian changes take on a particular importance in serial measurements when erroneous trends may become apparent due to sampling at different body times (Simpson, 1976). The importance of such factors in the variation of biochemical changes following alcohol abuse has not been established.

(b) Ethanol exhibits a rhythmicity in its rate of metabolism (see Chapter 3 Section 8) and this in turn may possibly influence the extent of biochemical changes consequent upon ethanol metabolism.

(c) Information relating to any direct effect of ethanol on the natural rhythms of biochemical parameters is scarce. The diurnal variation in serum iron, total iron binding capacity, and cortisol has been shown to be normal in alcoholics (Mendelson and Stein, 1966; Speck, 1970), whereas ethanol abolishes the episodic nature of testosterone secretion (Gordon and Southeren, 1977).

(d) After ingestion of a dose or doses of ethanol the response of various parameters is time-dependent, a factor which assumes particular importance in the context of the biochemical detection of alcohol abuse (see Chapter 6).

Several groups of workers have investigated blood, serum or urine biochemical values at short time intervals after consumption of ethanol (Mendelson, 1964; Mendelson and LaDou, 1964; Carey *et al.*, 1971; Freer and Statland, 1977a,b).

A time study of blood pyruvate, lactate and glucose, and serum uric acid and zinc is shown in Table 5.2. Blood lactate levels show the most dramatic changes, the levels falling by nearly 50% during the eight hour test period.

A
Hormones

Steroids	17-Hydroxy corticosteroid	
	Testosterone	
Amines	5-Hydroxytryptamine	
Proteins	ACTH	
	Human growth hormone	
	Insulin	
	Glucagon	
Electrolytes	Sodium	
	Potassium	
	Calcium	
	Chloride	
Glycosaminoglycans	Protein-bound carbohydrate	
	Hexosamine	
	Sialic acid	
Plasma proteins	Total protein	
	Albumin	
	Globulin	
	Albumin/globulin	
	γ-Globulin	
Enzymes	Alkaline phosphatase	
	Transaminase	
Carbohydrates	Glucose	
Fat metabolism	Triglycerides	
Bile metabolism	Bilirubin	
Protein metabolism	Urea nitrogen	

← 24h →

B
Hormones & metabolites

Catecholamines	Adrenaline	
	Noradrenaline	
	4-Hydroxy-3-methoxymandelic acid	
Steroids	Tetrahydrocorticosterone	
	Tetrahydrocortisol	
	17-Oxo steroid	
	Aldosterone	
	17-Hydroxy corticosteroid	
	Androsterone	
	Dehydroepiandrosterone	
	Etiocholanolone	
	Testosterone glucuronide	
	Epitestosterone glucuronide	
Product of protein metabolism	Urea	
Electrolytes	Sodium	
	Potassium	
	Sodium/potassium	
	Magnesium	
	Phosphate	
	Chloride	
	Calcium	
Miscellaneous	Volume	
	pH	
	Reducing substances	

← 24h →

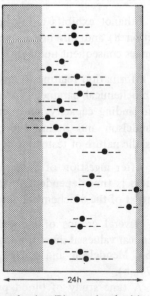

Fig. 5.5 – Timing of some variables in blood (A) and urine (B) associated with metabolic periodicity. ● , best estimate of phase (peak time); – – – –, 95% confidence limits; ⬜ , active; ▨ , recumbent.
Reproduced by permission from Simpson, *Essays in Medical Biochemistry*, The Biochemical Society and Association of Clinical Biochemists (1976).

Table 5.2
Blood chemistry values at short intervals after consumption of alcohol
(Time Study)*

Determination	Condition	Interval after last drink (hr)				
		0	1½	3	5	8
Blood pyruvate	Control	1.83	1.63	1.55	1.56	1.49
(mg/100ml)	Alcohol	1.61	1.62	1.87	1.76	1.78
Blood lactate	Control	5.87	5.47	5.03	6.51	5.80
(mg/100ml)	Alcohol	11.68	10.89	10.18	7.18	5.59
Serum uric acid	Control	5.5	5.6	5.6	5.6	5.8
(mg/100ml)	Alcohol	6.0	6.0	5.9	5.8	5.8
Blood glucose	Control	90	92	88	84	81
(mg/100ml)	Alcohol	90	74	75	79	76
Serum zinc	Control	80	80	84	91	97
(μg/100ml)	Alcohol	82	86	87	92	105

*Mean values from three subjects. Last drink of alcohol was at 11 pm.

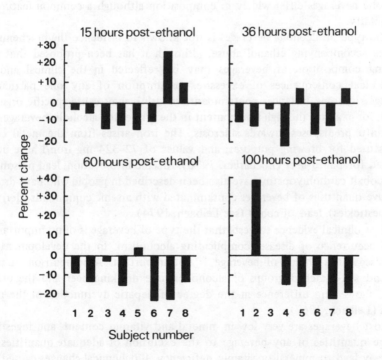

Fig. 5.6 – Percent changes (compared to baseline values) in aspartate transaminase
activity in serum of each of nine subjects 15, 36, 60 and 100h after ethanol.
Reproduced by permission from Freer and Statland, *Clinical Chemistry* (1977).

The studies of Freer and Statland (1977a,b) provide a further, and more spectacular, example of the time-dependence of serum biochemical values following ingestion of a dose of ethanol. Serum activities of aspartate amino-transferase in the eight subjects tested reveal an amazing pattern of change following administration of a dose of ethanol (0.75 g/kg) (Figure 5.6). Only subjects number four and six exhibited a constant trend in enzyme levels during the 100 h post-ethanol period. This study in particular illustrates the importance of time of testing in the observed changes in biochemical parameters following ethanol ingestion.

5.4 TYPE OF ALCOHOLIC BEVERAGE AND CONGENERS

An alcoholic beverage is a very complex mixture of substances. Most alcoholic beverages contain, in addition to ethanol and water, a large variety of organic alcohols, esters, aldehydes, acids, carbohydrates, proteins, amino acids, vitamins and minerals. Substances other than ethanol in alcoholic beverages, e.g. aldehydes, esters, are collectively known as congeners and these have been discussed in Chapter 4. Ranges of the constituents commonly found in beers, table wines, dessert and cocktail wines, and distilled spirits are presented in Table 5.3. Alcoholic beverages differ widely in composition although a common feature is their acidity.

The type of alcoholic beverages is not known to influence the biochemical changes accompanying ethanol abuse, although it has been proposed that the differing composition of beverages may be reflected in the clinical and/or biochemical consequences of excessive consumption of any one particular beverage. In some instances contaminants in drink may cause specific organic lesions, for example the high iron content in the fermented alcoholic beverages of the Bantu predisposes towards siderosis. The iron arises from the metal con-tainers used for brewing purposes, and values of 72–324 mg iron/l have been reported for Bantu beer (Bucharian, 1970). Arsenic intoxication, lead poisoning and a cobalt cardiomyopathy have also been described in people who have drunk excessive quantities of beverages contaminated with arsenic compounds (derived from pesticides), lead, or cobalt (see Lelbach, 1974).

Most clinical evidence suggests that the type of beverage is of no importance in the occurrence of diseases complicating alcoholism. In the development of liver disease the choice of beverage is not important. A comparison of two age- and sex-matched groups of alcoholics, one drinking beer and the other spirits, showed no difference in the degree of hepatic dysfunction of the two groups (Lelbach, 1967).

Most beverages are very low in mineral and vitamin content, and ingestion of large quantities of any beverage to the exclusion of adequate quantities of food may lead to mineral or vitamin deficiency. Biochemical changes caused by vitamin and/or mineral deficiency would serve to complicate the overall biochemical picture seen in an alcoholic.

Table 5.3
Chemical constituents of table wines

Component	Unit	Range			
ELECTROLYTES		Beers	Distilled spirits	Dessert and Cocktail wines	Table wines
Hydrogen ion	pH	3.90–4.70	3.7–6.9	3.14–4.18	2.84–4.07
Sodium	ppm	68–550	–	15–405	10–200
Potassium	ppm	130–1040	–	109–1420	180–1620
Magnesium	ppm	50–300	–	–	–
Iron	ppm	T–0.64	–	1.0–5.5	0–20
Copper	ppm	T–0.40	–	T–1.1	0–9
Calcium	ppm	20–70	–	32–72	29–99
Phosphate	ppm	50–350	–	–	–
ORGANIC ALCOHOLS, ESTERS, ALDEHYDES AND ACIDS					
Ethanol	%(Vol)	2.9–7.5	40–76	16.4–21.7	10.2–14.2
Methanol	ppm	0	0–1300	–	20–230
Higher alcohols	ppm	42–76	10–2650	156–900	140–417
Total Aldehydes	ppm	–	2–202	–	–
Acetaldehyde	ppm	2.3–19.5	–	15–217	5–292
Total esters	ppm	23–55	6–804	93–730	60–557
Total acids	ppm		4–810		
Acetic acid	ppm	–	–	150–540	220–1490
Lactic acid	%	0.08–0.50	–	–	0.1–0.5
Tartaric acid	%	–	–	0.29–0.89	0.4–1.1
VITAMINS					
Thiamine	µg/1	20–60	–	50–130	0–240
Riboflavin	µg/1	300–1200	–	110–240	60–220
Pantothenic acid	µg/1	400–900	–	120–240	70–450
Pyridoxine	µg/1	400–900	–	190–640	220–820
Nicotinic acid	µg/1	5000–20,000	–	880–2050	410–960
Biotin	µg/1	0–15	–	–	–
Cyanocobalamin (B_{12})	mµg/1	–	–	–	9–25
MISCELLANEOUS					
Total solids	%	2.79–6.10	0.003–1.85	3.8–13.5	1.7–8.3
Tannins	ppm	100–385	0–541	0.01–0.16	0.01–0.36
Amino acids	ppm	–	–	18–70	100–2000
Total carbohydrate	%	2.1–8.3	–	–	–
Protein	ppm	630–6160	–	–	–

T; trace

5.5 SOLUBILITY AND SOLVENT EFFECT OF ETHANOL

Many organic substances are soluble in ethanol and it is feasible that ethanol contained in alcoholic beverages may act, either as a solvent and so cause the dissolution of substances vital to cellular function, or as a solute and by its own dissolution in the lipid phase of cell membranes disrupt membrane structure and function.

Relative to other organic substances in serum, ethanol becomes the principal organic component above levels of approximately 30–40 mg/100 ml. This fact is most clearly demonstrated if ethanol concentration is expressed in molar terms. Fig 5.7 illustrates the concentrations of the main organic components of serum relative to ethanol at various ethanol levels. Blood alcohol levels as high as 780 mg/100 ml (177 mmol/l) have been recorded in live subjects (Lindblad and Olssen, 1976) and at such levels the blood stream approximates to a suspension of cells in dilute ethanol with metabolically important organic substances such as glucose relegated to trace constituents. The prolonged *in vivo* perfusion of the body with dilute ethanol could initiate changes at the cellular level, which would eventually lead to biochemical changes in addition to those produced as a result of hepatic metabolism of ethanol. Evidence from studies of the effect of ethanol on cell structure, membrane stability, permeability, action potential, and active transport processes would support this possibility (Kalant, 1971; Lundquist, 1975).

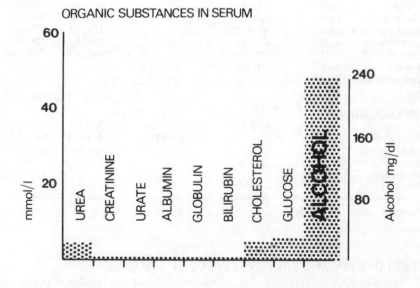

Fig. 5.7 – Relative molar levels of the major substances and alcohol (range 0–240 mg/dl) in serum.

Acute doses of ethanol (1 g/kg body weight) have been shown to cause haemorrhagic errosions of jejunal villi (Gottfried *et al.*, 1976). Chronic doses cause ultrastructural abnormalities, dilation of endoplasmic reticulum and cisternae of the Golgi apparatus, and also cause focal cytoplasmic degradation in villus and crypt cells in both the jejunum and ileum (Rubin *et al.*, 1972). Motility of the duodenum, jejunum and ileum is altered by *i.v.* or oral ethanol and this may also be a manifestation of the solvent/solute properties of ethanol (Pirola and Davis 1970; Robles *et al.*, 1974).

Ultrastructural changes have been observed in biopsy specimens taken from peripheral muscle of subjects who had consumed 225 g ethanol/day for 28 days. Since very little ethanol metabolism occurs in muscle these changes have been interpreted as due to a direct toxic effects (or solvent effect?) of ethanol (Song and Rubin, 1972).

Bone marrow cells may also be directly affected by ethanol. Vacuolisation of bone marrow red cell precursors is a characteristic but transient finding in recently intoxicated alcholics (Lindenbaum, 1977). Similar vacuoles have been demonstrated in marrow cells of infants born to mothers receiving *i.v.* ethanol (Logez and Montoya, 1971).

The permeability of cell membranes to sodium and potassium ions and the activity of cellular enzyme systems have been shown to be affected by biologically significant levels of ethanol (Kalant, 1971). Ethanol inhibits the activity of (Na^+-K^+)-activated ATPase in various tissues, thus causing an impairment of the Na/K pump (Sun and Samorajski, 1975; Baraona and Lindenbaum, 1977).

Malabsorption of many important substances, e.g. fat (Roggin *et al.*, 1969; Mezey *et al.*, 1970), thiamine (Tomasulo *et al.*, 1968; Thomson *et al.*, 1970), folic acid (Halsted *et al.*, 1967), vitamin B_{12} (Roggin *et al.*, 1969; Lindenbaum and Pezzimenti, 1973), sodium and water (Halsted *et al.*, 1971, 1973; Krasner *et al.*, 1974; Mekhjian *et al.*, 1974). L-methionine (Israel *et al.*, 1969) and xylose (Mezey *et al.*, 1970) has been demonstrated in alcoholics. The solvent and solute effects of ethanol may also be augmented by effects arising from the hypertonicity of body fluids containing large amounts of ethanol.

5.6 NUTRITIONAL STATUS

Ethanol can impair nutritional status in a number of ways by: (i) replacing vitamin- and mineral-rich foodstuffs, (ii) impairing absorption of vitamins and minerals and (iii) interfering with the conversion of vitamins to their active metabolites (see Chapter 7, Section 15). Changes in nutritional status may then influence other biochemical parameters and so have a bearing on the overall biochemical picture encountered in a person abusing ethanol.

Ethanol is a source of energy and provides 7.1 Kcal/g. Thus 150-200g of ethanol (Approximately 1 pint of 86 proof spirits) would represent about half of the daily caloric requirement. Ethanol, by replacing other foodstuffs as a source of calories, can lead to a decreased intake of nutritive proteins, minerals and vitamins, although alcoholic beverages do contain small amounts of essential nutrients (see Section 5.5).

Recommended daily vitamin allowances are collected in Table 5.4. An adequate intake of niacin, for example, could be obtained from a moderate intake (1.51) of certain types of beers. In contrast the recommended daily allowance of vitamin B_1 (thiamine) could only be obtained by ingesting a very large quantity (281) of beer (Vitale and Coffey, 1971). Clinical signs (glossitis, anaemia, peripheral neuropathy) and laboratory evidence (folate, thiamine, B_1 levels) of vitamin deficiencies are regularly encountered in alcoholics. Deficiencies of vitamin A, C and E have also been described (see Chapter 7, Section 15).

Table 5.4
Recommended daily vitamin allowances for adults.

VITAMIN	ALLOWANCE/DAY
THIAMINE (VITAMIN B_1)	1.0-1.4 mg
RIBOFLAVIN (VITAMIN B_2)	1.5-1.7 mg
NIACIN	13-18 mg
FOLATE	0.4 mg
PANTOTHENIC ACID	10-15 mg
VITAMIN B_6	2.0 mg
VITAMIN B_{12}	5 μg
ASCORBATE (VITAMIN C)	55-60 mg

Vitamins play key roles in a multitude of biochemical transformations in man. Deficiencies can lead to the impairment of such transformations, and any consequent biochemical abnormalities will be superimposed on those already present due directly to alcohol abuse. For example, thiamine and pantothenic acid are involved in glucose metabolism and in the maintenance of NADPH levels. The latter is required for many transformations, e.g. steroid biosynthesis–thus abnormalities in adrenocortical function may be secondary to vitamin deficiency rather than due to ethanol abuse (Noble, 1973). Any biochemical changes due to hypovitaminosis are only likely to be encountered in the non-hospitalised alcoholic due to the widespread practice of administering prophylactic doses of multivitamin preparations to alcoholics admitted to hospital. Electrolyte deficiencies are also encountered in alcoholics as a result of reduced intake. Beer drinkers, for example, may develop a hyponatraemic hypoosmolal syndrome. The daily requirement for sodium is approximately 100-200 mmol. Beer contains 1-2 mmol/l. Thus in alcoholics drinking large quantities of beer and eating little or no food, sodium intake may fall seriously short of the daily requirement and hyponatraemia may develop. Hilden and Svendsen (1975) have described hyponatraemia (98-107 mmol/l) in a group of beer drinkers imbibing 5 l/day.

As well as vitamin and mineral deficiency due to long term malnutrition, food restriction can have various metabolic effects depending upon the period of restriction (Dietze *et al.*, 1976). Reduced food intake among alcoholics may occur for any of a number of reasons, e.g. decreased intake due to anorexia or altered taste secondary to zinc depletion, malabsorption due to the toxic effect of ethanol on intestinal mucosa, diarrhoea, or steatorrhoea (Leevy and Zetterman, 1975).

Metabolic effects due solely to food restriction include a decrease in blood glucose and insulin levels and a rise in glucagon levels. Glycogenolysis, gluconeogenesis and lipolysis increase, and increased lipolysis in turn raises the free fatty acid levels. Free fatty acids are then used as an energy source for tissues. Prolonged fasting produces a decline in gluconeogenesis from amino acids due to an inhibition of proteolysis of skeletal muscle and also a decrease in the utilisation of free fatty acids and *pari passu* a rise in ketone bodies (acetoacetate, beta–hydroxybutyrate, acetone) (Dietze *et al.*, 1976). These complex disturbances of intermediary metabolism due to malnutrition may complicate and contribute to the biochemical abnormalities seen in an alcoholic. For example Wolfe *et al.*, (1976) have studied the metabolism of free fatty acids, amino acids, and carbohydrates following an infusion of ethanol in individuals fasted for differing periods of time. They noted significant differences in fatty acid transport, splanchnic storage of fat, and production of ketone bodies.

The inter-relationships and respective rôles of nutrient deficiencies and the metabolic and toxic effects of ethanol in the development of altered intermediary metabolism are, as yet, not fully characterised.

5.7 ENDOCRINE EFFECTS OF ETHANOL

The clinical endocrinology of alcohol abuse has received scant attention and is not well understood. Ethanol may induce alterations in steroid and peptide hormone levels and these in turn give rise to alterations in the levels of other substances. In considering the mechanism(s) of the effect of ethanol on the endocrine system, several factors must be taken into account; namely the dose of ethanol, the direct effect of alcohol upon an endocrine organ, the sedative effect of alcohol, stress, and the clinical status of the patient i.e. intoxicated or withdrawn.

A summary of substantiated and proposed endocrine changes following alcohol abuse is shown in Figure 5.8. These changes are discussed in more detail in Chapter 7 Sections 7 and 8.

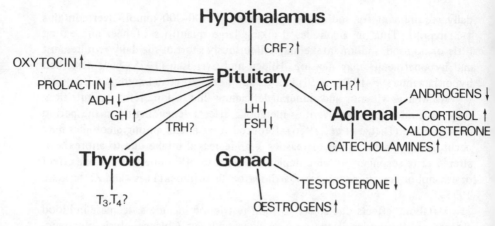

Fig. 5.8 – Endocrine effects of ethanol.

5.8 STRESS DUE TO INTOXICATION

The stress associated with intoxication is another factor which may contribute to and complicate the biochemical changes seen in alcoholics. Post-stress metabolism is complex. Secretion of adrenaline, cortisol, ADH, glucagon, and thyroid hormones may be increased. Water and sodium retention, potassium loss and acidosis may occur. Protein catabolism increases whilst synthesis decreases. Reduced synthesis of important proteins (e.g. digestive enzymes, transport proteins) may further complicate the post-stress situation. Post-stress energy metabolism is characterised by decreased glucose utilisation and insulin effectiveness, and increased lipolysis and ketogenesis (Taggart and Carruthers, 1971; Schultis and Beisbarth, 1976). Some aspects of the disturbances in, for example, carbohydrate metabolism have been attributed to stress due to intoxication rather than ethanol itself. The extent to which other biochemical changes encountered in the alcoholic are stress-related is not known.

5.9 DISEASE DUE OR SECONDARY TO ALCOHOL ABUSE

Another important factor which complicates the biochemical sequelae of alcohol abuse is disease. Various diseases are commonly associated with alcohol abuse, most notably liver disease. The biochemical disturbances characteristic of such diseases will occur in the alcoholic alongside disturbances due solely to alcohol ingestion and metabolism. The range of diseases encountered in alcoholics is discussed in Chapter 2.

5.10 GENETIC FACTORS

Genetic factors may contribute to the range and complexity of the biochemical changes which accompany alcohol abuse. Evidence in support of the operation of genetic factors comes from many different types of study (Lelbach, 1974; Anon, 1977).

Inter- and intrapersonal differences (Vesell, 1972; Wagner and Patel, 1972) and ethnic differences in the rate of elimination of ethanol from blood (Dietrich and Collins, 1977), the distribution and properties of the hepatic isoenzymes of ADh (Smith *et al.*, 1971; Wartburg *et al.*, 1974; Branden *et al.*, 1975; Li *et al.*, 1977), and the incidence of the flushing reaction (Wolff, 1973) have been cited as evidence for the operation of genetic factors in alcohol metabolism and tolerance.

Non-secretion of the ABH blood group substances (Swinson and Madden, 1973) the prevalence of the S antigen and the SS phenotype of complement, C3. and the linkage between the D gene of the Rh system and alcoholism are also believed to have a genetic basis (Hill, *et al.*, 1975).

Comparisons of the frequency of alcoholism in relatives of alcoholics strongly support the familial nature of this disorder. Family studies (Tarter *et al.*, 1977) and studies of grandsons of alcoholics (Kaij and Dock, 1975), twin studies (Partanen *et al.*, 1966) and studies of sons and daughters of alcoholics brought up in a non-alcoholic environment (Goodwin *et al.*, 1974, 1977) have all shown an increased prevalence of alcoholism, thus pointing to a genetic predisposition towards alcoholism.

Further evidence for the operation of genetic factors is seen in the striking differences between individuals in their tolerance and susceptibility to the effects of ethanol (Omenn and Moutulsky, 1972). Some individuals are able to consume regularly large quantities of ethanol over periods of years or decades without showing any adverse effects (e.g. normal liver histology), whilst others develop severe liver damage. For example a centenarian described by Steinmann (1966) had consumed large quantities of ethanol during most of his life, yet at postmortem no cirrhosis was detected. The reason for the obvious tolerance of such people to the adverse effects of ethanol is not known. Genetically predetermined constitutional factors may serve to protect such individuals from the effects of ethanol.

5.11 ANALYTICAL INTERFERENCES

A wide range of drugs and drug metabolites is known to interfere with analytical procedures employed in the determination of substances of clinical interest. Ethanol, acetaldehyde or components of alcoholic beverages present in biological specimens may, by interfering with an analytical method, falsely raise or lower the value for a particular determination. The influence of ethanol, acetaldehyde and other components of alcoholic beverages on the analytical methods utilised in the clinical laboratory have not been fully characterised and it is possible that some of the biochemical effects produced by ethanol may be artefactual. For example, ethanol interferes with certain types of glucose determination and with calcium determinations employing calcium specific electrodes, whilst acetaldehyde interferes with the methodology of ketone determinations (Young *et al.*, 1975). As well as ethanol, alcoholics or test subjects may be abusing other drugs or receiving drugs for therapeutic purposes. Such drugs or their metabolites may interfere with analytical procedures, e.g. diazepam therapy in alcoholics, can lead to an apparent elevation of urinary 5-hydroxyindole acetic acid (5-HIAA) *via* interference of diazepam in the analytical procedure for 5-HIAA (Clark and Kricka, 1977).

The contribution of analytical interferences by ethanol, acetaldehyde and components of beverages to the biochemical changes observed following ethanol abuse requires further study.

5.12 SUMMARY

The fact that ethanol is metabolised almost exclusively by the liver, the site of many essential metabolic transformations, explains in part the range and complexity of the biochemical disturbances accompanying alcohol abuse. Hepatic metabolism of ethanol leads to an alteration in the cytoplasmic NAD/NADH ratio which in turn influences the equilibrium of all NAD-dependent reactions. Competitive inhibition of aldehyde dehydrogenase by acetaldehyde, the primary metabolite of ethanol, may also reduce the conversion of various aldehydes to alcohols.

Table 5.5
Influence of ethanol on blood, serum or plasma levels of various substances or groups of substances*

I	**Elevated levels** Copper, Hydrogen ion, AlaT, AspT, AP, LDH, CK, IgA, IgG, IgM, Uric acid, GH, LH, Secretin, Gastrin, Cortisol, Oestrogens, Bilirubin, Lipoproteins, Triglycerides, Lactate, β-Hydroxybutyrate, Acetoacetate, Acetate, Catecholamines, Renin.
II	**Depressed levels** Potassium, Magnesium, Calcium, Zinc, Phosphate, Oxytocin, ADH, Testosterone, Pyruvate, Vitamin A, B, B_6, C, E, Folate.
III	**Variable response to ethanol** Sodium, Chloride, Iron, Albumin, Haptoglobin, Caeruloplasmin, Prolactin, FSH, Insulin, Aldosterone, Glucose, FFA, Vitamin D.

*The reader is directed to chapter 7 for a fuller account of the effects of ethanol on the levels of various substances in body fluids.

There are many factors which may influence the biochemical changes encountered in the alcoholic e.g. nutritional status, extent and duration of abuse. Factors such as time of testing, solubility and solvent effects of ethanol, endocrine effects of ethanol and genetic susceptibility are incompletely understood and poorly characterised. Experimental design and reporting of biochemical studies involving either administration of ethanol to healthy subjects or to alcoholics should, where possible, take account of these factors.

A summary of the major changes in the levels of substances in blood, serum or plasma following ethanol abuse is presented in Table 5.5. The changes are divided into three broad categories–(i) substances which are commonly depressed by ethanol (ii) elevated and (iii) those substances for which the changes are variable. It is intended that this tabulation will provide a broad overview of the biochemical changes in blood, serum or plasma which may be encountered in an alcoholic. In Chapter 7, which is intended for reference purposes, a detailed account of the effect of alcohol on individual biochemical parameters is presented.

5.13 REFERENCES

Abbot, R. R., Conboy, J. L., and Rekate, A. C. (1963) Liver function in alcoholism. *J. Mich. Med. Soc.*, **62**, 990.

Anon. (1977) How important are genetic influences on alcohol dependence? *Br. Med. J.*, **2**, 1371-1372.

Bang, N. U., Iversen, K., Jagt, T., and Madsen, S. (1958) Serum glutamic oxalacetic transaminase activity in acute and chronic alcoholism. *J. Am. Med. Assoc.*, **168**, 156-160.

Belfrage, P., Berg, P., Cronholm, T., Elmquist, D., Hägerstrand, I., Johannson, B., Nilsson-Ehle, P., Norden, G., Sjövall, J., and Wiebe, T. (1973) Prolonged administration of ethanol to young healthy volunteers: Effects on biochemical, morphological and neuro-physiological parameters. *Acta Med. Scand.*, **Suppl. No. 2**. 5-43.

Brohult, J. and Reichard, H. (1965) Liver damage after a dose of alcohol. *Lancet*, **ii**, 78-79.

Buchanan, W. M. (1970) Experimental production of 'Bantu' siderosis using home brewed beer. *S. Afr. J. Med. Sci.*, **35**, 15-21.

Carey, M. A., Jones, J. D., and Gastineau, C. F. (1971) Effect of moderate alcohol intake on blood chemistry values. *J. Am. Med. Assoc.*, **216**, 1766-1769.

Childs, A. W., Kivel, R. M., and Lieberman, A. (1963) Effects of ethyl alcohol on hepatic circulation, sulfobromophthalein clearance, and hepatic glutamic oxaloacetic transaminase production in man. *Gastroenterology*, **45**, 176-181.

Clark, P. M. S. and Kricka, L. J. (1977) Interference by diazepam in the determination of 5-hydroxyindole-3-acetic acid. *Ann. Clin. Biochem.*, **14**, 233-234.

Dietze, G., Wicklmayer, M., and Mehnert, H. (1976) Physiology of metabolism during starvation. *In* Parenteral Nutrition (Ahnefeld, F. W., Burri, C., Dick, W., and Halmagyi, M. *eds.*) pp. 17–30, Springer-Verlag, Berlin.

Dimberg, R., Hed, R., Kallner, G. and Nygren, A. (1967) Liver-muscle enzyme activities in the serum of alcoholics on a diet poor in carbohydrates. *Acta Med. Scand.*, **181**, 227–232.

Freer, D. E., and Statland, B. E. (1977a) The effects of ethanol (0.75 g/kg body weight) on the activities of selected enzymes in sera of healthy young adults: 1. Intermediate-term effects. *Clin. Chem.*, **23**, 830–834.

Freer, D. E., and Statland, B. E. (1977b) Effects of ethanol (0.75 g/kg body weight) on the activities of selected enzymes in sera of healthy young adults: 2. Inter-individual variations in response of γ-glutamyltransferase to repeated ethanol challenges. *Clin. Chem.*, **23**, 2099–2102.

Galambos, J. T., Asade, M., and Shanks, J. Z. (1963) The effect of intravenous ethanol on serum enzymes in patients with normal or diseased liver. *Gastroenterology*, **44**, 267–274.

Goldberg, D. M., and Watts, C. (1965) Serum enzyme changes as evidence of liver reaction to oral alcohol. *Gastroenterology*, **49**, 256–261.

Goodwin, D. W., Schulsinger, F., Møller, N., Hermansen, L., Winokur, G., and Guze, S. B. (1974) Drinking problems in adopted and nonadopted sons of alcoholics. *Arch. Gen. Psychiatry*, **31**, 164–171.

Goodwin, D. W., Schulsinger, F., Knop, J., Mednick, S., and Guze, S. D. (1977) Alcoholism and depression in adopted-out daughters of alcoholics. *Arch. Gen. Psychiatry*, **34**, 751–755.

Gordon, G. G. and Southren, A. L. (1977) Metabolic effects of alcohol on the endocrine system. *In* Metabolic Aspects of Alcoholism (Lieber, C. S. *ed.*) pp. 249–302. MTP Press Ltd., Lancaster.

Gottfried, E. B., Korsten, M. A. and Lieber, C. S. (1976) Gastritis and duodenitis induced by alcohol: an endoscopic and histologic assessment. *Gastroenterology*, **70**, 890 (Abstr.).

Halsted, C. H., Criggs, R. C., and Harris, J. W. (1967) The effect of alcoholism on the absorption of folic acid (^{3}H-PGA) evaluated by plasma levels and urine excretion. *J. Lab. Clin. Med.*, **69**, 116–131.

Halsted, C. H., Robles, E. A., and Mezey, E. (1971) Decreased jejunal uptake of labeled folic acid (^{3}H-PGA) in alcoholic patients: Roles of alcohol and nutrition. *N. Engl. J. Med.*, **285**, 701–706.

Halsted, C. H., Robles, E. A. and Mezey, E. (1973) Intestinal malabsorption in folate-deficient alcoholics. *Gastroenterology*, **64**, 526–532.

Hed, R., Nygren, A., and Sundblad, L. (1972) Muscle and liver serum enzyme activities in healthy volunteers given alcohol on a diet poor in carbohydrates. *Acta Med. Scand.*, **191**, 529–534.

Hilden, T., and Svendsen, T. L. (1975) Electrolyte disturbance in beer drinkers. *Lancet*, **ii**, 245–246.

Hines, J. D., and Cowan, D. H. (1970) Studies on the pathogenesis of alcohol induced sideroblastic bone-marrow abnormalities. *N. Engl. J. Med.,* **283,** 441-446.

Israel, Y., Valenzuela, J. E., Salazar, I., and Ugarte, G. (1969) Alcohol and amino acid transport in the human intestine. *J. Nutr.,* **98,** 222-224.

Jenkins, J. S., and Connolly, J. (1968) Adrenocortical response to ethanol in man. *Br. Med. J.,* **ii,** 804-805.

Kaij, L. and Dock, J. (1975) Grandsons of alcoholics. *Arch. Gen. Psychiatry,* **32,** 1379-1381.

Kalant, H. (1971) Absorption, diffusion, distribution, and elimination of ethanol: Effects on biological membranes. *In* Biology of Alcoholism, (Kissin, B., and Begleiter, H. *eds.*) Vol 1, pp. 1-62, Plenum Press.

Krasner, N., Cochran, K. M., Thompson, C. G., Carmichael, H. A., and Russel, R. (1974) Effects of ethanol on small intestinal absorption. *Gut,* **15,** 831 (Abstr.).

Leevy, C. M., and Zetterman, R. K. (1975) Malnutrition and alcoholism - An overview. *In* Alcohol and Abnormal Protein Biosynthesis (Rothschild, M. A., Oratz, M., and Schreiber, S. S. *eds.*) pp. 3-15, Pergamon Press, Oxford.

Lelbach, W. K. (1967) Zur leberschädigen Wirkung verschiedener Alkoholiker. *Dtsch. Med. Wochenschr.,* **92,** 233-238.

Lelbach, W. K. (1974) Organic pathology related to volume and pattern of alcohol use. *Res. Adv. Alcohol Drug Probs.,* **1,** 93-198.

Li, T.-K., Bosron, W. F., Dafeldecker, W. P., Lange, L. G., and Vallee, B. L. (1977) Isolation of II-alcohol dehydrogenase of human liver: Is it a determinant of alcoholism? *Proc. Natl. Acad. Sci.,* **74,** 4378-4381.

Lieber, C. S., Jones, D. P., and DeCarli, L. M. (1965) Effects of prolonged ethanol intake. Production of fatty liver despite adequate diets. *J. Clin. Invest.,* **44,** 1009-1021.

Lieber, C. S., and DeCarli, L. M. (1977) Metabolic effects of alcohol on the liver. *In* Metabolic Aspects of Alcoholism (Lieber, C. S. *ed.*) pp. 31-79, MTP Press Ltd., Lancaster.

Lindblad, B., and Olsson, R. (1976) Unusually high levels of blood alcohol? *J. Am. Med. Assoc.,* **236,** 1600-1602.

Lindenbaum, J., and Pezzimenti, J. F. (1973) Effects of B_{12} and folate deficiency on small intestinal function. *Clin. Res.,* **21,** 518.

Lopez, R., and Montoya, M. F. (1971) Abnormal bone marrow morphology in the premature infant associated with maternal alcohol infusion. *J. Pediat.,* **79,** 1008.

Lundquist, F. (1975) Interference of ethanol in cellular metabolism. *Ann. N. Y. Acad. Sci.,* **252,** 10-20.

Mekhijian, H. S., May, E. S., and Sury, T. (1974) The effect of ethanol on human jejunal absorption. *Clin. Res.,* **22,** 604 (Abstr.).

Mendelson, J. H. (1964) Experimentally induced chronic intoxication and withdrawal in alcoholics, Part X. Conclusion and implications. *Q. J. Stud. Alcohol*, **Suppl. No. 2,** 117-126.

Mendelson, J. H., and LaDou, J. (1964) Experimentally induced chronic intoxication and withdrawal in alcoholics, Part I. Background and experimental design. *Q. J. Stud. Alcohol*, **Suppl. No. 2,** 1-13.

Mendelson, J. H., and Stein, S. (1966) Serum cortisol levels in alcoholic and non-alcoholic subjects during experimentally induced ethanol intoxication. *Psychosom. Med.*, **28,** 616-626.

Mezey, E., Jow, E., Slavin, R. E., and Tobon, F. (1970) Pancreatic function and intestinal absorption in chronic alcoholism. *Gastroenterology*, **59,** 657-664.

Müting, D. (1971) Alkohol and Leber. *Arztl. Praxis.*, **23,** 3699.

Noble, E. P. (1973) Alcohol and adrenocortical functions of animals and man. *In* Alcoholism (Bourne, P. G., and Fox, R. *eds.*) pp. 105-135, Academic Press.

Omenn, G. S., and Motulsky, A. G. (1972) A biochemical and genetic approach to alcoholism. *Ann. N. Y. Acad. Sci.*, **197,** 16-23.

Partanen, J., Bruun, K., and Markkanen, T. (1966) *Inheritance of Drinking Behaviour*, Finnish Foundation for Alcohol Studies, Helsinki.

Philips, G. B., and Safrit, H. F. (1971) Alcoholic diabetes. Induction of glucose intolerance with alcohol. *J. Am. Med. Assoc.*, **217,** 1513-1519.

Pirola, R. C., and Davis, A. E. (1970) Effects of intravenous alcohol on motility of the duodenum and of the sphincter of Oddi. *Aust. Ann. Med.*, **19,** 1.

Reid, N. C. R. W., Brunt, P. W., Bias, W. B., Maddrey, W. C., Alonso, B. A., and Iber, F. L. (1968) Genetic characteristics and cirrhosis; A controlled study of 200 patients. *Br. Med. J.*, **2,** 463-465.

Robles, E. A., Mexey, E., Halsted, C. H., and Schuster, M. M. (1974) Effect of ethanol on motility of the small intestine. *Johns Hopkins Med. J.*, **135,** 17-24.

Roggin, G. M., Iber, F. L., Kater, R. M. H., and Tobon, F. (1969) Malabsorption in the chronic alcoholic. *Johns Hopkins Med. J.*, **125,** 321-330.

Rubin, E., and Lieber, C. S. (1968) Alcohol-induced hepatic injury in non-alcoholic volunteers. *N. Engl. J. Med.*, **278,** 869-876.

Rubin, E., Rybak, B. J., Lindenbaum, J., Gerson, C. D., Walker, G., and Lieber, C. S. (1972) Ultrastructural changes in the small intestine induced by ethanol. *Gastroenterology*, **63,** 801-814.

Schultis, K., and Beisbarth, H. (1976) Pathobiochemistry of post-stress metabolism. *In* Parenteral Nutrition (Ahnefeld, F. W., Burri, C., Dick, W., and Halmagyi, M. *eds.*) pp. 31-44, Springer-Verlag, Berlin.

Seligson, D., Wadstein, S. S., Gige, B., Mekoway, W. H., and Sborov, V. M. (1953) Some metabolic effects of ethanol in humans. *Clin. Res.*, **1,** 86.

Simpson, H. W. (1976) A new perspective: Chronobiochemistry. *In* Essays in Medical Biochemistry (Marks, V., and Hales, C. N. *eds.*) Vol 2, pp. 115-187, The Biochemical Society and Association of Clinical Biochemists, London.

Song, S. K., and Rubin, E. (1972) Ethanol produces muscle damage in human volunteers. *Science (Wash. D. C.)*, 175, 327-328.

Speck, B. (1970) Die Tagesschwankungen des Serumeisens und der latenten Eisenbindungskapazität bei Hepatitis, Leberzirrhose, Alkoholismus, Hämochromatose und aplastischer Anämie. *Schweiz. Med. Wochenschr.*, 100, 303-305.

Steinmann, B. (1966) Uber Hundertjährige. *Gerentol. Clin.*, 8, 23.

Sun, A. Y., Samorajski, T. (1975) The effects of age and alcohol on $[Na^+ + K^+]$ - ATPase activity of whole homogenate and synaptosomes prepared from mouse and human brain. *J. Neurochem.*, 24, 161-164.

Swinson, R. P. (1972) Genetic polymorphism and alcoholism. *Ann. N. Y. Acad. Sci.*, 197, 129-133.

Swinson, R. P., and Madden, J. S. (1973) ABO blood groups and ABH substance secretion in alcoholics. *Q. J. Stud. Alcohol*, 34, 64-70.

Taggart, P., and Carruthers, M. (1971) Endogenous hyperlipaemia induced by emotional stress of racing drivers. *Lancet*, i, 363-366.

Tarter, R. E., McBride, H., Buonpane, N., and Schneider, D. U. (1977) Differentiation of alcoholics. *Arch. Gen. Psychiatry*, 34, 761-768.

Taskinen, M.-R., and Nikkilä, E. A. (1977) Nocturnal hypertriglyceridemia and hyperinsulinaemia following moderate evening intake of alcohol. *Acta Med. Scand.*, 202, 173-177.

Thomson, A. D., Baker, H., and Leevy, C. M. (1970) Patterns of ^{35}S-thiamine hydrochloride absorption in the malnourished alcoholic patient. *J. Lab. Clin. Med.*, 76, 34-45.

Tomasulo, P. A., Kater, R. M. H., and Iber, F. L. (1968) Impairment of thiamine absorption in alcoholism. *Am. J. Clin. Nutr.*, 21, 1340-1344.

Truit, E. B., and Walsh, M. J. (1971) The role of acetaldehyde in the actions of ethanol. *In* The Biology of Alcoholism (Kissin, B., and Begleiter, H. *eds.*) Vol 1, pp. 161-195, Plenum Press.

Vesell, E. S. (1972) Ethanol metabolism: Regulation by genetic factors in normal volunteers under a controlled environment and the effect of chronic ethanol administration. *Ann. N. Y. Acad. Sci.*, 197, 79-88.

Vitale, J. J., and Coffey, J. (1971) Alcohol and vitamin metabolism. *In* The Biology of Alcoholism (Kissin, B., and Begleiter, H. *eds.*) pp. 327-352, Plenum Press.

Wartburg, J. P., von (1971) The metabolism of alcohol in normals and alcoholics: Enzymes. *In* The biology of Alcoholism (Kissin, B., and Begleiter, H. *eds.*) Vol 2, pp. 63-102, Plenum Press.

Wolfe, B. M., Havel, J. R., Marliss, E. B., Kane, J. P., Seymour, J., and Ahuja, S. P. (1976) Effects of a 3-day fast and of ethanol on splanchnic metabolism of FFA, amino acids, and carbohydrates in healthy young men. *J. Clin. Invest.*, 57, 329-340.

Wolff, P. H. (1973) Vasomotor sensitivity to alcohol in diverse mongoloid populations. *Am. J. Human Genetics,* **25**, 193–199.

Young, D. S., Pestaner, L. C., and Gibberman, V. (1975) Effects of drugs on clinical laboratory tests. *Clin. Chem.,* **21**, 1D–432D.

CHAPTER 6

Biochemical Tests for the Detection and Assessment of Alcohol Abuse

6.1 INTRODUCTION

It is often very difficult to establish how much ethanol a person has consumed and over what period of time. One or more of a number of biochemical tests have been either advocated or are currently employed to detect alcohol abuse (Table 6.1), and this chapter reviews those presently advocated.

An effective biochemical test or biochemical marker for ethanol abuse should ideally possess the following characteristics:

(i) Prolonged excessive ingestion of ethanol should lead to a significant and persistent change in the test parameter.

(ii) The alteration in the test parameter should be detectable for a period of time after cessation of drinking. Thus the alcoholic or heavy drinker who was abstinent for a day or several days prior to testing would not escape detection.

(iii) The test parameter should not be significantly affected by acute ingestion of ethanol in a social or occasional drinker, thus reducing or eliminating the possibility of a false result.

(iv) Concurrent disease (especially liver disease), and dietary factors other than ethanol, should not markedly affect the test parameter.

(v) The biochemical test should be analytically convenient and reliable and performed on a readily available biological specimen such as blood, serum or urine.

None of the currently available biochemical tests for ethanol abuse fulfill all of these criteria, being either inconvenient to perform or susceptible to false positive or negative results. As yet no simple and reliable biochemical test to distinguish the ethanol abuser from the non-abuser is available.

6.2 BLOOD ETHANOL AND SERUM OSMOLALITY

The measurement of blood ethanol is the most direct method for following the success of treatment of the ethanol abuser. It may also be useful in the initial diagnosis of ethanol abuse and as an adjunct to techniques of investigating

Table 6.1
Biochemical Tests and Markers for Alcohol Abuse.

Blood or breath ethanol
Serum osmolality

Blood lactate/pyruvate
Galactose tolerance test
Urinary biogenic amine metabolites
Plasma steroids

Plasma alpha-amino-n-butyric acid/leucine

Serum gamma-glutamyl transferase
Erythrocyte delta-aminolaevulinic acid dehydratase
Serum glutamate dehydrogenase

Biochemical profile coupled with pattern analysis

Serological markers

Urinary D-glucaric acid

Mean corpuscular volume

Aminopyrine breath test
Urinary coproporphyrin
Urinary zinc

liver disease (Hamlyn *et al.*, 1975). Measurement of ethanol in breath using a
'Breathalyzer' or similar devices is also of value as a means of detecting ethanol
ingestion. Blood ethanol levels are best measured by gas chromatographic
methods (Payne, 1975), because these are subject to fewer interferences. Enzymatic and chemical methods are also available for the estimation of blood
ethanol concentrations (Sunshine and Hodnett, 1971). Indirectly, blood ethanol
concentrations have been estimated by measuring the serum osmolality (Redetzki
et al., 1972). It has been shown that there is a direct relationship between blood
ethanol concentration and serum osmolality as measured by depression of the
freezing point. The increased osmolality is due mainly to the presence of ethanol,
but may also be due in part to an elevation of lactate levels and possibly due to
the presence of congeners. This simple technique has been advocated for the
rapid clinical evaluation of alcohol intoxication.

Blood ethanol levels, however, may not reflect the severity of alcohol abuse, or distinguish between intermittent and prolonged alcohol abuse. A further problem is that the devious alcoholic may abstain from drinking immediately prior to testing, thus having no blood alcohol, and so may avoid detection.

6.3 TESTS BASED ON THE ALTERED HEPATIC NAD/NADH RATIO

Many biochemical tests have sought to detect ethanol abuse indirectly *via* assessment of the hepatic NAD/NADH ratio. Excessive ethanol metabolism in the liver causes an increase in NADH levels in the hepatocyte (Forsander, 1970). As explained in Chapter 5, this alteration in the NAD/NADH ratio has a profound effect on many NAD-dependent metabolic transformations. Measurement of the levels of metabolites in serum or urine which are sensitive to the NAD/NADH ratio has been employed as a means of detecting ethanol abuse.

6.3.1 Blood Lactate/Pyruvate Ratio

The blood lactate/pyruvate ratio is sometimes used as an index of ethanol abuse. Ethanol metabolism generates NADH in the hepatocyte, and this leads to an increase in blood lactate levels as compared with pyruvate levels (Figure 6.1). However other factors, such as exercise, carbohydrate metabolism and thiamine status, may alter the lactate/pyruvate ratio (Park and Grubler, 1969; Henderson, 1971); the last two factors also being altered in alcoholics. Hepatic vein catheterisation studies have shown that ethanol raised the lactate/pyruvate ratio from a value of 25.1 to 156.6 (Lundquist *et al.*, 1962; Tygstrup *et al.*, 1965). The change in the ratio of these metabolites is so great that it can also be detected in peripheral blood. The sampling and analysis of blood for lactate and pyruvate is inconvenient, blood must be immediately deproteinised because otherwise significant changes in pyruvate and lactate levels will occur (Drewes, 1974).

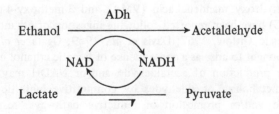
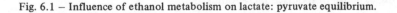

Fig. 6.1 − Influence of ethanol metabolism on lactate: pyruvate equilibrium.

6.3.2 Galactose Tolerance Test

The galactose tolerance test has been used for the diagnosis of alcoholism and alcoholic fatty liver disease. This test is based on the inhibitory effect of ethanol on the conversion of galactose to glucose. The enzyme UDP-galactose-4-epimerase which catalyses this transformation requires catalytic amounts of NAD and is strongly inhibited by NADH. Increased formation of NADH as a consequence of hepatic ethanol metabolism inhibits the enzyme and thus reduces the conversion of galactose to glucose. The test involves i.v. administration of galactose and subsequent monitoring of either the blood glucose or galactose levels. If ethanol has been ingested there will be little rise in blood glucose levels and decreased hepatic elimination of galactose, as evidenced by an increased half-life of galactose in blood (Tygstrup and Lundquist, 1962; Salaspuro, 1967).

In a healthy non-alcoholic subject, a dose of ethanol, 3.0 mmol/kg body weight, has been shown to reduce the hepatic galactose elimination capacity by 50%. The presence of steatosis or cirrhosis, however, lessens the inhibitory effect of ethanol (Lindskov and Bach-Mortensen, 1973).

Another form of the test involves administration of ^{14}C-labelled galactose and measurement of expired $^{14}CO_2$. Patients with alcoholic cirrhosis have been shown to excrete labelled carbon dioxide at one half to one third the rate of normals (Shreeve et al., 1976), reflecting the decreased conversion of galactose to glucose and glucose to carbon dioxide. This test for ethanol abuse, like the lactate/pyruvate test, is relatively inconvenient, time consuming, and is complicated by the presence of liver disease.

6.3.3 Biogenic Amine Metabolites

There are several reports of alterations in the urinary excretion of amines and their metabolites following ingestion of ethanol (see Chapter 7 section 14), but the diagnostic value of such changes has not been extensively investigated.

Increased urinary excretion of tryptamine (Maynard and Schenker, 1962), and complementary reductions and elevations respectively in the urinary excretion of the serotonin metabolites 5-hydroxyindole-3-acetic acid (5-HIAA) (Olsen et al., 1960; Rosenfeld, 1960) and 5-hydroxytryptophol (Feldstein et al., 1964; Davis et al., 1966, 1967, 1969), and of the norepinephrine metabolites 3-methoxy-4-hydroxy mandelic acid (VMA) and 3-methoxy-4-phenylethylene glycol (MHPG) have been reported following ingestion of ethanol (Davis et al., 1967; Smith and Gitlow, 1967; Davis et al., 1969; Ogata et al., 1971). Such changes are thought to arise as a consequence of hepatic ethanol metabolism.

Excessive production of acetaldehyde and/or NADH may interfere with the hepatic metabolism of aldehydes by competitive inhibition of aldehyde dehydrogenase and/or promotion of reductive pathways, respectively. This results in changes in amine metabolism — reduced metabolites being increased at the expense of oxidised metabolites.

Akhter and coworkers (1978) have studied the urinary excretion of the amine metabolites tryptamine, 5-HIAA, VMA and MHPG in alcoholics, patients with non-alcoholic liver disease and healthy controls. Significant differences were found between healthy controls and the alcoholics in respect of urinary levels of tryptamine, MHPG, and the ratio tryptamine/5-HIAA in random urine specimens (Figure 6.2), although these parameters did not correlate with serum

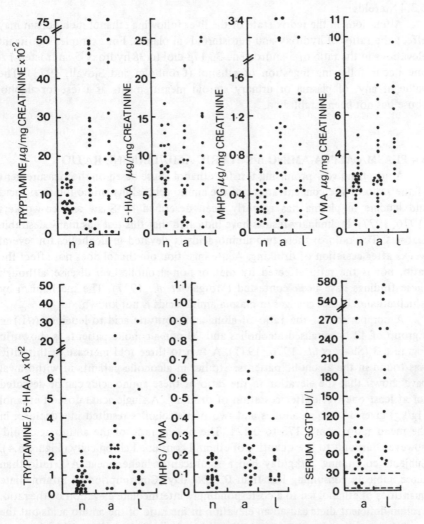

Fig. 6.2 – Urinary biogenic amines and metabolites and serum gamma-glutamyl transferase in healthy controls (n), alcoholics (a) and patients with non-alcoholic liver disease (l).
Reproduced by permission from Akhter *et al.*, Journal of Studies on Alcohol (1978)

GGT levels. The best discrimination between the three groups of patients studied was afforded by the ratio tryptamine/5-HIAA and it has been suggested that this parameter may be of use as a screening test for alcohol abuse.

Although the test has the advantage of using random urine specimens, the analytical methods are tedious to perform and subject to drug interference.

6.3.4 Steroids

Alterations in the redox state of the liver following ethanol metabolism may affect the ratios of hydroxy-and ketosteroids in plasma. For example, significant elevations in the ratio of 5-androstene-3β,17β-diol to 3β-hydroxy-5-androsten-17-one occur following ingestion of ethanol (Crönholm and Sjovall, 1973). The value, if any, of plasma or urinary steroid measurements as a test for alcohol abuse has not been established.

6.4 PLASMA ALPHA-AMINO-n-BUTYRIC ACID/LEUCINE RATIO

A novel and very promising test for ethanol abuse based on the measurement of the ratio of the concentrations of the amino acids alpha-amino-n-butyric acid and leucine in plasma has recently been described by Shaw and co-workers (1976, 1977). Preliminary results have indicated that this test has many desirable features. The ratio of these two amino acids is elevated in alcoholics for several weeks after cessation of drinking. Acute ingestion of ethanol does not affect the ratio, nor is the ratio affected by diet or non-alcoholic liver disease, although these findings have been contested (Morgan et al., 1977). The mechanism by which ethanol causes changes in plasma amino acids is not known.

A comparison of the ratio of alpha-aminobutyric acid to leucine (A/L) in a group of 42 hospitalised alcoholics and 20 non-alcoholic patients is shown in Figure 6.3 (Shaw et al., 1976, 1977). A two to three fold increase in this ratio was found in the alcoholic patients. Studies in alcoholic patients in withdrawal have shown that the elevation in the ratio of these amino acids can be detected for at least one week after cessation of drinking. A single acute dose of ethanol (1g/kg) given to two alcoholics and two non-alcoholics resulted in a decrease in the mean ratio from 0.173 to 0.121. The plasma ratio of the amino acids did, however, respond to the quantity of ethanol consumed chronically (Figure 6.4). Subjects consuming 2g/kg/day had a significantly higher mean A/L ratio than those subjects consuming less than 0.2g/kg/day. Consumption of intermediate quantities of ethanol led to a correspondingly intermediate elevation of the ratio. Protein-deficient diets caused an elevation in the ratio of the amino acids but the magnitude of the elevation was similar in hospitalised alcoholics with either long term (52 weeks) or short term (2 weeks) dietary protein deficiency. These results indicated that the ratio was not significantly altered by differences in nutritional status.

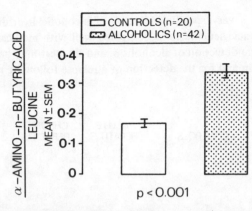

Fig. 6.3 – Increased plasma alpha-aminobutyric acid/leucine ratio amongst 42 hospitalised alcoholics compared to 20 non-alcoholic controls. All alcoholics fulfilled major National Council for Alcoholism criteria of alcoholism and the majority had been drinking heavily until admission.
Reproduced by permission from Shaw *et al.*, Currents in Alcholism: Biochemical and Clinical Studies. Vol. 1. Grune and Stratton (1977)

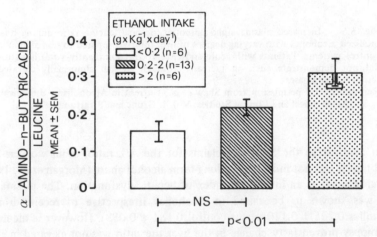

Fig. 6.4 – Increased plasma alpha-aminobutyric acid/leucine ratio in relation to average daily ethanol intake among 25 methadone maintenance patients. A significant increase was present among subjects consuming more than 2g/kg/day compared to those consuming less than 0.2g/kg/day; and intermediate elevation was present among those consuming 0.2–2g/kg/day. Recency of alcohol consumption was similar for all subjects who consumed alcohol on a daily basis.
Reproduced by permission from Shaw *et al.*, Currents in Alcoholism: Biological, Biochemical and Clinical Studies. Vol. 1. Grune and Stratton (1977)

The effect of liver disease on the ratio is illustrated in Figure 6.5. In acute and chronic hepatitis the ratio is not significantly different from control values, whilst in alcoholic liver disease a considerable elevation occurs. The ratio would therefore appear to a very specific indicator of alcoholic liver disease. Plasma alpha-aminobutyric acid/leucine ratio compares well with medical and psychological criteria for the detection of alcoholism, and this test may be a very useful marker for alcoholism and for the detection of a relapse following rehabilitation.

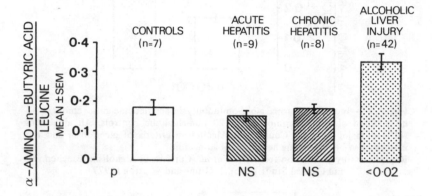

Fig. 6.5 – Increased plasma alpha-aminobutyric acid/leucine ratio among hospitalized alcoholics with varying degrees of liver injury compared to non-alcoholic control patients. Patients with acute and chronic (predominantly viral) hepatitis did not demonstrate such an increase although all had abnormally elevated serum transaminases.
Reproduced by permission from Shaw *et al.*, Current in Alcoholism: Biological, Biochemical and Clinical Studies: Vol. 1. Grune and Stratton (1977)

In contrast to the foregoing claims for the A/L ratio, other workers have found that it was not indicative of long-term alcohol abuse (Morgan *et al.*, 1977). Instead it acted as an insensitive index of hepatic-dysfunction. The plasma A/L ratio was shown to be raised in alcoholics irrespective of recent drinking (alcoholics 0.225 ± 0.110 versus control 0.181 ± 0.058). However in alcoholics with biopsy-proven fatty change in the liver the ratio was not elevated in either a drinking or a non-drinking group. Patients with more severe liver disease did have elevated plasma A/L ratios irrespective of recent drinking, and this was taken as evidence that the ratio was indicating liver damage rather than alcoholism. Support for this suggestion was provided by the finding of significantly elevated plasma A/L ratios in patients with non-alcoholic liver disease.

One minor problem is that the analytical determination of these amino acids involves an amino acid analyser. This methodology would prove inconvenient in many laboratories and a faster, more simple method of analysis would be advantageous.

In view of the controversial nature of this test and the analytical problems, further studies are needed to clarify its value as a test for alcohol abuse.

6.5 ENZYMES

Ethanol may cause changes in serum enzyme levels by induction, tissue damage, or a combination of both. Extent of elevation of enzyme levels provides some indication of the degree of induction and/or magnitude of tissue damage and may thus be equated with extent and duration of ethanol abuse.

6.5.1 Gamma-Glutamyl Transferase (Transpeptidase)

Serum levels of gamma-glutamyl transferase (GGT) are perhaps the most widely used biochemical test for assessing ethanol abuse (see also Chapter 7 Section 3 and the review by Rosalki (1975)). The application of serum GGT as a test for ethanol abuse is complicated, however, by various diseases and certain types of drug therapy and drug abuse.

A rise in serum GGT activity following ethanol abuse occurs as a result of hepatic induction of the enzyme, although hepatocellular damage and cholestasis may also contribute to the increased serum activity. Ethanol is not the only drug which can induce GGT, and increased activities of this enzyme have been recorded in drug addicts using singly or in combination heroin, morphine, cocaine, physeptone, LSD, amphetamines, barbiturates or cannabis. Elevated levels have been reported in patients receiving anticonvulsant therapy and also in patients receiving warfarin in combination with barbiturates or phenazone (Whitfield et al., 1972). In a group of alcoholics and drug dependents studied by Patel and O'Gorman 1975), 48% of the alcoholics and 50% of the drug dependents had elevated serum GGT levels (Figure 6.6).

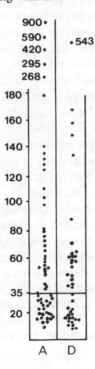

Fig. 6.6 – Serum gamma-glutamyl transferase activities (IU/L) in 67 alcoholics (A) and 40 drug dependents (D). (The upper limit of the normal range is indicated by a horizontal line).
Reproduced by permission from Patel and O'Gorman, *Journal of Clinical Pathology* (1975)

Activity of GGT is located mainly in the kidney, prostate, pancreas and liver (approximate relative activities 100: 30: 15: 10). Diseases affecting the liver and pancreas and also the cardiovascular system can cause significant elevations in serum GGT activity. Such causes must be ruled out when employing GGT as a marker for ethanol abuse (Rosalki and Zilva, 1977).

Generally, GGT values average two to three times the upper limit of the reference interval in hospitalised and up to two times the upper limit in out-patient alcoholics, although levels as high as twenty times the upper limit of the reference interval have been recorded (Rosalki and Rau, 1972; Rosalki, 1975). Acute ingestion of ethanol by healthy individuals leads to a rise in GGT levels, which gradually return to normal values during a period of a few days (Rosalki, 1975; Freer and Statland, 1977a,b).

A correlation has been described between alcohol intake and GGT activity even at low levels of alcohol consumption (Figure 6.7). However, whilst the mean GGT activity of the different drinking populations was found to differ, there was considerable overlap in the GGT activity of the populations (Rollason *et al.*, 1972). Serum GGT levels have been found to fall during abstinence, and hence its measurement may be useful in determining the success of treatment of alcoholism. A group of 44 patients was studied by Lamy *et al.*, (1975) during a two year period following a 'cure' for alcoholism. In the 29 patients who did not resume drinking the GGT levels were 148 ± 184 mU/ml (mean ± S.D.) at the beginning of the 'cure', 21 ± 14 after one year and 19 ± 13 after two years. In the remaining 15 patients, who resumed drinking less than one year after the 'cure', serum GGT levels were 140 ± 161 at the beginning of the 'cure', and 166 ± 164 and 162 ± 163 after one and two years, respectively. Similarly, other workers (Wietholtz and Colombo, 1976) have highlighted the usefulness of GGT deter-minations in the evaluation of recovery from alcoholism and in the detection of relapses. Of the 90 chronic alcoholics studied by Wietholtz and Colombo (1976) 79 (88%) had elevated GGT levels at the beginning of the alcohol withdrawal course, whilst aspartate and alanine aminotransferase were elevated in 34% and 23% of the patients, respectively. During a 30-day withdrawal period GGT levels returned to normal except in the 14 patients who relapsed. In these patients GGT levels rose immediately after the new intake of ethanol.

The effect of duration of ethanol abuse on GGT and other enzymes such as alanine and aspartate aminotransferase has been investigated by Skude and Wadstein (1977). A study of 182 chronic alcoholics showed that the highest values of these enzymes were encountered after 5–20 years of well-documented alcoholism (Figure 6.8). Long-standing alcohol abusers showed a tendency to normalisation of the serum GGT activities. It is interesting to note that in 14 (8%) of the alcoholics studied (5 had been alcoholics for more than 20 years, 3 had delirium tremens, and together they had been admitted to hospital 74 times due to alcoholism in the previous five years), that all of the tests were normal.

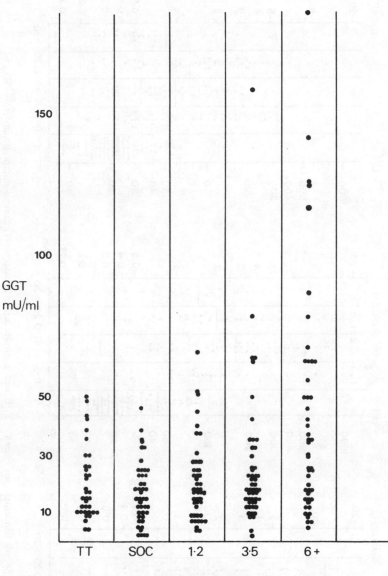

Fig. 6.7 — Gamma-glutamyl transferase in different drinking groups. (TT, tee-total; soc, social drinkers; 1-2, 1-2 drinks per day; 3-5, 3-5 drinks per day; 6+, greater than 6 drinks per day).
    Reproduced by permission from Rollason *et al.*, *Clinica Chimica Acta* (1972)

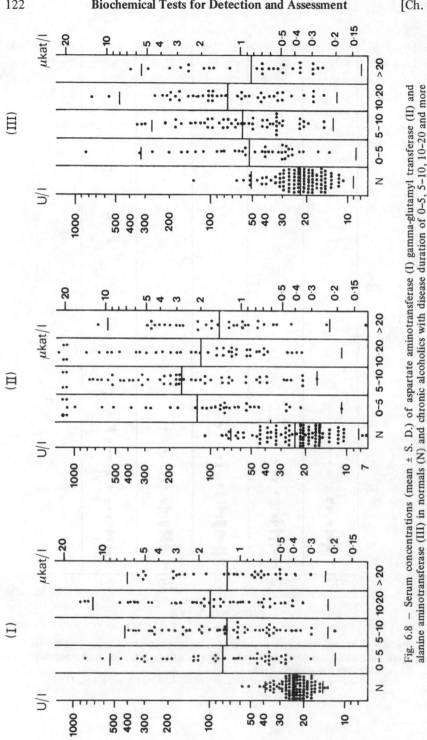

Fig. 6.8 – Serum concentrations (mean ± S. D.) of aspartate aminotransferase (I) gamma-glutamyl transferase (II) and alanine aminotransferase (III) in normals (N) and chronic alcoholics with disease duration of 0–5, 5–10, 10–20 and more than 20 years. Reproduced by permission from Skude and Wadstein, *Acta Medica Scandinavica* (1977)

The reason for the tendency towards normalisation of enzyme values in the group with the longest-standing alcoholism, and the normal enzyme levels detected in 8% of the alcoholics, is obscure. It may be that some alcoholics have an inherent resistance to ethanol, or it may be related to dietary or genetic factors.

Drinking pattern has also been shown to affect serum GGT values. In daily drinkers, the so-called inability-to-abstain or delta-alcoholics, there is a higher incidence (75 versus 46% of raised GGT levels as compared with bout drinkers, i.e. those with loss of control or delta alcoholism (Wiseman and Spencer-Peet, 1977). These results indicate that daily-drinking alcoholics would be more likely to be detected than bout drinkers by serum GGT measurements. In the latter group, the closer the sample is taken to drinking the more likely the chance of finding an abnormal result. Since serum GGT levels fall when consumption of ethanol stops then serial samples may be useful in investigating a patient with a suspected ethanol abuse problem.

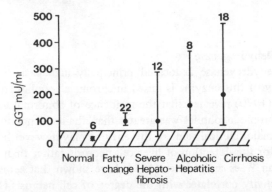

Fig. 6.9 – Relationship of serum gamma-glutamyl transferase (GGT) to the type of histological liver damage. GGT level is expressed as mean ± 1 S. D. calculated from the logarithmic distribution (n indicated above each bar and normal range indicated by shaded area).

Reproduced by permission from Wu, *American Journal of Gastroenterology* (1976)

Alcoholic liver disease can be a cause of elevated serum GGT levels in the alcoholic. The extent of elevation of GGT levels correlates to some extent with the type of histological damage (Wu *et al.*, 1976). In a group of 66 alcoholic patients who had admitted to drinking in excess of 80g ethanol per day for at least several years and who had clinical and/or biochemical evidence of liver disease, the mean serum GGT was highest in those patients with the most severe histological damage, i.e. cirrhosis (Figure 6.9). Serum GGT in combination with other serum enzymes such as aspartate or alanine aminotransferase has also been employed in discriminatory processes for separating patients with various types of alcoholic liver disease.

6.5.2 Delta-Aminolaevulinic acid Dehydratase

Ethanol has an effect on the activity of several enzymes of haem biosynthesis. The activity of δ-aminolaevulinic acid (ALA) synthase (EC 2.3.1.37) is raised whilst the activities of ALA dehydratase (porphobilinogen synthase; EC 4.2.1.24) and ferrochelatase (EC 4.99.1.1) decreased. A study by Krasner and colleagues (1974) has indicated that ALA dehydratase may be a useful index of ethanol abuse. Activity of this enzyme in erythrocytes is decreased for several days after withdrawal, normal activity not being reached until approximately 7 days after withdrawal. Measurement of this enzyme was found to be more reliable than gamma-glutamyl transferase as an index of ethanol abuse. The effect of ethanol on ALA dehydratase activity is thought to be mediated by changes in glutathione levels consequent on altered NADH levels. Increased NADH levels lead to the conversion of glutathione to its reduced form, the latter causing an inhibition of ALA dehydratase activity (Moore *et al.*, 1971). Further research is required in order to establish the value of this enzyme as a diagnostic test for alcohol abuse.

6.5.3 Glutamate Dehydrogenase

Glutamate dehydrogenase is located principally in hepatic mitochondria. The serum activity of this enzyme is raised in chronic alcoholics and a study by Konttinen *et al.*, (1970) revealed that the incidence of abnormal values for this enzyme in 100 chronic alcoholics was greater than the incidence for GGT (47% versus 43%). The major clinical value of this enzyme may however be as a reliable biochemical test for the detection of liver cell necrosis rather than as a test for alcohol abuse. Van Waes and Lieber (1977) have shown that serum glutamate dehydrogenase activity correlates with the degree of cell necrosis (Figure 6.10) and discriminates efficiently between patients with and without alcoholic hepatitis.

6.6 BIOCHEMICAL PROFILING COUPLED WITH PATTERN ANALYSIS

Many laboratories perform biochemical profile investigations: such profiles consist of 'groups of investigations performed on patients and which include some discretionary tests but in addition, others that the laboratory finds convenient to perform because of the way the analytical work is organised' (Whitby *et al.*, 1975). A profile might typically consist of sodium, potassium, urea, creatinine, urate, calcium, albumin, globulin, bilirubin, alkaline phosphatase, aspartate aminotransferase, cholesterol, and glucose determinations.

A convenient and yet largely unexplored approach to the detection of alcohol abuse involves the mathematical analysis of biochemical profile results to determine if any parameter or combination of parameters might provide information on alcohol intake or abuse. This particular approach has obvious

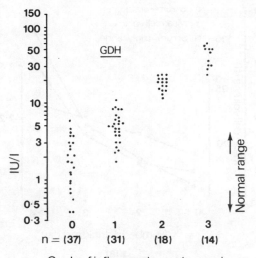

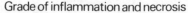

Grade of inflammation and necrosis

Fig. 6.10 – Correlation of glutamate dehydrogenase (GDH) with degree of liver cell necrosis in 100 alcoholics (O- absence of necrosis and parenchymal inflammation; 1- occasional cell drop-out; 2-scattered foci of necrotic cells in the parenchyma with polynuclear infiltration predominently in the centrolobular region; 3-diffuse parenchymal necrosis with polymorphonuclear infiltrates).
Reproduced by permission from Van Waes and Lieber, *British Medical Journal* (1977)

advantages because it does not involve the introduction of any new tests into the laboratory.

A preliminary report from Bagrel and Siest (1978) has indicated that the activity of alanine aminotransferase and the GGT/urea ratio may constitute an index of ethanol consumption. Other investigators have noted the association between ethanol intake and the incidence of abnormal results for certain components of biochemical profiles (Whitehead *et al.*, 1978; Whitfield *et al.*, 1978). The latter group have reported that in subjects admitting to more than six drinks per day the incidence of abnormalities was, in males and females respectively: GGT 45 and 28%; triglyceride 19 and 10%; urate 38 and 4%; aspartate aminotransferase 18 and 6%. No associations were found between ethanol intake and plasma bilirubin, alkaline phosphatase, or albumin. The reason for the sex-related differences in the incidence of abnormalities is not known.

Similarly, in a study of 2,034 male subjects, elevated levels of serum GGT, triglyceride, urate and aspartate aminotransferase were associated with ethanol intake (Whitehead *et al.*, 1978). Figure 6.11 illustrates the relationship between daily ethanol intake and these four parameters in a sub-group of 146 subjects. Elevations of serum GGT and aspartate aminotransferase produced by high

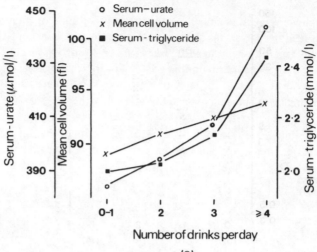

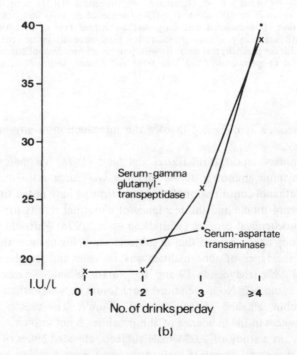

Fig. 6.11 – Serum urate and triglycerides (A) and serum gamma-glutamyl transferase, mean cell volume and aspartate aminotransferase (B) related to daily alcohol intake in a group of 146 subjects.

Reproduced by permission from Whitehead *et al.*, *Lancet* (1978) ethanol intake were much greater than those for either urate or triglycerides. In an otherwise healthy person the finding of both an elevated serum GGT and an elevated serum aspartate aminotransferase would be strongly indicative of a high ethanol intake. The concurrent finding of a high serum urate level would serve as confirmatory evidence that the enzyme elevations were indeed due to ethanol. Thus, out of the 2,034 subjects screened in this study there were 85 (4.2%) with elevations of both enzymes and 70.7% of this sub-group had concurrent elevation of serum urate. The combination of these three findings is indicative of a high ethanol intake but does not necessarily imply that the subjects are ethanol-dependent. Such results would however, alert the clinician to a possible excessive intake of ethanol.

A biochemical profile can provide additional information if the results are subjected to a form of pattern analysis such as discriminant function analysis and the results interpreted with the aid of a computer. This approach has already been used to advantage in diagnostic and prognostic procedures (Solberg, 1975; Wilding et al., 1977). The two-dimensional plot of the serum enzymes activities shown in Figure 6.12 is an example of a form of pattern analysis. The simple expedient of plotting the two serum enzyme values for each of the subjects and the use of the upper limits of the reference intervals for the enzymes has separated the subjects into four groups-one group with normal enzymes, two groups

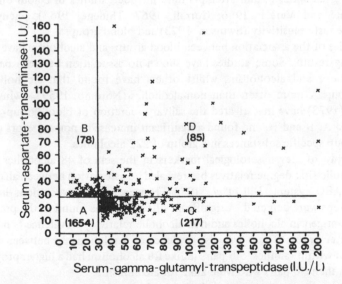

Fig. 6.12 – Serum gamma-glutamyl transferase and serum aspartate amino-transferase in whole group of 2034 subjects. A-both enzymes normal, B-serum aspartate transaminase raised, C-serum gamma glutamyl transpeptidase raised, D-both enzymes raised.

Reproduced by permission from Whitehead et al., Lancet (1978) with an elevation of only one enzyme, and a further diffuse group with elevations of both enzymes. Thus discrimination has been achieved between the patients, but there is a very poor separation between the four groups. Better discrimination could be achieved by employing more than two parameters to characterise the subjects, thus effecting a separation of various groups of subjects in a multi-dimensional space. This approach has been investigated, and preliminary results indicate that the combination of biochemical profiling and discriminant function analysis may have great potential as a screening test for alcohol abuse (Wilding, 1978).

6.7 SEROLOGICAL MARKERS

A prospective approach to the problem of detecting the alcohol abuser is to identify those people within the community with a possible genetic predisposition towards alcoholism. This approach contrasts with the various biochemical tests such as GGT which are retrospective in nature.

Many studies have indicated the familial nature of alcoholism. The incidence of alcoholism amongst relatives of alcoholics is higher than in the general population (Goodwin, 1971; Goodwin et al., 1973, 1974; Kaij and Dock, 1975; Tartar et al., 1977), and studies of adoptees (Goodwin et al., 1973, 1974) have also indicated a possible genetic predisposition towards ethanol abuse. The encouraging findings of these studies have stimulated the search for a 'genetic marker' for alcoholism, and attempts have included studies of colour blindness, (Curz-Coke and Varela, 1966; Gorrell, 1967; Thulene, 1967), phenyl thio-carbamide taste sensitivity (Swinson, 1973) and blood groups.

Studies of the association between blood groups and alcoholism have yielded conflicting results. Some studies have shown no association between particular blood groups and alcoholism, whilst others have found that alcoholics have blood group A more often than non-alcoholics (Nordmo, 1959). Swinson and Madden (1973) have investigated the salivary secretion of blood group–specific substances A, B and H, and found a significant increase in non-secretors of these blood group specific substances in a group of 222 alcoholics.

A study of eleven serological markers in the sera of 48 alcoholics and 46 non-alcoholic first degree relatives has revealed no association between alcoholism and the ABO system (Hill et al., 1975). However, two associations involving blood groups were detected. A significant difference was found in the prevalence of the S antigen in alcoholics and non-alcoholic relatives, prevalence being lower in the latter group. There was also evidence of a relationship between Rh and alcoholism within families. Sib pairs unlike for alcoholism had a higher proportion of like Rh then sib pairs who were alike for alcoholism.

These authors also studied five genetically determined serum proteins (alpha$_1$-antitrypsin, complement C3, Gm(a) gamma-globulin, haptoglobin, and group-specific component). Only in the case of complement C3 was an association discovered between a serum protein and alcoholism. All of the alcoholics and their non-alcoholic relatives had an SS phenotype when analysed for the serum protein complement C3 (normal prevalence rate of this phenotype 50%). This association is suprising and confirmation and further studies are warranted.

6.8 MEAN CORPUSCULAR VOLUME

A very high incidence of elevated mean corpuscular volume (MCV) has been noted in alcoholics (Ungar and Johnson, 1974; Wu *et al.*, 1974; How and Davidson, 1978). The mechanism responsible has not been established, although it seems probable that it is a direct effect of ethanol on the bone marrow (Lindenbaum and Lieber, 1969).

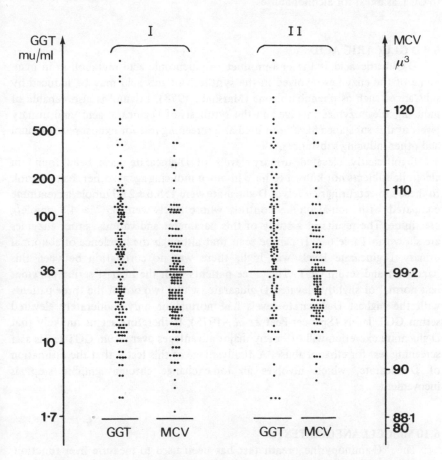

Fig. 6.13 — Comparison of gamma-glutamyl transferase (GGT) and mean corpuscular volume (MCV) for the detection of ethanol abuse in (I) alcoholics who had previously undergone detoxication (II) alcoholics not 'weaned' during a rest cure or in a hospital.

Reproduced by permission from Baglin *et al.*, *Clinica Chimica Acta* (1976)

The observed elevation of the MCV in drinkers has suggested that the MCV might be a useful screening procedure for ethanol abuse. More recently, however a comparison has been made of the relative efficiency of MCV and GGT in the detection of ethanol abuse (Figure 6.13). This comparison revealed that the incidence of elevated serum GGT values was greater than the incidence of elevated MCV: 67% versus 44% in alcoholics not previously 'weaned' during a rest cure or in hospital and 53% versus 44% in alcoholics who had previously undergone treatment for alcoholism (Baglin et al., 1976). Other studies have confirmed that there is an higher incidence of GGT elevation than of MCV in drinkers (Whitfield et al., 1978), and MCV would therefore appear to be inferior to GGT as a test for alcohol abuse.

6.9 D-GLUCARIC ACID

D-Glucaric acid is the end-product of glucuronic acid metabolism in man. Some of the enzymes involved in the synthesis of this acid may be induced by substances such as phenobarbitone (Marshall, 1978). Ethanol is also capable of inducing the enzymes involved in the synthesis of D-glucaric acid, and urinary levels of this substance have been used as a screening test for exposure to ethanol and other inducing substances.

Significantly elevated urinary levels of D-glucarate have been found in alcoholic subjects not known to have imbibed inducing agents other than ethanol. In these subjects urinary levels of D-glucarate were $158.6 \pm 21.7 \, \mu$mole/g creatinine compared with non-alcoholic controls whose levels were $65.7 \pm 4.6 \, \mu$mole/g creatinine. The results of a study of this parameter and various serum enzymes are shown in Table 6.2; It can be seen that although the incidence of abnormal urinary D-glucarate levels was high, there was no correlation between this parameter and serum GGT. The three patients with the highest serum enzymes had normal or slightly elevated D-glucarate, whilst two out of the three patients with the highest D-glucarate levels had normal or only moderately elevated serum GGT levels (Spencer-Peet et al., 1975). It therefore seems unlikely that D-glucarate excretion will offer any major advantages over serum GGT levels as a screening test for ethanol abuse. A disadvantage of this test is that the estimation of D-glucarate, which involves an ion-exchange chromatographic step, is incovenient.

6.10 MISCELLANEOUS TESTS

The ^{14}C-aminopyrine breath test has been used to measure liver function, and has also been proposed as a method of measuring enzyme induction. Lewis et al., (1977) studied a group of 20 alcoholics without cirrhosis and found the 2 hour excretion of $^{14}CO_2$ (derived from hepatic metabolism of the ^{14}C-methyl groups of aminopyrine to $^{14}CO_2$) was significantly elevated compared with

Table 6.2

Serum enzymes and urinary excretion of D-glucaric acid in 25 alcoholic patients.
Reproduced by permission from Spencer-Peet *et al.*, *British Journal of Addiction*
(1975)

Estimation	Range	%Abnormal	Mean	S.E.M.	Correlation with GGT
*Gamma-glutamyl transferase (GGT)	31–3,500	75	530	160	
**Aspartate amino-transferase	8–60	64	26.75	2.6	r = 0.45 p < 0.05
**Alanine amino-transferase	4–60	36	16.7	2.85	r = 0.51 p < 0.05
†Alkaline phosphatase	4–22	8	9.0	0.77	r = 0.19 not significant
††D-glucaric acid excretion	57–481	56	158.6	21.7	r = 0.12 not significant

*I.U./l at 37°C; **I.U./l at 25°C, †King-Amstrong Units/100 ml.; ††μmol per g. creatinine.
S.E.M. standard error of the mean.

healthy controls. All of the alcoholics had been drinking over 10 pints (6 litres)
of beer or its equivalent for at least two years. The $^{14}CO_2$ excretion correlated
with the serum GGT in those patients with normal serum alkaline phosphatase
levels, but elevated $^{14}CO_2$ excretions were also found in subjects taking other
enzyme-inducing drugs, e.g. barbiturates. The possible value of this test as a test
for alcohol abuse has not been fully assessed.

Ethanol also affects the urinary excretion of porphyrins, particularly
coproporphyrin (see Chapter 7, Section 10). The response seems to be dose-
dependent, but independent of the degree of liver dysfunction. It has been
proposed (Orten and Sardesai, 1971) that the measurement of coproporphyrin/
creatinine ratios could be used as a test for alcoholism.

An increase in urinary zinc excretion has been noted in alcoholics and in
healthy persons following ingestion of ethanol (see Chapter 7, Section 2).
Although serum and urinary zinc estimations have been suggested as a possible
test for alcohol abuse, the results have been unpromising (Helwig *et al.*, 1966;
Helwig, 1969).

6.11 SUMMARY

A variety of biochemical tests has been advocated for the detection and
monitoring of alcohol abuse but, apart from the measurement of serum GGT

activity, few of the tests have gained widespread application. Most tests have sought to detect alcohol abuse by monitoring changes in the redox state of the liver or enzyme induction caused by ethanol. A problem common to many of the tests is that liver disease, or ingestion of other drugs, may mimic the changes brought about by ethanol.

GGT activity is the most widely used and the most useful test for the detection of alcohol abuse. The level of this enzyme is increased in alcoholics, decreases on abstinence, and increases on resumption of drinking. Measurement of GGT is analytically convenient and reliable. However, GGT results should be interpreted with caution because some drinking alcoholics show no rise in GGT whilst chronic alcoholics, although having an elevated GGT initially, may on continued drinking regain a normal level. In other situations elevations of GGT may be due to induction by drugs, pancreatic disease, or non-alcoholic liver disease rather than to alcohol abuse.

No test for alcohol abuse which fulfills all the criteria outlined in the Introduction to this Chapter is yet available. It is to be hoped, however, that a better understanding of the biochemical changes associated with alcohol abuse, and the mechanisms of such changes will facilitate the development of simpler and more reliable tests for alcohol abuse. Plasma amino acids and the combination of biochemical profiling with pattern or discriminant function analysis would seem to be potentially the most promising tests for alcohol abuse.

6.12 REFERENCES

Akhter, M. I., Clark, P. M. S., Kricka, L. J., and Nicholson, G. (1978) Urinary metabolites of tryptophan, serotonin and norepinephrine. *J. Stud. Alcohol*, **39**, 833-841.

Baglin, M. C., Bernot, J. L., Bremond, J. L., Lamy, J., Leroux, M. E., and Wall, J. (1976) Efficacite comparee du volume globulaire moyen (VGM) et de la gamma-glutamyltransferase (γ-GT) serique comme tests de triage des buveurs excessifs d'alcool. *Clin. Chim. Acta*, **68**, 321-326.

Bagrel, A., and Siest, G. (1978) Detection of chronic alcoholics: Multiparametric analysis of biological data and of the psychosocial context. Abstracts, xth International Clinical Chemistry Congress, Mexico, p.88.

Cronholm, T. and Sjövall, J. (1973) Effects on steroid metabolites in plasma. *Acta Med. Scand. Suppl.*, **52**, 32-37.

Cruz-Coke, R., and Varela, A. (1966) Inheritance of alcoholism. *Lancet*, **ii**, 1282-1284.

Davis, V. E., Cashaw, J. L., Huff, J. A., and Brown, M. (1966) Identification of 5-hydroxytryptophol as a serotonin metabolite in man. *Proc. Soc. Exp. Biol. and Med.*, **122**, 890-893.

Davis, V. E., Brown, H., Huff, J. A., and Cashaw, J. L. (1967) The alteration of serotonin metabolism to 5-hydroxytryptophol by ethanol ingestion in man. *J. Lab. Clin. Med.*, **69**, 132-140.

Davis, V. E., Huff, J. A., and Brown, H. (1969) Alcohol and biogenic amines. *In* Biochemical and Clinical Aspects of Alcohol Metabolism (Sardesai, V. M. *ed.*) pp. 95-104, Charles C. Thomas, Springfield, Ilinois.

Drewes, P. A. (1974) Carbohydrate derivatives and metabolites. *In* Clinical Chemistry (Henry, R. J., Cannon, D. C., and Winkelman, J. W. *eds.*) 2nd *edn.*, pp. 1327-1369, Harper and Row.

Feldstein, A., Hoagland, H., Wong, K., and Freeman, J. (1964) Biogenic amines, biogenic aldehydes and alcohol. *Q. J. Stud. Alcohol*, **25**, 218-225.

Forsander, O. A. (1970) Influence of ethanol on the redox state of the liver. *Q. J. Stud. Alcohol*, **31**, 550-570.

Freer, D. E., and Statland, B. E. (1977a) The effects of ethanol (0.75g/kg body weight) on the activities of selected enzymes in sera of healthy young adults; 1. Intermediate-term effects. *Clin Chem.*, **23**, 830-834.

Freer, D. E., and Statland, B. E., (1977b) Effects of ethanol (0.75g/kg body weight) on the activities of selected enzymes in the sera of healthy young adults: 2. Inter-individual variations in response of γ-glutamyltransferase to repeated ethanol challenges. *Clin. Chem.*, **21**, 2099-2102.

Goodwin, D. W. (1971) Is alcoholism hereditary. *Arch. Gen. Psychiatry*, **25**, 545-549.

Goodwin, D. W., Schulsinger, F., Hermansen, L., Guze, S. B., and Winokur, G. (1973) Alcohol problems in adoptees raised apart from alcoholic biological parents. *Arch. Gen. Psychiatry*, **28**, 238-243.

Goodwin, D. W., Schulsinger, F., Moller, N., Hermansen, L., Winokur, G., and Guze, S. B. (1974) Drinking problems in adopted and non-adopted sons of alcoholics. *Arch. Gen. Psychiatry*, **31**, 164-169.

Helwig, H. L. (1969) Zinc levels in serum and urine of alcoholics. *In* Biochemical and Clinical Aspects of Alcohol Metabolism (Sardesai, V. M., *ed.*) pp. 40-44, Charles C. Thomas, Springfield, Illinois.

Helwig, H. L., Hoffer, E. M., Thielen, W. C., Alcocer, A. E., Hotelling, D. R., Rogers, W. H., and Lench, J. (1966) Urinary and serum zinc levels in chronic alcoholism. *Am. J. Clin. Pathol.*, **45**, 156-159.

Gorrell, G. J. (1967) Inheritance of alcoholism, *Lancet*, **i**, 274.

Hamlyn, A. N., Brown, A. J., Sherlock, S., and Baron, D. N. (1975) Casual blood-ethanol estimations in patients with chronic liver disease. *Lancet*, **i**, 345.

Henderson, A. R. (1971) A source of error in blood pyruvate determinations. *J. Clin. Pathol. (Lond.)*, **24**, 475.

Hill, S. Y., Goodwin, D. W., Cadoret, R., Osterland, K., and Doner, S. M. (1975) Association and linkage between alcoholism and eleven serological markers. *J. Stud. Alcohol.*, **36**, 981-922.

How, J., and Davidson, R. J. (1978) Alcoholism and blood picture *Lancet,* **i,** 564.

Kaij, L. and Dock, J. (1975) Grandsons of alcoholics. *Arch. Gen. Psychiatry,* **32,** 1379-1381.

Konttinen, A., Härtel, G., and Louhija, A. (1970) Multiple serum enzyme analysis in chronic alcoholics. *Acta Med. Scand.,* **188,** 257-264.

Krasner, N., Moore, M. R., Thompson, G. G., McIntosh, W., and Goldberg, A. (1974) Depression of erythrocytes 5-aminolaevulinic acid dehydratase activity in alcoholics. *Clin. Sci. Mol. Med.,* **46,** 415-418.

Lamy, J., Baglin, M-C., Ferrant, J-P., and Weill, J. (1975) Emploi de la mesure de la γ-glutamyltranspeptidase serique pour controler le succes des cures de desintoxication anti-alcoolique. *Clin. Chim. Acta.,* **60,** 103-107.

Lewis, K. O., Nicholson, G., Lance, P., and Paton, A. (1977) Aminopyrine breath test in alcoholic liver disease and in patients on enzyme inducing drugs. *J. Clin. Pathol. (Lond.),* **30,** 1040-1043.

Lindenbaum, J., and Lieber, C. S. (1969) Haematologic effects of alcohol in man in the absence of nutritional deficiency. *N. Eng. J. Med.,* **281,** 333-338.

Lindskov, J., and Bach-Mortensen, N. (1973) The diagnostic value of the inhibitory effect of ethanol on galactose elimination in liver disease. *Acta. Med. Scand.,* **194,** 491-496.

Lundquist, F., Tygstrup, N., Winkler, K., Mellemgaard, K., and Munck-Peterson, S. (1962) Ethanol metabolism and production of free acetate in the human liver. *J. Clin. Invest.,* **41,** 955-961.

Marshall, W. J. (1978) Enzyme induction by drugs. *Ann. Clin. Biochem.,* **15,** 55-64.

Maynard, L. S., and Schenker, V. J. (1962) Monoamine oxidase inhibition by ethanol *in vitro. Nature (Lond.),* **196,** 595-596.

Moore, M. R., Beattie, A. D., Thompson, G. G., and Goldberg, A. (1971) Depression of γ-amino laevulinic acid dehydrase activity by ethanol in man and rat. *Clin. Sci.,* **40,** 81-88.

Morgan, M. Y., Milsom, J. P., and Sherlock, S. (1977) Ratio of plasma alpha amino-n-butyric acid to leucine as an empirical marker of alcoholism: Diagnostic value. *Science (Wash. D. C.),* **197,** 1183-1185.

Nordmo, S. H. (1959) Blood groups in schizophrenia, alcoholism and mental deficiency. *Am. J. Psychiatry,* **116,** 460-461.

Ogata, M., Mendelson, J. H., Mello, N. K., and Majchrowicz, E. (1971) Adrenal function and Alcoholism. II Catecholamines. *Psychosom. Med.,* **33,** 159-179.

Olsen, R. E., Gursey, D., and Vester, J. W. (1960) Evidence for a defect in tryptophan metabolism in chronic alcoholism. *N. Eng. J. Med.,* **263,** 1169-1174.

Orten, J. M., and Sardesai, V. M. (1971) Protein, nucleotide and porphyrin metabolism. *In* The Biology of Alcoholism (Kissin, B., and Begleiter, H. eds.) Vol 1. pp. 229-261, Plenum Press, New York.

Ortmans, H., and Eisenberg, K. (1976) Bedeutung, biochemischer Messwerte bei Diagnostik und Verlaufskontrolle alkoholbedingter Leberekrankungen. *Med. Klin.*, **71**, 380–384.

Park, D. H., and Gubler, C. J. (1969) Studies on the physiological functions of thiamine. V Effects of thiamine deprivation and thiamine antagonists on blood pyruvate and lactate levels and activity of lactate dehydrogenase and its isoenzymes in blood and tissue. *Biochem. Biophys. Acta*, **177**, 537–543.

Patel, S., and O'Gorman, P. (1975) Serum enzyme levels in alcoholism and drug dependency. *J. Clin. Path. (Lond.)*, **28**, 414–417.

Payne, J. P. (1975) Measurement of alcohol in body tissues. *Proc. R. Soc. Med.*, **68**, 375–377.

Redetzki, H. M., Koerner, T. A., Hughes, J. R., and Smith, A. G. (1972) Osmometry in the evaluation of alcohol intoxication. *Clin. Toxicol.*, **5**, 343–363.

Rollason, J. G., Pincherle, G., and Robinson, D. (1972) Serum gamma glutamyl transpeptidase in relation to alcohol consumption. *Clin. Chim. Acta*, **39**, 75–80.

Rosalki, S. B. (1975) Gamma-glutamyl transpeptidase. *Adv. Clin. Chem.*, **17**, 53–107.

Rosalki, S. B. (1976) Plasma enzyme changes and their interpretation in patients receiving anticonvulsant and enzyme inducing drugs. *In* Anti convulsant Drugs and Enzyme Induction (Richens, A. and Woodford, F. P. *eds.*) p. 27, Elsevier, Amsterdam.

Rosalki, S. B., and Rau, D. (1972) Serum γ-glutamyl transpeptidase activity in alcoholism. *Clin. Chim. Acta*, **39**, 41–47.

Rosalki, S. B., and Zilva, J. F. (1977) Serum γ-glutamyltransferase and alcoholism. *Lancet*, **ii**, 1183–1184.

Rosenfeld, G. (1960) Inhibitory influence of ethanol on serotonin metabolism. *Proc. Soc. Exp. Biol. Med.*, **103**, 144–149.

Salaspuro, M. P. (1967) Application of the galactose tolerance test for the early diagnosis of fatty liver in human alcoholics. *Scand. J. Clin. Lab. Invest.*, **20**, 274–280.

Shaw, S., and Lieber, C. S. (1976) Characteristic plasma amino acid abnormalities in the alcoholic: Respective roles of alcoholism nutrition and liver injury. *Clin. Res.*, **24**, 291A.

Shaw, S., Stimmel, B., and Lieber, C. S. (1976) Plasma alpha amino-n-butyric acid to leucine ratio: An empirical biochemical marker of alcoholism. *Science (Wash. D. C.)*, **194**, 1057–1058.

Shaw, S., Stimmel, B., and Lieber, C. S. (1977) Plasma amino-n-butyric acid/ leucine; A biochemical marker of alcohol consumption. Applications for the detection and assessment of alcoholism. *In* Currents in Alcoholism: Biological, Biochemical and Clinical Studies (Seixas, F. A., *ed.*) Vol 1, pp. 17–31, Grune and Stratton Inc., New York.

Shreeve, W. W., Shoop, J. D., Ott, D. G., and McInter, B. B. (1976) Test for alcoholic cirrhosis by conversion of (^{14}C)-or (^{13}C) Galactose to expired carbon dioxide. *Gastroenterology*, 71, 98-101.

Skude, G., and Wadstein, J. (1977) Amylase, hepatic enzymes and bilirubin in serum of chronic alcoholics *Acta. Med. Scand.*, 201, 53-58.

Smith, A. A., and Gitlow, S. (1967) Effect of disulfiram and ethanol on the catabolism of norepinephrine in man. *In* Biochemical Factors in Alcoholism (Maickel, R. P. *ed.*) pp. 53-59, Pergamon Press, Oxford.

Solberg, H. E. (1975) Discriminant analysis in clinical chemistry. *Scand. J. Clin. Lab. Invest.*, 35, 705-712.

Spencer-Peet, J., Wood, D. C. F., Glatt, M. M., and Wiseman, S. M. (1975) Urinary D-glucaric acid excretion and serum gamma-glutamyl transpeptidase activity in alcoholism. *Br. J. Addict.*, 70, 359-364.

Sunshine, I., and Hodnett, N. (1971) Methods for the determination of ethanol and acetaldehyde. *In* Biology of Alcoholism (Kissin, B., and Begleiter, H. *eds.*) Vol 1, pp. 545-573, Plenum Press, New York.

Swinson, R. P. (1973) Phenylthiocarbamide taste sensitivity in alcoholism. *Brit. J. Addict.*, 68, 33-36.

Swinson, R. P., and Madden, J. S. (1973) ABO blood groups and ABA substance secretion in alcoholics. *Q. J. Stud. Alcohol*, 34, 64-70.

Tarter, R. E., McBride, H., Buonpane, N., and Schneider, D. U. (1977) Differentiation of alcoholics. *Arch. Gen. Psychiatry*, 34, 761-768.

Thulene, H. C. (1967) Inheritance of alcoholism. *Lancet*, i, 274-275.

Tygstrup, N. and Lundquist, F. (1962) The effect of ethanol in galactose elimination in man. *J. Lab. Clin. Med.*, 59, 102-109.

Tygstrup, N., Winkler, K., and Lundquist, F. (1965) The mechanism of the fructose effect on the ethanol metabolism of the human liver. *J. Clin. Invest.*, 44, 817-830.

Unger, K. W., and Johnson, Jr., D. (1974) Red blood cell mean corpuscular volume: a potential indicator of alcohol usage in a working population. *Am. J. Med. Sci.*, 267, 281-289.

Van Waes, L., and Lieber, C. S. (1977) Glutamate dehydrogenase: a reliable marker of liver cell necrosis in the alcoholic. *Br. Med. J.*, 2, 1508-1510.

Whitby, L. G., Percy-Robb, I. W., and Smith, A. F. (1975) *Lecture Notes on Clinical Chemistry*, p. 1. Blackwell Scientific Publications, Oxford.

Whitfield, J. B., Moss, D. W., Neale, G., Orme, M., and Breckenbridge, A. (1972) Changes in plasma γ-glutamyl transpeptidase activity associated with alterations in drug metabolism in man. *Br. Med. J.* 1, 316-318.

Whitfield, J. B., Hensley, W. J., Bryden, D., and Gallagher, H. (1978) Incidence of some biochemical abnormalities in heavy drinkers, and prediction of alcohol intake from the biochemical profile. Abstracts, xth International Clinical Chemistry Congress, Mexico, p. 49.

Whitehead, T. P., Clark, C., and Whitfield, A. G. W. (1978) Biochemical and haematological markers of alcohol intake. *Lancet*, **i**, 978-981.

Wietholtz, H., and Colombo, J. P. (1976) Das Verhalten der γ-Glutamyltranspeptidase und anderer Leberenzyme in Plasma während der Alkohol-Entziehungskur. *Schweiz. Med. Wochenschr.*, **106**, 981-987.

Wilding, P. (1978) Personal communication.

Wilding, P., Bradwell, A. R., Holder, R. L., Morriss, P., Sturdee, D., and Whitehead, T. P. (1977) Applications of discriminant analysis in clinical chemistry. *In* Advances in Automated Analysis. Technicon International Congress, 1976. pp. 51-54, Mediad Inc., Tarrytown, New York.

Wiseman, S. M., and Spencer-Peet, J. (1977) The effect of drinking patterns on enzyme screening tests for alcoholism. *Practitioner*, **219**, 243-245.

Wu, A., Chanarin, I., Levi, A. J. (1974) Macrocytosis of chronic alcoholism. *Lancet*, **i**, 829-831.

Wu, A., Slavin, G., and Levi, A. J. (1976) Elevated serum gamma-glutamyltransferase (transpeptidase) and histological liver damage in alcoholism. *Am. J. Gastroenterol.*, **65**, 318-323.

CHAPTER 7

Effects of Alcohol Intake on Individual Biochemical Parameters

7.1 INTRODUCTION

This chapter presents an account of the effect of ethanol and ethanol abuse on individual biochemical parameters. The coverage is rigorously restricted to the biochemical changes induced by alcohol in man and covers the literature from 1965 to the middle of 1978. For many of the biochemical parameters presented, alcohol produces a range of disturbances, i.e. elevated, lowered, no change. This is a manifestation of the complex interactions of factors such as duration of abuse, extent of abuse, type of alcoholic beverage, solvent effects of ethanol, and the presence of disease secondary to ethanol abuse. These factors have been covered in Chapter 5.

No attempt has been made to standardise the units used for the various biochemical parameters covered in this chapter. Both conventional and S.I. (Systeme International) units are used and conversion scales are provided in the Appendix.

7.2 WATER AND ELECTROLYTES

7.2.1 Water

Administration of ethanol results in a water diuresis during the first few hours after ingestion when ethanol levels are rising, which is then followed by a period of water retention. Diuresis is not sustained by elevated blood ethanol levels, presumably because increased blood osmolality following the initial diuresis promotes anti-diuretic hormone (ADH) release (Perman, 1961; Merzon and Khorunzhaya 1970; Beard and Knott, 1971; Ogata *et al.*, 1968, 1971a).

Few studies have been made of the effect of chronic ethanol ingestion on fluid balance. Kissin and co-workers (1965) and Beard and Knott (1971) have found an increase in total body water (TBW) in chronic alcoholics, in the absence of diarrhoea and vomiting.

In contrast, other studies (Shaw *et al.*, 1974; MacSweeney, 1975) have reported that the values for TBW, intra-cellular water (ICW) and extra-cellular water (ECW) in alcoholics were not significantly different from control values, whilst another study (Beard and Knott, 1968) on a group of alcoholics in acute withdrawal has shown that the alcoholics were in a state of iso-osmotic over-hydration (Table 7.1).

Other workers have found blood and plasma volumes to be increased in chronic alcholics in withdrawal. This was attributed to 'rebound' increases in ADH following long suppression of the hormone by continous drinking (Sereny et al., 1966).

The mechanism by which ethanol exerts its diuretic effect involves inhibition of the release of ADH by the supraoptical-hypophysial system (see Section 7.7.6). Enhanced water excretion is compensated by increased consumption and an associated shift of water from the intracellular to the extra-cellular compartment (Wartburg and Papenberg, 1970).

Studies of eccrine sweat gland function (Zazgornik et al., 1972) have revealed that weight loss due to sweating following thermal stress is significantly greater (p > 0.05) in alcoholics (weight loss 1.02 ± 0.54% body weight) than in controls (0.81 ± 0.15). This was attributed to a possible overhydration of the alcoholic patients due to habitual excessive fluid intake.

7.2.2 Sodium, Potassium and Chloride

Recent studies on levels of sodium, potassium, and chloride in serum, plasma, urine, sweat, saliva, vitreous humour, red blood cells, csf, brain and muscle of alcoholics and of healthy controls following exposure to ethanol, are collected in Tables 7.2, 3 and 4.

Hyper-, hypo- and normonatraemia have all been described in alcoholic patients. In alcoholics without liver disease, significant retention of sodium has been reported during withdrawal (Sereny et al., 1966). However, recent studies of exchangeable sodium have shown no differences between alcoholics and healthy controls (MacSweeney, 1975; Shaw et al., 1974).

Generally, serum potassium levels and urinary excretion of potassium are depressed in alcoholic patients. A study of 50 alcoholics in acute withdrawal has shown only 8/50 of the alcoholics had normal (4.0–4.5 mmol/l) serum potassium levels, the remainder of the alcoholics having potassium levels in the range 1.6–4.0 mmol/l (Vetter et al., 1967). Hypokalaemia has also been observed during experimentally induced intoxication in alcoholics (Ogata et al., 1968). No difference has been found, however, between values of total body potassium in alcoholics and controls (MacSweeney, 1975; Shaw et al., 1974).

Both normo- and hypochloraemia have been described in alcoholics (Table 7.2)

Alterations in electrolyte levels in alcoholics have been variously ascribed to altered renal excretion, decreased absorption in the small intestine (Krasner et al., 1976; Mekhjian and May, 1977), and diminished dietary intake (Shishov et al., 1972).

Table 7.1

Total, Extra-cellular and Intracellular Water in Alcoholics.

		PATIENTS	
		number	clinical details	Reference
TBW	males 42.86 (44.35)* females 33.18 (32.47) 1	21 males and 15 females	alcoholics, abstinent for 2 weeks prior to study	Shaw, *et al.*, 1974. MacSweeney, 1975.
ICW	males 24.22 (25.33) females 17.02 (18.57) 1			
ECW	males 18.40 (18.99) females 14.86 (15.05) 1			
TBW	565 ± 9.4 ml/kg	30	chronic alcoholics in acute withdrawal	Beard and Knott, 1968.
ICW	319 ± 8.9			
ECW	246 ± 3.8			
Interstitial water	205 ± 4.6			
Plasma water	41 ± 0.9			
Blood	75 ± 1.5			

*control values in parenthesis

Table 7.2
Sodium Levels in Alcoholic Patients

Mean levels ± SD or range	Reference interval (normal range) or control values	Number of subjects	Clinical details	Reference*
serum 141 ± 3.6 mmol/l urine 6.7 ± 5.4 mmol/h		30	acute alcoholic	1
serum 139 ± 2.4 mmol/l urine 141 ± 65 mmol/l sweat 118 ± 19 mmol/l	144 ± 4.0 210 ± 39 117 ± 17	25	chronic alcoholic	2
serum 142 ± 2.1 mmol/l csf 146.8 ± 2.3 mmol/l	145 ± 3.6 148 ± 1.9	9	alcoholic with delirium tremens	3
serum 140 ± 4.56 mmol/l		6	chronic alcoholic	4
serum 140 ± 4.6 mmol/l		44	alcoholic intoxicated	5
brain 67.4 mmol/kg wet weight 31.4 mmol/kg dry weight 85.4 mmol/kg water	63.6 291 81.5	25	alcoholic	6
exchangeable 18.40 mmol 14.86 mmol	18.99 15.05	21 (males) 15 (females)	alcoholic (2 week abstention)	7,8
plasma 142 ± 0.7 mmol/l rbc 14.3 ± 0.42 mmol/l urine 154 ± 18 mmol/24h		30	chronic alcoholic in acute withdrawal	9
serum 138.1 ± 4.95 mmol/l	135 – 152	29	chronic alcoholic with seizures	10
csf 142.2 ± 5.33 mmol/l serum 139.4 ± 4.43 mmol/l csf 144.6 ± 4.24 mmol/l	146.1 – 149.9	22	chronic alcoholic	

Table 7.2 (*continued*)

Sample	Reference interval (normal range) or control values	Mean levels ± SD or range	Number of subjects	Clinical details	Reference
muscle		120.4 ± 9.7 mmol/kg fat free dry weight	20	alcoholic	11
plasma	normal	172.3 ± 15.5	19	healthy controls given alcohol 1.5 g/kg bw	12
vitreous humour serum	131–151 mmol/l	100–152 mmol/l	20	alcoholic	13

*1. Sullivan et al., 1969. 2. Zagornik et al., 1972. 3. Schnaberth et al., 1972. 4. Levy et al., 1973. 5. Redetzki et al., 1972. 6. Shaw et al., 1970. 7. MacSweeney, 1975. 8. Shaw et al., 1974. 9. Beard and Knott, 1968. 10. Meyer and Urban, 1977. 11. Flink et al., 1969. 12. Ylikhari et al., 1974a. 13. Sturner and Coe, 1973.

Table 7.3
Potassium Levels in Alcoholic Patients

Sample	Reference interval (normal range) or control values	Mean levels ± SD or range	Number of subjects	Clinical details	Reference
serum	—	4.5 ± 1.1 mmol/l	30	acute alcoholic	1
urine	—	3.1 ± 2.6 mmol/h			
serum	4.5 ± 0.5	3.9 ± 0.2 mmol/l	25	chronic alcoholic	2
sweat	5.3 ± 0.7	5.2 ± 1.3 mmol/l			
urine	81 ± 1	46 ± 26 mmol/l			
serum	4.14 ± 0.2	3.62 ± 0.11 mmol/l	9	alcoholic with delirium tremens	3
csf	3.09 ± 0.05	3.36 ± 0.24 mmol/l			

Table 7.3 (*continued*)

		n		description	ref
serum	4.9 ± 0.45 mmol/l	6		chronic alcoholic	4
serum	4.0 ± 0.5 mmol/l	44		alcohol intoxicated	5
serum	3.36 ± 0.96 mmol/l	39	3.6 – 5.5	chronic alcoholic with seizures	6
csf serum csf	2.75 ± 0.19 mmol/l 4.16 ± 0.34 mmol/l 2.8 ± 0.33 mmol/l	28 22 22	3.0 – 3.2	chronic alcoholic	6
muscle	277.7 ± 18.9 mmol/kg ffdw	20	381.4 ± 6.5	alcoholic	7
plasma	3.9 ± 0.1 mmol/l	30		chronic alcoholic in acute withdrawal	8
rbc urine	91.0 ± 1.51 mmol/l 61 ± 11 mmol/24h				
vitreous humour	4.0 – > 10 mmol/l	20		alcoholic	9
brain	66.3 mmol/kg wet weight 309 mmol/kg dry weight 84.5 mmol/kg water	25	73.5 337 94.2	alcoholic	10
plasma	normal	19		healthy controls given alcohol 1.5 g/kg bw	11
total body	3247 mmol 2148 mmol	21 (males) 15 (females)	3394 2210	alcoholic (2 week abstention)	12,13

*1. Sullivan et al., 1969. 2. Zazgornik et al., 1972. 3. Schnaberth et al., 1972. 4. Levy et al., 1973. 5. Redetzki et al., 1972. 6. Meyer and Urban, 1977. 7. Flink et al., 1971. 8. Beard and Knott, 1968. 9. Sturner and Coe, 1973. 10. Shaw et al., 1970. 11. Yiikihari et al., 1974. 12. MacSweeney, 1975. 13. Shaw et al., 1974.

Table 7.4
Chloride Levels in Alcoholic Patients

Sample	Mean Levels ± SD or range	Reference interval (normal range) or control values	Number of of patients	Clinical details	Reference*
serum csf	109.4 ± 3.4 mmol/l 124.0 ± 4.4 mmol/l		9	alcoholic with delirium tremens	1
serum	94 ± 1.41 mmol/l		5	chronic alcoholic	2
serum	99 ± 5.0 mmol/l		44	alcohol intoxicated	3
vitreous humour serum	118–131 mmol/l 68–88 mmol/l	105–132	20	alcoholic	4
brain	56.9 mmol/kg wet weight 266 mmol/kg dry weight 72.6 mmol/kg water	62.2 285 79.6	25	alcoholic	5
exchangeable	2216 mmol 1822 mmol	2305 1819	20 (males) 15 (females)	alcoholic (2 week abstention)	6,7
serum	351–357 mg%	450–550	50	chronic alcoholic	8
plasma rbc urine	103 ± 13 mmol/l 59 ± 1 mmol/l 120 ± 13 mmol/24h		30	chronic alcoholic in acute withdrawal	9

Table 7.4 (*continued*)

	normal				
plasma	normal		19	healthy controls given alcohol 1.5 g/kg bw	10
serum	100 ± 3.8 mmol/l		30	acute alcoholic	11
serum	97.2 ± 2.94	97–107	29	chronic alcoholic with seizures	12
csf	115.3 ± 6.17	120–128			
serum	98.3 ± 5.02		22	chronic alcoholic	
csf	117.7 ± 3.48				

*1. Schnaberth et al., 1972. 2. Levy et al., 1973. 3. Redetzki et al., 1972. 4. Sturner and Coe, 1973. 5. Shaw et al., 1970. 6. MacSweeney, 1975. 7. Shaw et al., 1974. 8. Ibragimov, 1976. 9. Beard and Knott, 1968. 10. Yikihari et al., 1974. 11. Sullivan et al., 1969. 12. Meyer and Urban, 1977.

A diminished dietary intake has been implicated as the cause of hyponatraemia (108-127 mmol/l) seen in a group of subjects who consumed large amounts of beer and little or no ordinary food. Beer contains typically 1-2 mmol of sodium per litre. Daily consumption of beer in this group was 5 litres, hence sodium intake at 5-10 mmol was totally inadequate (Hilden and Svendsen, 1975).

7.2.3 Osmolality

Serum osmolality is increased in alcohol intoxication and the measurement of serum osmolality has been advocated as a simple method of estimating blood alcohol (Redetzki et al., 1972). A study of 565 cases of acute trauma (236 had measurable blood alcohol) has shown that there is a relationship between blood alcohol and serum osmolality. By regression analysis the correlation between serum osmolality and blood alcohol was found to fit the equation $y = 2.6x-750$ with a correlation coefficient of 0.88 (Champion et al., 1975). Hypo-osmolality, together with hypo-natraemia and hypokalaemia, has been reported in alcoholics with a considerable intake of beer taken with little or no food (Hilden and Svendsen, 1975).

Urine osmolality is depressed by ethanol. Compared to a control group (mean urine osmolality 601.1 ± 24 mOsm/kg), the loading of healthy subjects with various amounts of ethanol dramatically decreased the urine osmolality due to an inhibition of ADH. Alcohol loaded subjects exhibited the following mean values-216.3 ± 59.9 (blood alcohol 50-100 mg/100 ml), 161.4 ± 37.5 (200-250 mg/100 ml) and 143.0 ± mOsm/kg (300-400 mg/100 ml) (Cobo and Quintero, 1969).

7.2.4 Magnesium

A magnesium deficiency syndrome has been described repeatedly in alcoholic patients, especially during alcohol withdrawal, and in patients with delirium tremens or rum fits (Delaney et al., 1966; Sullivan et al., 1966, 1969; Jones et al., 1969; Wolfe and Victor, 1969; Hines and Cowan, 1970; Lim and Jacob, 1972; Medalle and Waterhouse, 1973; Meyer and Urban, 1977).

Biochemical findings in alcoholics include low serum, red blood cell, c.s.f. muscle, and ultra-filterable magnesium levels; also an increased urinary excretion of magnesium and low values for exchangeable magnesium. Balance studies have shown that alcoholics retain more magnesium than non-alcoholics following an infusion of magnesium sulphate or acetate (Flink et al., 1969).

Kinetics of exchange of radio magnesium have been found to be normal in a group of chronic alcoholics with liver dysfunction and with low serum magnesium during withdrawal (Dimich and Wallace, 1969).

Studies involving the administration of alcohol to both healthy volunteers and alcoholic patients have indicated that alcohol is the cause of the hypomagnesaemia and magnesium diuresis observed in alcoholics. Magnesium excretion is reported to be most marked when blood alcohol levels are rising. Excretion is normal, however, when blood ethanol levels are high (approx. 300 mg/100 ml) but stable (Mendelson et al., 1969).

Although administration of ethanol (0.75 g/kg) significantly reduces blood concentrations of magnesium in healthy volunteers (Plaza de los Reyes et al., 1968), other factors such as lactic acidosis, starvation ketoacidosis, protein caloric malnutrition, vomiting, and decreased dietary intake may also be of importance in the development of hypomagnesaemia in the alcoholic.

Increased urinary excretion of magnesium in alcoholic patients is commonly accompanied by increases in urinary excretion of lactate. It has been proposed that soluble chelates of magnesium and lactate prevent renal reabsorption of magnesium, thus facilitating the excretion of magnesium. However, infusion of lactate into either chronic alcoholic patients or normal subjects is not accompanied by an increase in magnesium excretion indicating that increased lactate and magnesium excretion are not directly related (Sullivan et al., 1966).

Although hypomagnesaemia is the most common finding, hypermagnesaemia in alcoholics has been reported (Delaney et al., 1966).

7.2.5 Calcium

Hypocalcaemia has been reported to occur in chronic alcoholic patients (Ibragimov, 1967; Medalle and Waterhouse, 1973) although acute ingestion in normal controls has no effect on either ionised or total calcium levels (Earll et al., 1976).

Estep et al., (1969) have reported that alcoholic patients with hypocalcaemia and hypomagnesaemia do not respond to parathyroid hormone (PTH). However correction of the hypomagnesaemia by intravenous infusion of magnesium sulphate restores the normal response to PTH and serum calcium levels rise. Similarly, serum calcium levels in an alcoholic patient with both hypocalcaemia and hypomagnesaemia were not corrected by administration of either ergo-cholecalciferol or dihydrotachysterol. Magnesium repletion, however, corrected both magnesium and calcium levels (Medalle et al., 1976).

The hypocalcaemia may arise in part as a result of diminished intestinal absorption of calcium. The absorption of ^{47}Ca has been shown to be reduced in chronic alcoholics with or without cirrhosis as compared to healthy controls (Vodoz et al., 1977). A positive correlation has also been found between serum 25-hydroxy Vitamin D and ^{47}Ca absorption and it has been proposed that deficiency of 25-hydroxy Vitamin D causes the reduced calcium absorption (Luisier et al., 1977).

7.2.6 Zinc

Zinc deficiency is of considerable importance in view of the zinc requirement of several essential enzyme systems. In particular the enzyme alcohol dehydrogenase is a zinc metallo-enzyme, and a deficit of zinc could possibly lead to an impairment of the activity of this enzyme and subsequent impairment of ethanol metabolism.

Low levels of serum zinc have been reported in several studies of alcoholic patients (Table 7.5), levels being particularly low in alcoholics with liver disease (Sullivan, 1968). Administration of alcohol to healthy volunteers has revealed no striking abnormalities in serum zinc in an 8 hour period following ingestion, although an increased urinary excretion of zinc was noted (Carey *et al.*, 1971). A similar increase in urinary zinc excretion (Sullivan and Lankford, 1965; Zazgornik, 1973) and in zinc clearance has been reported in alcoholics (Sullivan and Heaney, 1970).

Studies of the zinc content of heart tissue obtained at autopsy from patients dying of 'beer drinkers' myocardiopathy' have shown reduced levels (9.3 ± 3.5 μg/g) as compared to controls (12.9 ± 4.5 μg/g) (Sullivan *et al.*, 1968).

The concentration of zinc in sweat has not been extensively investigated. No significant difference was found between the concentration of zinc in the sweat of a group of alcoholics and of healthy controls following exposure in a hot chamber (Zazgornik, 1973).

Sullivan and Heaney (1970) have investigated the metabolism of ^{65}Zn in a small group of alcoholics with severe hepatic dysfunction. Results of this study indicated that there was a diminution of pool size and turnover of zinc in the alcoholic patients.

Attempts to utilise measurements of serum zinc and urinary excretion of zinc as screening tests for alcohol abuse have not been successful (Helwig, 1967; Helwig *et al.*, 1966).

7.2.7 Copper

Hypercupraemia, together with decreased urinary and faecal excretion of copper, and elevated caeruloplasmin levels, have been described in alcoholics and alcoholic patients with cirrhosis (Sviripa, 1972). A study of copper levels in liver tissue from chronic alcoholics has found no significant difference between the levels in the alcoholics (57.9 ± 112.8 ppm dry weight) and controls (109.4 ± 207.6) (Jaross *et al.*, 1972).

7.2.8 Phosphate

Phosphate has many functions, and there are many factors which influence its metabolism and blood levels. So, not surprisingly, changes in blood phosphate levels are generally non-specific. There have been few reports of phosphate metabolism in alcoholics. Most studies report hypophosphataemia in alcoholics (Medalle and Waterhouse, 1973; Territo and Tanaka, 1974; Knochel, 1977). In a study by Territo and Tanaka (1974) hypophosphataemia was found to be associated with low levels of red blood cell ATP and 2,3–DPG, and hemolytic anaemia. Non-diabetic ketoacidosis, pancreatitis, hematemesis, altered sensorium and pneumonia were concomitant findings in these patients. The authors suggest

Table 7.5
Serum Zinc Levels in Alcoholic Patients

Mean Levels ± SD (range) μg/100 ml	Reference interval (normal range) or control values μg/100 ml	Number of subjects	Clinical Details	Reference*
107 ± 14	136 ± 13	22	alcoholics	1
82 – 105	80 – 97	12	healthy controls given alcohol	2
98 ± 13		24	cirrhosis	3
101 ± 19		28	no abnormal liver function tests	3
36 – 92	—	10	severe hepatic dysfunction	4
91 ± 36.0 (40 – 218)	91 ± 16.7 (55 – 149)	36	no abnormal liver function tests	5
63 ± 14 (42 – 89)	26 ± 13	19	alcoholic cirrhosis	6

*1. Zazgornik, 1973. 2. Carey et al., 1971. 3. Zazgornik et al., 1970. 4. Sullivan and Heany, 1970. 5. Helwig et al., 1966. 6. Halsted et al., 1968.

that the cause of the hypophosphataemia is unclear but that the presence of an acidosis, and hence compensatory renal phosphate loss, and poor diet might account for it. The changes in red blood cell 2, 3-DPG and ATP may be accounted for by the hypophosphataemia and the acidosis.

Knochel (1977) reviews the causes of hypophosphataemia in alcoholics: they are alcohol *per se,* magnesium deficiency, alcoholic hypocalcaemia, and keto-acidosis. The mechanisms by which these operate are discussed. Ethanol may effect urinary excretion of phosphate, whilst changes in calcium and magnesium metabolism caused by alcohol may also tend to phosphaturia. Finally, ketoacidosis may lead to increased catabolism of organic phosphates and hence to increased loss in the urine.

Hyperphosphataemia in a chronic alcoholic has also been associated with magnesium deficiency and hypocalcaemia (Medalle and Waterhouse, 1973). They observed a patient with hypomagnesemia who presented with tetany, hypocalcaemia and hyperphosphataemia which were all corrected by magnesium repletion alone. These biochemical abnormalities could be mistaken for pseudo-hypoparathyroidism, hypoparathydroidism and renal failure. However the subsequent clinical course and renal function tests ruled this out. So magnesium depletion should be considered in all cases of coexisting hypocalcaemia and hyperphosphataemia, particularly where there are reasons to suspect magnesium deficiency, such as in cases of alcoholism. The mechanism of the hyperphos-phataemia in this patient was not understood.

7.2.9 Iron

Disturbances of iron metabolism in alcoholism (Wartburg and Papenberg, 1970; Hawkins and Kalant, 1972) have been variously ascribed to: a direct toxic effect of alcohol on haem synthesis (Hourihane and Weir, 1970), negative vitamin balance (Eichner and Hillman, 1971), liver damage, altered iron absorption (Davis and Badenoch, 1962; Charlton *et al.,* 1964; Sorensen, 1966), and intake of large amounts of iron contained in some alcoholic beverages (Wartburg and Papenberg, 1970; Flink, 1971). These changes in iron metabolism are found with the various types of anaemia associated with alcoholism. However there are other factors which will determine the haematological status of the alcoholic, such as associated liver disease, gastrointestinal bleeding, haemolysis, inadequate red cell production and the timing of the investigation (Kimber *et al.,* 1965). Alcohol associated disease may also influence iron metabolism. Rüdiger *et al.,* (1970) found that in Zieve's Syndrome with haemolysis the serum iron levels are grossly raised. Chronic liver disease and chronic pancreatitis may also con-tribute to iron overload (Davis and Badenoch, 1962; Callender and Malpas, 1963).

Generally, there seem to be three disorders of iron metabolism associated with alcoholism; firstly iron deficiency anaemia, and secondly megaloblastic anaemia with high levels of serum iron. The proportion of these two found in alcoholics varies from study to study. Thirdly haemochromatosis and siderosis can be associated with alcoholism.

Decreased levels of serum iron have been found in alcoholics, particularly those with GIT bleeding and liver disease (Kimber et al., 1965), occasionally in those with acute blood loss (Eichner and Hillman, 1971) and in those alcoholics in whom an obvious cause of blood loss is their frequent donations to blood banks (Eichner et al., 1972). A normal plasma iron clearance and increased amounts of iron in the liver, (Kimber et al., 1965) have been found to be associated with this decrease in serum iron levels.

Increased levels of serum iron have also been observed. Speck (1970) found that though the serum iron levels were increased in alcoholics, the diurnal variation in serum iron was intact. His patients also showed a diurnal variation in latent iron binding capacity (a measure of percentage unsaturation) so that a practically constant but subnormal total iron binding capacity resulted. Krasner et al., (1976) found serum iron levels greater than 150 μg % in five out of ten alcoholics they studied, whilst Eichner and Hillman (1971) in a study of a group of 65 alcoholics found a similar incidence of increased serum iron levels. The percentage saturation of transferrin was also increased. A gradual rise in serum iron levels has been found in healthy volunteers with experimental alcohol intoxication. These levels fell sharply on recovery (Lindenbaun and Lieber, 1969a).

Other studies discussed by Hawkins and Kalant (1972) suggest that such disturbances in iron metabolism are secondary to the effect of alcohol on pyridoxine metabolism.

In a study of alcoholics from both high and low socioeconomic groups, iron deficiency anaemia was the commonest cause of anaemia (Eichner et al., 1972). These workers also found some alcoholics suffering from megaloblastic anaemia with normal or high serum irons and plentiful iron stores. The high levels of serum iron may have been due to the recycling of short lived red blood cells found in megaloblastic anaemia. This anaemia may result from folate deficiency in the diet, which is found in alcoholics or from insensitivity to folate due to ethanol. When treated with folic acid, it was found that serum iron levels and iron stores fell, and some patients became iron deficient (Eichner et al., 1972). This fall in serum iron levels in both normals and alcoholics on treatment and/or withdrawal from alcohol has been observed by other authors (Waters et al., 1966; Lindenbaum and Lieber, 1969a, Eichner and Hillman, 1971). Böttiger (1973) suggests that this fall corresponds to a change from ineffective to effective erythropoiesis. Hourihane and Weir (1970) found high levels of serum iron which fell dramatically on treatment. These patients were, however, well nourished and not suffering from folate deficiency. It was therefore suggested that ethanol interferes with normal haem synthesis. The sudden fall in serum iron is thought to indicate the onset of effective erythropoiesis. Finally, it is postulated (Hourihane and Weir, 1970) that the low levels of serum iron found in alcoholics on occasion may result purely from measuring the iron after withdrawal when this dramatic fall has taken place.

In contrast to the view that there are many types of anaemia found in alcoholics, Eichner and Hillman (1971) postulate the following evolution of an alcoholic anaemia:

Stage 1: Negative vitamin balance

Stage 2: Megaloblastic conversion, severe vitamin deficiency

Stage 3: Sideroblastic conversion, pyridoxine deficiency. This stage is also affected by iron availability

Stage 4: Early resolution, when alcohol is stopped or diet improved. Serum iron also falls

Stage 5: Late resolution

These authors therefore suggest that haematological findings should be related to the clinical course of the alcoholic rather than to the aetiology of the disease.

Haemochromatosis has also been associated with alcoholism. It has been suggested that this results from the ingestion of large amounts of iron found in some alcoholic beverages (Wartburg and Papenberg, 1970; Flink, 1971). These authors postulate that because iron uptake and storage are strongly regulated in the normal organism ethanol must play an additional toxic role. There are two possibilities:

(1) There is evidence that ethanol enhances iron absorption of ferric iron in normal subjects whilst there was no effect on the absorption of ferrous or haemoglobin iron. This effect was not seen in four achlorhydric subjects, so that it was postulated that ethanol enhanced ferric iron absorption *via* stimulation of gastric hydrochloric acid production rather than by a direct effect on intestinal transport (See also Jacobs *et al.*, 1971). Similarly, iron deficient subjects given doses of iron and alcohol, showed increases in serum iron levels (Sörensen, 1966) greater than when given iron alone. These results have not always been supported by other workers (Wartburg and Papenberg, 1970). Celeda *et al.*, (1977) using whole body counter techniques found that alcohol ingestion gave rise to a diminution in absorption of organic but not inorganic iron.

Finally Callender and Malpas (1963) found increased iron absorption (in the form of ferrous sulphate and haemoglobin) in alcoholic cirrhotics. Therefore these results suggest that alcohol influences iron absorption, though whether this leads to haemochromatosis is not clear.

(2) Liver damage enhances pathological iron deposition, so that alcoholic liver damage may then predispose to haemochromatosis (Wartburg and Papenberg, 1970).

7.2.10 Acid-Base

Thomas in 1898 noted a mild acidosis following ethanol ingestion and this was later followed by the observation that this acidosis was related to increased lactic acid levels (see Oliva, 1970). Latterly, there have been three main areas of interest in the acid-base status of alcohol abuse, namely the effect of ethanol on the acid-base state of healthy volunteers, the acid-base status of alcoholics, and the role of acid-base disturbances in hangover.

The effect of ethanol on healthy subjects was studied by Räiha and Mänpää (1964) who showed that ethanol gave rise to a decrease in blood pH (7.41 → 7.38 Δ pH 0.03), base excess (4.2 → 0.04 mmol/l, Δ base excess 4.16) and standard bicarbonate (26 → 23.2 mmol/l, Δ standard bicarbonate 2.8) over a period of four hours. Their subjects were healthy volunteers who were allowed to eat during the period of the study. They concluded that the acidosis produced by ethanol in these non-fasted individuals, was unlikely to be due to ketone bodies. Their study did not show whether the acidosis was of renal origin and they suggested that it might be accounted for by increased production of lactate and/or acetate. Similarly moderate ethanol intake in human subjects led to an increase in the degree of post excercise lacticacidaemia (Krebs et al., 1969a). The lactic acidosis associated with the oral intake of alcohol is usually mild. However, intravenous alcohol may be given in the treatment of premature labour. Ott et al., (1976) reported a case of severe lactic acidosis under such conditions. The following results were obtained:

arterial pO_2 59 mm Hg, pCO_2 31 mm Hg, pH 7.05, HCO_3 8.5 mEq/l, 75% O_2 saturation, serum lactate 6.3 mEq/l (normal < 2 mEq/liter). Serum beta-hydroxybutyrate was 0.1 mEq/l (minimally elevated).

Five other patients treated with alcohol for premature labour were also found to have mild elevations of serum lactate levels.

The acidosis found in alcoholic subjects, after the consumption of ethanol, has often been thought to be due to the increased production of lactate. In a study of nine patients who were admitted for alcoholic delirium, their acid-base status was assessed by measuring both blood and csf levels of lactate, pyruvate, electrolytes, pH and pCO_2, during the course of their illness (Schnaberth et al., 1972). An increase in the levels of lactate and pyruvate were found, reflecting the underlying tissue hypoxia. It was postulated that the csf acidosis caused an increase in respiration, thus giving rise to a respiratory alkalosis. The clinical severity of the condition was found to parallel the behaviour of the metabolic changes in the csf. Similarly in a study of the use of osmometry in the evaluation of alcohol intoxication (Redetzki et al., 1972) a raised blood lactate was found in those patients admitted who showed signs of alcohol intoxication. However it has been shown that acetate may also contribute to the acidosis found in alcoholics after the ingestion of alcohol (Lundquist et al., 1962; Redetzki et al., 1972).

The role of ketone bodies in the metabolic acidosis of alcoholism is incompletely understood. In a study of nine non-diabetic individuals who admitted to excessive alcohol intake, it was concluded that the metabolic acidosis in these patients was caused by elevated plasma levels of ketone bodies. Ketoacidosis has also been found in non-diabetic alcoholic patients (Dillon et al., 1940).

More recently Levy et al., (1973) described six episodes of ketoacidosis in non-diabetic alcoholic subjects. All had suffered from protracted vomiting and fasting, all had a marked acidosis with a mean arterial pH of 7.16. The arterial pCO_2 levels were low indicating compensatory mechanisms. Increased levels of beta-hydroxybutyrate, acetoacetate and lactate were found, whilst insulin levels were decreased and free fatty acids and cortisol increased.

These results of metabolic acidosis in alcoholics however have not been confirmed by studies on alcoholics during ethanol withdrawal (Wolfe and Victor, 1969; Beard and Knott, 1971). In these cases a combined metabolic/respiratory alkalosis was found.

Studies on the acid-base status of hangover have shown a correlation between metabolic acidosis and the severity of hangover (Ylikahri et al., 1974a,b). It was shown that the concentrations of lactic acid, ketone bodies and free fatty acids were highest in those with the most severe hangovers. The correlation between the degree of acidosis and the intensity of hangover was significant. Several mechanisms for this acidosis have been proposed (Ylikahri et al., 1974a,b): (1) that ethanol causes depression of the respiratory centre giving rise to increased blood pCO_2, and hence a respiratory acidosis; (2) that ethanol causes a rise in lactate, acetate, free fatty acids, and ketone levels in blood and hence a metabolic acidosis; (3) that the endocrine effects of ethanol may cause an acidosis. The metabolic acidosis caused by any of these three factors may be followed by a compensatory respiratory alkalosis. It was also noted that during hangover the acidosis is mainly metabolic, and that during alcoholic withdrawal there is a combined metabolic/respiratory alkalosis.

Few studies of oxygen status of alcoholics have been made and no significant differences in arterial pO_2 between alcoholics and normals have been found (Schnaberth et al., 1972).

7.3 ENZYMES

Acute and chronic ethanol abuse result in changes in the activities of a great number of enzymes in both tissues and in serum. Specific changes in activity occur in the enzymes concerned with ethanol metabolism e.g. MEOS (see Chapter 3) and ethanol may also induce other enzymes, e.g. GGT. The changes in activities of other enzymes are less specific and result from the toxic effects of ethanol upon various organs and tissue.

Multiple serum enzyme analyses have been performed in both alcoholics and social drinkers in order to assess the effect of ethanol on the more commonly determined serum enzymes and the relative value of individual enzyme determinations in ethanol abuse. Results of some of these studies are collected in Table 7.6.

Table 7.6

Serum and Plasma Enzymes in Healthy Volunteers, Alcoholics and Alcoholics with Liver Disease

Levels	Clinical Details	References*
Alanine aminotransferase		
N	healthy volunteer given ethanol	1–3
N, E	alcoholic	4,5–15
E	alcoholic liver disease	16
Alkaline phosphatase		
N	healthy volunteer	2
N, E	alcoholic	4–7,9,11,14,17–21
E	alcoholic liver disease	4,16
Alpha-amylase		
N	healthy volunteer	22
E	alcoholic	14,15,18,23
Aminoacid arylamidase		
E	alcoholic	24
Arginase		
E	alcoholic	25
Acid phosphatase		
N	alcoholic	24

Table 7.6 *(continued)*

Levels	Clinical Details	References*
Aryl sulphatase A		
E	alcoholic	26
Aryl sulphatase B		
E	alcoholic	26
Aspartate aminotransferase		
N	healthy volunteer	1,3
E	alcoholic	4,5,6,9,11–15,17,18,20,21,23,27
E	alcoholic with liver disease	16
Beta-Glucuronidase		
E	alcoholic	28
Cholinesterase		
E	alcoholic	29
Creatine phosphokinase		
N, E	healthy volunteer	1,19,30
E	alcoholic	6,14,31–34
E	alcoholic with muscle syndrome	35,36

Table 7.6 (*continued*)

Levels	Clinical Details	References*
Delta-aminolaevulinic acid dehydratase		
D	alcoholic	37
Dipeptidyl arylamidase I		
N	alcoholic	24
Dipeptidyl arylamidase II		
E	alcoholic	24
Fructose-6-phosphate kinase		
N	alcoholic with Zieves syndrome	38
Gamma-glutamyl transferase		
N, E	social drinker	39
N, E	alcoholic	4,5,9,11,15,19,21,37,40–44
E	alcoholic with liver disease	16
Glucose-6-phosphate dehydrogenase		
N	alcoholic with Zieves syndrome	38
Glucose-6-phospho-gluconate dehydrogenase		
E	alcoholic with Zieves syndrome	38

Table 7.6 *(continued)*

Levels	Clinical Details	References*
Glutamate dehydrogenase		
N, E	alcoholic	4,14
E	alcoholic with liver disease	4
Glutathione reductase		
E	alcoholic	45
N	alcoholic with Zieves syndrome	38
Guanase (guanine deaminase)		
N, E	alcoholic	11,14
Hexokinase		
*N	alcoholic with Zieves syndrome	38
Hydroxybutyrate dehydrogenase		
N, E	alcoholic	6
Isocitric dehydrogenase		
E	healthy volunteer	3
N, E	alcoholic	41,46
Lactate dehydrogenase		
N, E	alcoholic	6,8,14,25,31,32
N, E	alcoholic with myopathy	32

Table 7.6 (*continued*)

Levels	Clinical Details	References*
Leucine aminopeptidase		
N	alcoholic, alcoholic with withdrawal	4,37
N, E	alcoholic	14,19,28
N, E	alcoholic with liver disease	4
Lysozyme		
N, E	alcoholic	48,49
5-Nucleotidase		
N, E	alcoholic	5
Ornithine carbamoyl transferase		
N, E	healthy volunteer	50
N, E	alcoholic	11,14,41
Pepsinogen (Group I)		
N, D	alcoholic	51
3-Phospho-glyceromutase		
N	alcoholic with Zieves syndrome	38
Pyridoxal phosphokinase		
*N, D	alcoholic	52

Table 7.6 *(continued)*

Levels	Clinical Details	References*
Pyridoxine phosphate oxidase		
*N	alcoholic	52
Transketolase		
+*D	alcoholic	53,54
D	alcoholic with liver damage	14
Triose-phosphate isomerase		
N, E	alcoholic with Zieves syndrome	38
Trypsin		
+N	alcoholic	55

KEY: N, normal levels; E, elevated levels; D, depressed levels; *red blood cell; +duodenal aspirate.

1. Hed *et al.*, 1972
2. Freer and Statland, 1977a
3. Goldberg and Watts, 1965
4. Adjarov and Iwanow, 1973
5. Boone *et al.*, 1974
6. Smith and Layden, 1972
7. Jaross *et al.*, 1972
8. Smith *et al.*, 1971

9. Rosalki and Rau, 1972
10. Williams and Girdwood, 1970
11. Konntinen et al., 1968
12. Devenyi et al., 1970
13. Wietholtz and Colombo, 1976
14. Konttinen et al., 1970
15. Skude and Wadstein, 1977
16. Ortmans and Eisenberg, 1976
17. Dinoso et al., 1971
18. Mezey et al., 1970
19. Pojer et al., 1972
20. Mezey and Tobon, 1971
21. Wiseman and Spencer-Peet, 1977
22. Fisher et al., 1965
23. Augustine, 1967
24. Vanha-perttula and Kalliomaki, 1973
25. Rothfeld et al., 1970
26. Rinderknecht et al., 1970a
27. Irsigler et al., 1971
28. Goldbarg et al., 1966
29. Ozkan et al., 1968
30. Paterson and Lawrence, 1972
31. Nygren, 1971
32. Lafair and Myerson, 1968
33. Nygren, 1966
34. Rinderknecht et al., 1970b
35. Nygren, 1967
36. Perkoff et al., 1966
37. Krasner et al., 1974
38. Rudiger et al., 1970
39. Rollason et al., 1972
40. Lamy et al., 1975
41. Patel and O'Gorman, 1975
42. Zein and Discombe, 1970
43. Baglin et al., 1976
44. Wu et al., 1976
45. Rosenthal et al., 1973
46. Beard and Knott, 1968
47. Nygren and Sundblad, 1971
48. Pezzimenti and Lindenbaum, 1972
49. Liu, 1973
50. Vestal et al., 1977
51. Samloff et al., 1975
52. Lumeng and Li, 1974
53. Markkanen and Peltola, 1971a
54. Markkanen and Peltola, 1971b
55. Carlsson and Dehlin, 1972

The 'intermediate-term' effects of ethanol (0.75 g/kg body weight) on six serum enzymes have been described by Freer and Statland (1977a) in nine apparently healthy young adults. During the period 10–100 hours after the completion of ethanol consumption the serum activities of aspartate and alanine aminotransferase, gamma-glutamyl transferase, lactate dehydrogenase, creatine phosphokinase and alkaline phosphatase were monitored and the mean percentage changes are illustrated in Figure 7.1. The most notable changes are the 25% increase in gamma-glutamyl transferase, 12% increase in alanine aminotrans-ferase, and the 12% decrease in the mean aspartate aminotransferase activity at 60h. These three enzymes showed similar time courses, the mean maximum change being either an increase or a decrease in activity occurring at 60h and then returning to near baseline values by 100h after ethanol.

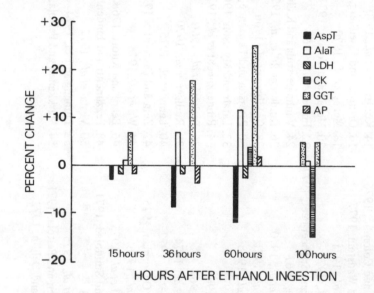

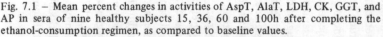

Fig. 7.1 – Mean percent changes in activities of AspT, AlaT, LDH, CK, GGT, and AP in sera of nine healthy subjects 15, 36, 60 and 100h after completing the ethanol-consumption regimen, as compared to baseline values.
Reproduced by permission from Freer and Statland, *Clinical Chemistry* (1977a)

A number of comparisons have been published of the activities of several serum enzymes in heavy drinkers, alcoholics and chronic alcoholics and the results of these studies are summarised in Table 7.7. Such multiple enzyme studies have sought to establish the value of individual enzymes as indicators of liver cell damage or early alcoholic liver disease. Generally, GGT has provided a sensitive and specific screening test for liver involvement which proved superior to such other tests of liver function as the aminotransferases and alkaline phosphatase.

Table 7.7
Multiple Enzyme Studies in Alcoholics

Enzyme (Serum)	% of Alcoholics Showing Abnormal Responses			
	Study A	Study B	Study C	Study D
Gamma glutamyltransferase	48	54	75	69
Alanine aminotransferase	30	43	19	53
Aspartate aminotransferase	24	64	31	73
Alkaline phosphatase	10	23	5	–
Creatine phosphokinase	–	43	–	–
Ornithine carbamoyl transferase	24	56	–	–
Isocitrate dehydrogenase	39	–	–	–
Guanase	–	20	–	–
Glutamate dehydrogenase	–	47	–	–
Amylase	–	8	–	6
Leucine aminopeptidase	–	22	–	–
Lactate dehydrogenase	–	49	–	–

(Study A: Patel and O'Gorman (1975); B: Konttinen et al., (1970a); C: Rosalki and Rau (1972); D: Skude and Wadstein (1977)

7.3.1 Aspartate (AspT) and Alanine Aminotransferase (AlaT)

The enzyme aspartate aminotransferase is present in most tissue but especially in muscle, cardiac muscle, erythrocytes and the lung. Alanine aminotransferase is present in the liver in high concentration and to a lesser extent in skeletal muscle, kidney and heart.

The serum activities of these enzymes are frequently raised in alcoholics with liver involvement. However, they may also be raised in alcoholics with muscular complaints (Hed et al., 1962). The incidence of elevated values of serum AlaT and AspT in heavy drinkers and alcoholics is shown in Figure 7.2.

In healthy individuals ethanol has opposite effects on AspT and AlaT. The pattern of serum enzyme activities during the period 15–100h after three consecutive evenings of ethanol consumption (0.75 g/kg) is depicted in Figure 7.2. At 60h, post-ethanol the percentage change in the mean activity of AspT was decreased by 12%, whilst for AlaT it was increased by 12%. This striking difference in the effect of ethanol on the activity of these two enzymes is due to the differing organ specificities and cellular location of the enzymes, to their differing biological half-lives, and to altered synthesis and cellular release.

7.3.2 Gamma-glutamyl transferase (GGT) (E.C. 2:3:2:2)

Estimation of serum GGT activity has been extensively employed as a biochemical test for alcohol abuse and this topic is covered in more detail in a review by Rosalki (1975) and in Chapter 6.

Elevations in serum GGT activity occur as a result of hepatic induction of the enzyme, although hepatocellular damage or cholestasis often contribute to

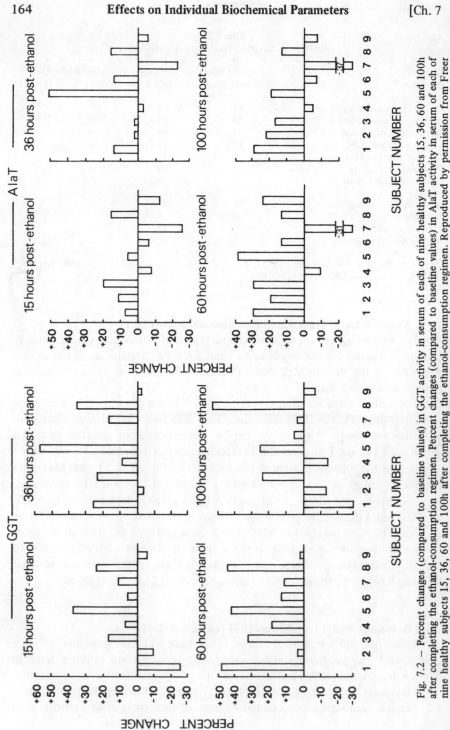

Fig. 7.2 — Percent changes (compared to baseline values) in GGT activity in serum of each of nine healthy subjects 15, 36, 60 and 100h after completing the ethanol-consumption regimen. Percent changes (compared to baseline values) in AlaT activity in serum of each of nine healthy subjects 15, 36, 60 and 100h after completing the ethanol-consumption regimen. Reproduced by permission from Freer and Statland, *Clinical Chemistry* (1977a)

the increased serum activity. The effect of a single or multiple challenges by
ethanol in healthy volunteers has been investigated by Freer and Statland
(1977a,b). Figure 7.1 illustrates the result of a single challenge of ethanol
(0.75 g/kg body weight), and it can be seen that ethanol causes a rise in GGT
activity which is maximal 60 hours after withdrawal of ethanol. Multiple challenges with ethanol have revealed a marked intra- and inter-individual variation
in GGT response. The mean percentage changes in activity of this enzyme
during a 27 day period, which included 4 periods of ethanol ingestion, are
illustrated in Figure 7.3. Inter-individual variation in the GGT response is shown
in Table 7.8. Variations in enzyme response ranged from +1 to +57% of the
base line values, and it has been suggested that these differences reflect individual differences in 'threshold tolerance' to ethanol and stress. The initial

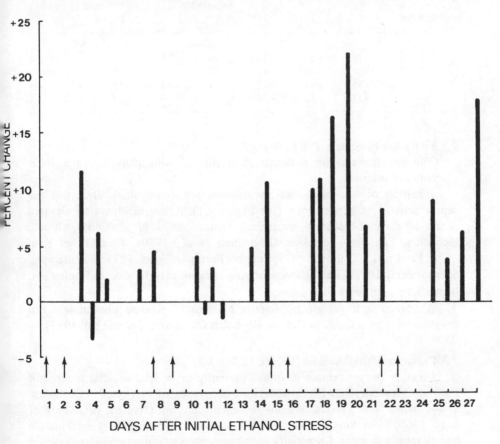

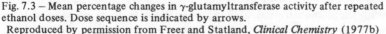

Fig. 7.3 – Mean percentage changes in γ-glutamyltransferase activity after repeated
ethanol doses. Dose sequence is indicated by arrows.
Reproduced by permission from Freer and Statland, *Clinical Chemistry* (1977b)

acute alteration of serum GGT (ranging from a 3% decrease to a 34% increase of baseline value) as a response to the initial challenge by ethanol may be dose-related with each individual having a specific threshold. Chronic elevation of GGT in response to subsequent and repeated challenges is then superimposed on the acute response. Minimal changes in serum GGT activity which may sometimes be encountered, following ethanol ingestion, may thus indicate that the 'threshold tolerances' of such persons are set unusually high.

Table 7.8

Peak Percentage Changes in GGT Activity as Compared with Baseline for Each Subject During Each Week of the Study.
Reproduced by permission from Freer and Statland *Clinical Chemistry* **(1977b).**

Week No.	Subject No.							
	1	2	3	4	5	6	7	8
				% change				
1	+26	+34	+13	+14	+6	+9	0	−3
2	+34	+24	+7	+15	+8	+3	−1	−13
3	+45	+45	+57	+24	+14	+12	+25	−4
4	+31	+13	+36	+19	+33	+4	+22	+1

7.3.3 Alkaline Phosphatase (E.C. 3:1:3:1)

The enzyme alkaline phosphatase is located principally in bone, liver, placenta and intestine.

Ingestion of ethanol by healthy volunteers does not markedly affect the serum activity of this enzyme (see Figure 7.1). A low incidence of elevated serum alkaline phosphatase levels has been reported in alcoholics, chronic alcoholics, and heavy drinkers (Konttinen *et al.,* 1970a; Rosalki and Rau, 1972; Patel and O'Gorman, 1975; Spencer-Peet and Wood, 1975; Wiseman and Spencer-Peet, 1977). Raised levels of this enzyme may be due to cholestasis, hepatitis or cirrhosis in such subjects.

Abnormal agar gel electrophoresis patterns of alkaline phosphatase iso-enzymes have been found in chronic alcoholics (Brohult and Sundbled, 1973).

7.3.4 Creatine Phosphokinase (CK) (E.C. 2:7:3:2)

Creatine phosphokinase is found primarily in skeletal muscle, heart, and the brain. Elevated serum CK activities have been repeatedly reported in alcoholics, in association with a reversible acute muscular syndrome (Nygren, 1966; Perkoff *et al.,* 1966; Rinderknecht *et al.,* 1970). Ultrastructural changes in skeletal muscle and elevations in serum CK activity have been observed during a four week period following the administration of 225g of ethanol to three non-alcoholic males. In one of the subjects CK values rose from a baseline value of 1.5 units during the control period to 11.8 units four weeks after administration of the dose of ethanol (Song and Rubin, 1972).

Several patterns of change of CK activities have been reported. In heavy drinkers CK levels were normal 24–48h after withdrawal of ethanol. This was then followed by a 4–5 day period during which CK levels rose to a maximum value and then returned to normal during a further week (Lafair and Myerson, 1968). In another group of acutely intoxicated alcoholics, the initially elevated serum CK levels returned to normal during a two week withdrawal period (Nygren, 1967).

In healthy individuals small doses of ethanol may cause a fall in serum CK activity (Paterson and Lawrence, 1972; Freer and Statland, 1977a), or may be without effect (Hed *et al.*, 1972). The course of mean serum CK levels in nine subjects during a 100h period following a dose of ethanol (0.75 g/kg) is illustrated in Figure 7.1. Initially there is a slight rise in the serum levels. This however is followed by a pronounced fall to a level 20% below the mean baseline value.

7.3.5 Lactate Dehydrogenase (LDH) (E.C. 1:1:1:27)

High concentrations of lactate dehydrogenase are found in heart, skeletal muscle, liver, kidney, brain, and erythrocytes. In alcoholics, elevated LDH levels arise from combination of liver and muscle damage. Isoenzyme studies have revealed that the LDH-1 and LDH-2 isoenzymes from muscle and LDH-5 isoenzyme from liver are frequently elevated both in intoxicated alcoholics and in healthy subjects who are given ethanol (Nygren and Sundblad, 1971; Nygren, 1971; Hed *et al.*, 1972).

The effect of ethanol on serum LDH in healthy controls is shown in Figure 7.1, and it can be seen that acute doses of ethanol have minimal effect on serum LDH levels.

7.4 PROTEINS

The study of serum proteins in alcoholic patients has not been extensive (Table 7.9). Many different proteins have been measured in the sera of alcoholics, but the number of alcoholic patients tested and the number of studies have been few, and the majority of studies have centred on alcoholics with liver disease. The liver is responsible for the synthesis of the majority of the serum proteins (except γ-globulins). Thus hepatic damage will be reflected by an inability to synthesize these proteins. Usually these changes are non-specific. The majority of studies reflect this, though a recent report of Wallerstedt *et al.*, (1977a) studied the coagulation factors and plasma proteins in abstinent chronic alcoholics. Their results were consistent with a post-inflammatory reaction, but not with liver dysfunction.

Other factors which cause changes in serum proteins in alcoholics include malabsorption, malnutrition and infection, though little is known about their significance.

Table 7.9
Levels of various serum proteins found in alcoholics.

Protein	Range (Mean ± SD)	Reference Interval (Normal value) or Control Value	No. of subjects	Clinical Details	Reference
Albumin	29.0 ± 4.2 g/l	–	12	alcoholic cirrhosis	1
	43 ± 7 g/l	35–55 g/l	11	chronic alcoholics without liver disease	2
	51.8 ± 6.3 g/l	–	42	–	3
	35–59 g/l	35–55 g/l	11	–	2
	27.23 ± 0.50 g/l***	43.47 ± 0.57 g/l***	91	alcoholic cirrhosis	4
	36.8 ± 4.5 g/l	35–56 g/l	48	–	5
	55.77 ± 5.31 rel %	58.59 ± 6.22*	–	chronic alcoholics	7
	27.83 ± 4.61 g/l	47.01 ± 3.54 g/l	35	alcoholic cirrhosis	6
Thyroxine Binding Pre-albumin	0.074 ± 0.005 g/l***	0.339 ± 0.008 g/l***	91	alcoholic cirrhosis	4
α-1-Antitrypsin	2.27 ± 0.10 g/l***	1.99 ± 0.05 g/l***	91	alcoholic cirrhosis	4
Alpha-1-Easily Precipitable Glycoprotein	140 ± 44	115 ± 19*	12	alcoholic cirrhosis	1
Alpha-1-Globulin	4.95 ± 1.05	4.73 ± 1.22*	–	chronic alcoholics	7
Alpha-2-Group Component	93 ± 20	117 ± 15*	12	alcoholic cirrhosis	1
Alpha-2-Globulin	11.68 ± 1.87	11.15 ± 1.79*	–	chronic alcoholics	7
Alpha₂-Macroglobulin	171 ± 61	122 ± 25*	12	alcoholic cirrhosis	1
	2.63 ± 0.12 g/l***	2.59 ± 0.12 g/l***	91	alcoholic cirrhosis	4

Protein					
Haptoglobin	0.90 ± 0.08 g/l***	1.51 ± 0.11 g/l***	91	alcoholic cirrhosis	4
	2.21 ± 0.94 g/l	2.3 g/l**	222	chronic alcoholic	13
	67 ± 63*	103 ± 44*	12	alcoholic cirrhosis	1
	0.69 ± 0.60 g/l	1.42 ± 0.57 g/l	34	alcoholic cirrhosis	6
	65.8 ± 45 mg/100ml	> 50 mg/100ml	7	alcoholic cirrhosis with hyperbilirubinaemia	11
Haemopexin	102 ± 29*	107 ± 13*	12	alcoholic cirrhosis	1
Orosomucoid	0.59 ± 0.034 g/l***	0.934 ± 0.041 g/l***	91	alcoholic cirrhosis	4
	0.63 ± 0.335 g/l***	0.81 ± 0.167 g/l***	34	alcoholic cirrhosis	6
Protein 9	118 ± 23*	121 ± 17*	12	alcoholic cirrhosis	1
Transferrin	91 ± 27*	110 ± 15*	12	alcoholic cirrhosis	1
C-Reactive Protein	0–0.2 g/l range	0.2 mg/100ml	–	alcoholic cirrhosis	12
Globulins	35.0 ± 7.5 g/l	33–56 g/l			5
	19–38 g/l	13–35 g/l			10
	19–50 g/l				
	24–40 g/l				
	24.6 ± 5.4 g/l	–	42		3
Beta-Globulins	11.99 ± 2.13	11.52 ± 2.19*		chronic alcoholics	7
Beta 1A-Globulin	0.708 ± 0.026 g/l***	0.916 ± 0.032 g/l***	91	alcoholic cirrhosis	4
	0.74 ± 0.21 g/l	0.91 ± 0.15 g/l	33	alcoholic cirrhosis	6
Gamma-Globulins	15.59 ± 3.11 g/l	13.97 ± 3.70*	42	chronic alcoholics	7
	24.6 ± 5.4 g/l	15–43 g/l			3
Sex steroid binding globulin	4.46 ± 0.50 (μg testosterone bound/100 ml plasma)	0.52 ± 0.29		chronic alcoholics	14

Table 7.9 (*continued*)

IgA	4.23 ± 1.48 g/l	—	27	alcoholics	9
	12.60 ± 5.8 g/l	—	15	alcoholics, death due to liver failure	9
	1–10 g/l (range)	0.30–1.35 g/l**	28	alcoholic cirrhosis	12
	6.94 ± 0.26 g/l***	2.22 ± 0.12 g/l***	91	alcoholic cirrhosis	4
	6.88 ± 2.25 g/l	1.970 ± 0.602 g/l	38	alcoholic cirrhosis	6
	3.77 ± 0.37 g/l	2.48 ± 0.90 g/l	8	alcoholics normal liver	
	3.96 ± 0.54 g/l	2.48 ± 0.90 g/l	7	alcoholics fatty liver	
	5.24 ± 0.42 g/l	2.48 ± 0.90 g/l	8	acute alcoholic hepatitis	8
	5.25 ± 0.98 g/l	2.48 ± 0.90 g/l	8	alcoholics fibrosis or cirrhosis	
	9.26 ± 0.77 g/l	2.48 ± 0.90 g/l	36	alcoholics with liver failure	
IgG	21.88 ± 0.68 g/l***	10.45 ± 0.26 g/l***	91	alcoholic cirrhosis	4
	12.80 ± 3.80 g/l	—	27	alcoholics	9
	26.01 ± 7.41 g/l	—	15	alcoholics death due to liver failure	9
	15.81 ± 1.73 g/l	13.10 ± 0.36 g/l	8	alcoholics normal liver	
	17.54 ± 2.22 g/l	13.10 ± 0.36 g/l	7	alcoholics fatty liver	
	19.25 ± 1.57 g/l	13.10 ± 0.36 g/l	8	acute alcoholics hepatitis	8
	20.42 ± 2.45 g/l	13.10 ± 0.36 g/l	8	alcoholics fibrosis or cirrhosis	
	26.02 ± 1.22 g/l	13.10 ± 0.36 g/l	36	alcoholics with liver failure	
	10–45 g/l (range)	6.0–14 g/l (range)	28	alcoholic cirrhosis	12
IgM	1.23 ± 0.78 g/l	—	27	alcoholics	9
	2.84 ± 0.90 g/l	—	15	alcoholics death due to liver failure	9
	1.88 ± 0.08 g/l***	1.23 ± 0.08 g/l***	91	alcoholic cirrhosis	4
	0.5–4.0 g/l (range)	0.3–1.2 g/l (range)	28	alcoholic cirrhosis	12

*relative percent **upper limit of normal range of reference serum ***standard error.

1. Murray-Lyon et al., (1972)
2. Halstead et al., (1971)
3. Redetzki et al., (1972)
4. Marasini et al., (1972)
5. Smith and Layden (1972)
6. Agostoni et al., (1969)
7. Jaross et al., (1972)
8. Iturriago et al., (1977)
9. Wilson et al., (1969)
10. Cowan and Hines (1971)
11. Fulop et al., (1971)
12. Lo Grippo et al., (1971)
13. Lamy et al., (1973)
14. Van Thiel et al., (1975)

7.4.1 Albumin and Pre-albumin

Both normal (Halstead *et al.*, 1971; Redetzki *et al.*, 1972) and low (Smith and Layden, 1972; LoGrippo, *et al.*, 1971; Agostoni *et al.*, 1969; Zakharov, 1968; Murray-Lyon *et al.*, 1972; Mezey and Tobon, 1971; Marasini *et al.*, 1972; Jaross *et al.*, 1972) levels of serum albumin have been reported in studies of alcoholic patients (Table 7.9). Generally low levels of albumin were found in alcoholics with cirrhosis, the low levels being attributable to reduced synthesis due to liver damage. Smith and Layden (1972) found that levels of serum albumin might rise to a small extent on abstinence.

These low levels of albumin found in alcoholics may have important effects on drug metabolism. In a study of tolbutamide use in alcoholics, an increase in drug clearance was found which correlated with decreased serum albumin levels. This increase in clearance was thought to be due to a decrease in protein binding (Thiessen *et al.*, 1976).

The concentration of thyroxine binding pre-albumin in serum is also severely reduced in alcoholic cirrhosis. In a study of 91 patients with alcoholic cirrhosis Marasini *et al.*, (1972) reported a mean serum level of 74 ± 49 mg/l compared to a control value of 339 ± 81 mg/l.

7.4.2 Globulins and Immunoglobulins

There have been several studies of the globulins and immunoglobulins in alcoholics, and the findings are summarised in Table 7.9. Decreased levels of globulins in alcoholics have been reported by few workers (Vier and Karapina, 1967; Ibragimov, 1967). The majority of studies in this area are concerned with the diffuse hypergammaglobulinaemia found in chronic alcoholics and alcoholics with cirrhosis (Cowan and Hines, 1971; Dinoso *et al.*, 1971; Akdamar *et al.*, 1972). This hypergammaglobulinaemia correlates with a proliferation of the antibody-synthesizing cells in the bone marrow, lymph nodes, spleen and the liver.

The cause of the raised immunoglobulins, especially IgG, has been attributed, to either a failure of the alcohol damaged liver to regulate synthesis, or as a result of an immunological reaction against antigens unmasked by liver injury (Wilson *et al.*, 1969). Smith and Layden (1972) found that globulins fell during treatment. It may also represent a response to be increased levels of oestrogens found in male alcoholics (see Section 7.8).

IgA

Elevated and severely elevated levels of serum IgA have been reported in alcoholics with fatty liver (Roser, 1970), and ascites (Murator *et al.*, 1971) and alcoholic cirrhosis (Lee, 1965; Feizi, 1968; Agostini *et al.*, 1969; Wilson *et al.*, 1969; LoGrippo *et al.*, 1971; Marisini *et al.*, 1972). The increase of IgA is most probably secondary to the cirrhosis rather than attributable to a direct effect of ethanol.

Iturriaga *et al.*, (1977) studied the relationship between serum IgA levels and liver disease. They studied three groups: alcoholics without liver damage, alcoholics with varying degrees of liver damage, and non-alcoholics with liver disease. The serum IgA concentration was increased in all groups of alcoholics and this increase was related to the severity of liver damage. IgA was also increased in the non-alcoholic group, but nevertheless both the degree of increase and the IgA/G ratios could still be used to distinguish these groups.

In contrast Wilson *et al.*, (1968) studied two patients with alcoholic cirrhosis in whom IgA was not detected in the serum. A trace amount of IgA was detected in external secretions. This deficiency may be associated with a predisposition to develop cirrhosis. An antibody to secretory IgA, not serum IgA, has also been detected in some patients with alcoholic cirrhosis (Wilson, 1972). The significance of this is not known.

IgG and IgM

Serum levels of IgG and IgM are also increased in those alcoholics with ascitic cirrhosis (Murator *et al.*, 1971) and cirrhosis (Lee, 1965; Feizi, 1968; Agostoni *et al.*, 1969; Wilson *et al.*, 1969; Roser, 1970).

These increases in immunoglobulins, particularly in IgG and IgA whilst showing individual variation, correlate with the severity of liver disease. The highest levels are found in these with active alcoholic cirrhosis (Hobbs, 1967; Gleichmann and Deicher, 1968; Wilson *et al.*, 1969). Wilson *et al.*, (1969) also studied levels of the sub-group γ G3 in alcoholics with liver disease. They found that variations in the γ G3 sub-group related to genetic differences in the Gm system. So they conclude that the capacity to increase the immunoglobulins in response to liver failure is in part genetically determined.

GASTRIC AUTO-ANTIBODIES

There have been some studies of the incidence of gastric autoantibodies and other autoantibodies, to determine whether there is an autoimmune basis for alcoholic gastritis.

Roberts and Taylor (1973) studied the incidence of gastric parietal cell antibodies, anti-thyroglobulin and antibodies to thyroid microsomes in alcoholics. They found that alcohol was the cause of the chronic gastritis and that the incidence of parietal cell antibody was unrelated to either the alcohol or the incidence and severity of the chronic gastritis. As there was also no increase in the incidence of anti-thyroglobulin there seems little evidence for an autoimmune process in alcoholic gastritis.

Similarly Pitchumoni *et al.*, (1975) found in a study of one hundred and fifty alcoholic men and women that there was no association of alcoholic gastritis with an increase in the incidence of parietal cell antibodies.

7.4.3 Alpha-Foetoprotein

Alpha-foetoprotein (AFP) has been detected in the serum of a patient with alcoholic hepatitis, during the acute phase of the illness. There was no evidence of malignant disease on investigation, and as the patient improved clinically the alpha-foetoprotein became undetectable.

Alcoholic hepatitis and hepatoma have similar clinical findings and hepatoma is commonly associated with cirrhosis. Miller *et al.*, (1975) therefore suggest that if AFP is detected in an alcoholic, a decrease with serial measurements should exclude the diagnosis of hepatoma. A further 89 serum samples from patients with alcoholic liver disease were analysed but failed to detect alpha-foetoprotein (Miller *et al.*, 1975).

7.4.4 Caeruloplasmin

Lo Grippo *et al.*, (1971) studied caeruloplasmin levels in patients with alcoholic cirrhosis. Both normal and elevated (above the mean serum level in 66% of patients and above mean $\pm$ 2 S. D. in 48%) values were found. There was no association with severity of liver disease, and similarly Murray-Lyon *et al.*, (1972) found increased levels of caeruloplasmin in alcoholic cirrhotics. This increase in caeruloplasmin may represent part of the 'acute phase reaction' – the inflammatory response to liver damage. Increases in caeruloplasmin have been reported in other liver diseases, though decreases can occur with severe parenchymal damage (Gault *et al.*, 1966; Walshe and Briggs, 1962). However, Sviripa (1972) found that there were disorders in copper metabolism in alcoholics with and without cirrhosis. He found decreased copper metabolism, increased retention of copper, and increased caeruloplasmin levels.

7.4.5 Carcinoembryonic Antigen

In a study by Moore *et al.*, (1971) carcinoembryonic antigen (CEA) was detected in the serum of 20 out of 46 patients with alcoholic liver disease. No malignancy of the gastrointestinal tract could be detected. The reason for the prescence of CEA in alcoholic liver disease is not clear. Moore *et al.*, (1971) suggest that a source might be the regenerating liver, especially since the liver is entodermally derived and is a source of CEA in the foetus. However, levels of CEA do not correlate well with the degree of regeneration found in these patients as judged histologically. A second possibility is that the antiserum used to measure CEA cross-reacts with other serum components, e.g. seromucoid, which may be increased in alcoholics. In conclusion, the detection of CEA in alcoholics should be interpreted with caution but a thorough investigation for malignancy should be carried out.

7.4.6 Haptoglobin

The reports of haptoglobin levels in alcoholics are confusing. This may well be because of the many factors influencing its metabolism. Haptoglobin is synthesized in the liver and hence liver function will affect its blood levels. Haptoglobin complexes with free haemoglobin and prevents its loss through the kidney. The complex is removed from the circulation by the reticulo-endothelial system and is subsequently degraded, the haem portion being conserved. Thus haemolysis will lead to a fall in serum haptoglobin levels. Haptoglobin is also involved in bile pigment formation. Levels generally rise when tissue breakdown increases, for example in infection, stress and trauma. Haptoglobin metabolism is also influenced by androgens and the menstrual cycle (De Torok and DeCrow, 1976). These factors may all influence the haptoglobin levels found in alcoholics.

Murray-Lyon et al., (1972) studying alcoholics with cirrhosis found no significant changes in serum haptoglobin levels. Similarly Fulop et al., (1971) found only two out of seven alcoholics with increased bilirubins and with decreased haptoglobin levels. However other workers (Agostoni et al., 1969) found that these changes correlated well with changes in albumin levels and others have concluded that the decreased levels reflected decreased synthesis of haptoglobin (Kallai et al., 1966; Piccinino et al., 1966). Marasini et al., (1972) concluded that there was either decreased synthesis of haptoglobin or a re-distribution in the extra-vascular space.

Sherwood (1972), studying patients with alcoholic liver disease and portal cirrhosis, came to different conclusions. It is difficult to recognise haemolytic disease in patients with chronic liver disease because the former may be obscured by the aberrant liver function. Sherwood (1972) therefore studied patients suffering from both diseases simultaneously, in order to assess the use of hapto-globin as an index of haemolysis in liver disease. He found that serum haptoglobin levels did not correlate with other measures of hepatic protein synthesis. He concluded that haptoglobin synthesis remains intact in alcoholic cirrhosis and that serum levels are a reliable guide to the recognition of haemolytic disease.

Pezzimenti and Lindenbaum (1972) describe two patients with decreased or absent serum haptoglobin associated with a folate deficiency secondary to the alcoholism.

Hyper-haptoglobinaemia has also been observed in chronic alcoholics. Lamy et al., (1973) found that 50% of a group of chronic alcoholics had serum haptoglobin levels above the upper limit of normal, and that these elevated levels persisted during three months of abstinence. The mechanism of this hyperhaptoglobinaemia is unclear. De Torok and De Crow (1976) analyzed serum haptoglobin levels both quantitatively and qualitatively in alcoholic and non-alcoholic groups. Genetic typing revealed no differences in the frequency of the Hp2 allele in either group. Thus the authors postulate the presence of a regulator gene, the activity of which may begin prior to the onset of drinking. The elevated haptoglobin may explain the iron overload found in alcoholics, because haptoglobin binds tightly and specifically with haemoglobin and hence is involved in iron conservation in the body.

7.4.7 Transferrin

Serum levels of transferrin are lowered in alcoholics with cirrhosis (LoGrippo *et al.*, 1971; Murray-Lyon *et al.*, 1972). The latter group has studied cirrhotic alcoholics and found 35% of the group to have transferrin levels below the lower limit of normal. This reduction in serum transferrin may be due to the livers decreased ability to synthesize proteins, or may be due to the poor nutritional state of the patient. It should be remembered that low serum levels of transferrin are found in the nutritional deficiency states e.g. Kwashiorkor (Murray-Lyon *et al.*, 1972). LoGrippo *et al.*, (1971) found that whilst transferrin was decreased in alcoholic cirrhosis levels were increased in obstructive jaundice – they concluded that transferrin levels might be used to distinguish the two.

7.4.8 Fibrin

Dettori *et al.*, (1977) studied fibrin formation in patients with severe alcoholic cirrhosis and increased prothrombin times. Their work on the physicochemical properties of the clot led them to conclude that in the later stages of alcoholic liver disease there is an altered synthesis of fibrinogen in the hepatocyte.

7.4.9 Protein Metabolism

McDonald and Margen (1976) studied the effects of wine and ethanol on the nitrogen balance of healthy volunteers. They found that both wine and ethanol gave rise to an increase in urinary urea and uric acid output. They concluded that ethanol may directly affect protein catabolism. There was no significant difference in faecal nitrogen excretion. This increase in urinary nitrogen might reflect increased protein degradation to provide additional energy, though decreased protein synthesis or enhanced catabolism might also play a part.

There is other evidence of altered protein metabolism due to alcohol. Studies in rats fed with ethanol (Baraona *et al.*, 1975) have shown an increase in liver protein. Although liver synthesis was increased there was no equivalent increase in release to the serum. Studies in humans (alcoholics with liver disease) suggest that once alcohol has been removed from the diet there is either increased or normal albumin synthesis. However, studies in rabbit have shown that alcohol may inhibit protein synthesis in the liver (Rothschild *et al.*, 1975).

Another study by Chowdhury *et al.,* (1977) found an increased loss of albumin in the faeces during alcohol ingestion. The loss was exaggerated when gastritis was also present. These results, whilst contrary to those of McDonald and Margen (1976), might explain in part the low levels of serum albumin in alcoholics.

7.5 AMINO-ACIDS

Several studies have indicated that the metabolism of amino-acids may be disturbed in alcoholics (Wartburg and Papenberg, 1970; Orten and Sardesai, 1971) Ning *et al.,* (1967) showed that patients with alcoholic hepatitis had normal concentrations of α-amino nitrogen but had an increased ratio of non-essential to branch chained essential amino-acids in their sera. There was a decrease in the serum concentrations of leucine, isoleucine, and valine with an increase in glutamic acid. The amino-acid pattern found was similar to that seen in Kwashiorkor or after hepatectomy, so reflecting the poor nutrition and liver dysfunction of alcoholics. The latter is important as the liver is a major site of amino-acid metabolism. Rosen *et al.,* (1977) studied serum amino-acid patterns in cases of hepatic encephalopathy of differing aetiology and found similar results to those of Ning *et al.,* (1967): the aromatic amino-acids, pheny-lalanine, tyrosine, and tryptophan as well as methionine, glutamate, and aspartate were increased in alcoholic hepatitis. The levels of the branched chain amino-acids, valine, leucine, and isoleucine were depressed. There is evidence both from human and animal studies that these changes in amino-acids are secondary to disorders in carbohydrate metabolism. Thus the catabolic state of the patient, especially in encephalopathy, and changes in insulin/glucagon levels, may affect the ability of liver, muscle and fat to utilise amino-acids as a source of energy. This will be reflected in changes in the branched chain amino-acids. The elevations in amino-acids are thought to reflect the degree of hepatic necrosis. These changes may in turn affect the level of neurotransmitters in the brain (Rosen *et al.,* 1977).

Similarly, alterations in serum amino-acid patterns have been found in alcoholics following an acute dose of ethanol, and also in delirium tremens (Wartburg and Papenberg, 1970). Siegel *et al.,* (1964) studied plasma amino-acid patterns in alcoholics and healthy volunteers given alcohol. Ethanol was found to depress the total blood amino-acids in the volunteers but not in the alcoholics. In the former, serine, threonine, methionine, leucine and alanine were depressed whilst glutamine was elevated. In alcoholics only serine was depressed whereas methionine, leucine, isoleucine and proline were elevated. From their work, these authors propose that there is a block in the glutamine synthetase system in alcoholics and that they may derive their endogenous glutamine by another metabolic route.

Mata *et al.*, (1975) studied the serum free proline and free hydroxyproline in patients with alcoholic liver cirrhosis. They found that levels of serum-free proline and free hydroxyproline were significantly higher in the alcoholics. Serum proline was particularly raised in cases of alcoholic hepatitis. Whilst these changes may be due to leakage from liver cells, it is more likely, bearing in mind the changes in hydroxyproline, that these changes reflect an alteration in collagen metabolism.

Similarly, urinary total hydroxyproline levels are increased in those drinking subjects with alcoholic cirrhosis as compared with alcoholics with normal livers, hepatofibrosis or fatty changes (Wu and Levi, 1975). These authors found that on withdrawal from alcohol there was an increased urinary excretion of hydroxyproline. The changes may reflect changes in collagen metabolism due to ethanol and may be of use in the diagnosis of alcoholism. Thus Shaw *et al.*, (1976, 1977) have shown that the plasma α-amino-n-butyric acid/leucine ratio is increased in alcoholics. The ratio does not indicate past alcoholism but may be useful in assessing the degree of alcoholism, and in detecting relapse during treatment. (see Chapter 6).

Ethanol has been shown to affect the intestinal transport of amino-acids. Orten (1963) showed in a non-alcoholic that ethanol promoted the ileal absorption of amino-acids usually absorbed slowly, e.g. glycine, L-glutamic and L-aspartic acids and L-threonine. However, amino acids usually absorbed rapidly were absorbed more slowly, e.g. L-isoleucine, L-arginine and L-methionine. Ethanol has also been shown to inhibit the intestinal absorption of L-methionine in normals (Israel *et al.*, 1969).

Orten and Sardesai (1971) also review the effects of alcohol on individual amino-acids. Briefly they are as follows:

Tryptophan. This amino-acid is involved in the synthesis of serotonin and hence 5-hydroxy-indole-3-acetic acid (5-HIAA) and nicotinic acid. Disturbances in both serotonin and nicotinic acid metabolism occur in alcoholics (see Sections 7.14 on biogenic amines and 7.15 on vitamins).

Tyrosine. Disturbances in norepinephrine and epinephrine metabolism are found in alcoholics (see Section 7.14 on biogenic amines) which are synthesized from tyrosine.

Glutamic acid. Ethanol has been shown to affect plasma glutamic acid levels (Orten and Sardesai, 1971). This may have important consequences as this amino-acid is a precursor of γ-aminobutyric acid (GABA) an inhibitor of neuro-transmitters in the brain.

Cysteine. The metabolic derivative of cysteine, taurine is excreted in excessive amounts by alcoholics (Orten and Sardesai, 1971).

Histidine. This amino-acid occupies a central position in the active site of alcohol dehydrogenase. A derivative of histidine, histamine has been implicated in some of the effects of ethanol, e.g. skin flushing.

Glycine. Ethanol has been shown to give rise to decreased hippuric acid excretion in healthy volunteers. This may reflect a decreased ability of the liver to conjugate glycine and benzoate to give hippurate, during ethanol metabolism.

Thus altered amino-acid patterns in alcoholics may not only result from liver dysfunction but may also result from poor nutrition and malabsorption. Any changes in amino-acid metabolism may have far reaching metabolic effects from altering protein synthesis and gluconeogenesis to the production of neurotransmitters.

7.6 NON-PROTEIN NITROGENOUS COMPOUNDS

7.6.1 Urea and Creatinine

Serum urea has been estimated in alcoholics in an investigation of osmometry in the evaluation of alcohol intoxication (Redetzki *et al.*, 1972). Normal values of urea nitrogen occurred in alcoholics unless there was concomittant vomiting and dehydration or renal impairment.

Urinary creatinine excretion has been found not to be affected by ethanol ingestion. This is important as urine creatinine levels may therefore be used to assess the adequacy of 24 hour collections. Urine creatinine levels are also used when studying catecholamine excretion in alcoholics. It is not definitely known whether ethanol-induced diuresis can enhance catecholamine excretion, and to allow for such an effect urinary catecholamine levels are usually reported per mg of creatinine.

7.6.2 Uric acid

Hyperuricaemia and decreased urinary excretion of uric acid are an indirect consequence of ethanol abuse. Excessive generation of NADH, due to hepatic metabolism of ethanol, leads to an increase in blood lactate levels, and a secondary hyperuricaemia arises due to competition between lactate and urate for excretion in the renal tubule Figure 7.4 (Lieber *et al.*, 1962; Lieber, 1965a, Bendersky, 1975).

Garrod (1876) first noted the association between excessive intake of alcoholic beverages and gouty attacks, and this has been supported by population surveys demonstrating a correlation between serum urate levels and ethanol intake (Evans *et al.*, 1968), and by studies on moderate drinkers (Saker *et al.*, 1967). The study of Olin *et al.*, (1973) revealed higher serum levels of urate in non-gouty drinkers as compared with non-gouty abstainers. Studies in alcoholics (Vogelberg *et al.*, 1971; Jaross *et al.*, 1972), in patients with hyperlipidaemia due to ethanol (De Gennes *et al.*, 1972), and in those suffering from alcohol intoxication (Redetzki *et al.*, 1972) have shown increased levels of serum urate. It has also been noted that the elevation in serum urate levels following alcohol ingestion is higher in the fasted compared with the non-fasted subject (Maclachlan and Rodnan, 1967). Table 7.10 summarises the uric acid levels found in various groups of alcoholics and controls.

An interesting study has been made of urate levels in the csf of alcoholics (Carlsson and Dencker, 1973). After an alcoholic debauche the patients showed significant and persistently increased levels of csf urate, although the serum urate was not raised. It was suggested that the changes reflected an increased catabolism of nucleic acids in the CNS due to a cellular toxic effect of ethanol, and such continued increased levels might explain the development of a chronic brain syndrome found in advanced chronic alcoholism.

Acute doses of ethanol have been shown to raise serum urate levels. Normal levels were regained by eight hours after ingestion (Carey *et al.*, 1971).

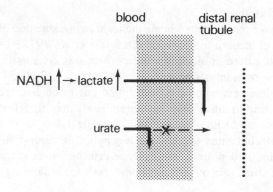

Fig. 7.4 – Effect of Lactate on the Renal Excretion of Urate.

7.7 PEPTIDE HORMONES

There have been very few studies on the effects of ethanol and ethanol abuse on peptide hormones. In many instances conflicting results have appeared and it is therefore difficult to draw any firm conclusions as to the effects of ethanol on certain peptide hormones. Study of the effects of ethanol on individual hormones is complicated by the intricate systems involving releasing hormones, inhibiting hormones and feed-back mechanisms which control peptide hormone levels (see Butt, 1975). To date little or no information is available on the effect of ethanol on releasing and inhibiting hormones.

The clinical significance of many of the changes is not known. An intriguing hypothesis has recently been proposed, however, which links the observed higher occurrence of cancers of the breast and thyroid, and malignant melanoma in drinkers with levels of several peptide hormones (Williams, 1976). The hypothesis, summarised in Figure 7.5, proposes that alcohol or other drugs stimulate anterior pituitary secretion of prolactin, thyroid-stimulating hormone (TSH) and melanocyte-stimulating hormone (MSH), and that under the stimulation of these hormones the three target tissues display increased mitotic activity and a

Table 7.10
Uric Acid Levels in Alcoholic Patients

	Mean ± SD or range	Reference interval (normal range) or control values	Number of subjects	Clinical details	
serum	5.0–14.6 mg/100 ml		4	alcoholic with diabetic ketoacidosis	Levy et al., 1973
serum	7.6 ± 2.7 mg/100 ml		32	alcohol intoxicated	Redetzki et al., 1972
serum csf	5.74 ± 0.27 mg/100 ml 4.44 ± 1.71 mg/100 ml	2.54 ± 0.5	52	alcoholic in withdrawal	Carlsson and Dencker, 1973
serum csf	4.81 ± 0.23 mg/100 ml 3.15 ± 0.99 mg/100 ml		13	sober alcoholic	
serum	5.5 mg/100 ml	5.3	12	healthy control given alcohol	Carey et al., 1971
serum	4.52 ± 1.35 mg/100 ml	3.73 ± 1.09	41	chronic alcoholic	Jaross et al., 1972

subsequent increased susceptibility to developing a malignancy. The observed effect of ethanol on serum prolactin (Zanaboni and Zanoboni-Muciaccia, 1976) has been cited as evidence in support of this hypothesis. Lack of any significant difference between the incidence of these cancers in a Mormon (drinking of ethanol proscribed) and a non-Mormon population has, however, been cited as confounding evidence (Lyon, *et al.*, 1976).

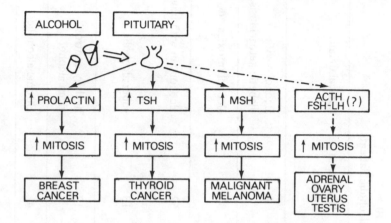

Fig. 7.5 – Alcohol Induced Pituitary Hypersecretion and Possible Cancer Promotion. Reproduced by permission from Williams, *Lancet* (1976)

ADENOHYPOPHYSEAL HORMONES

7.7.1 Growth Hormone (Somatotrophin)

Growth hormone (GH) plays a central role in regulating growth. It also promotes protein synthesis, stimulates amino acid uptake by cells, antagonises the insulin-mediated uptake of glucose, inhibits the synthesis of fat from carbohydrate and stimulates lipolysis. Secretion of GH is stimulated by stress, starvation and hypoglycaemia. GH secretion is supressed by hyperglycaemia.

Elevated serum levels of growth hormone have been reported in alcoholic patients in the acute, untreated phase of clinical alcoholic hypoglycaemia (Joffe *et al.*, 1975), in alcoholics with severe metabolic acidosis (Levy *et al.*, 1973), and in alcoholics with cirrhosis (Zanoboni and Zanoboni-Muciaccia, 1977). In healthy males very large elevations in growth hormone have been demonstrated following oral ingestion of 20% alcohol solutions (1.5 ml/kg). Eight out of the eleven healthy males studied exhibited raised levels, whilst the remaining three showed either an unchanged or depressed growth hormone level. Peak levels occurred 1–1.5h after ingestion and were typically 5–6 times the control values (Table 7.11), and normal levels were regained 2–3 hours after ingestion of the

Table 7.11

Effects of Ethanol Ingestion on Serum Growth Hormone Levels in 11 Subjects
Reproduced by permission from Bellet et al., Metabolism (1971) 20, 763–769.

Time after administration of test solution (min).	0	30	60	90	120	180
Mean GH concentration of control phase (ng/ml)	0.94 ± 0.57	0.83 ± 0.44*	1.00 ± 0.72	1.32 ± 1.40	1.22 ± 1.08	2.03 ± 1.88
Mean GH concentration of alcohol phase (ng/ml)	1.00 ± 0.67	3.08 ± 3.04	5.65 ± 5.99	5.94 ± 5.73	4.04 ± 4.73	2.13 ± 1.76
	n.s.	p <0.05	<0.05	<0.02	n.s.	n.s.
Plasma alcohol levels during alcohol consumption phase (mg/100 ml)	0	118.2 ± 40.3	130.2 ± 27.7	138.0 ± 29.3	139.8 ± 27.5	127.3 ± 36.2

*Values expressed as mean ± SD.
n.s.: Differences not statistically significant at 5% level on basis of paired comparison.

dose of alcohol. The mechanism by which ethanol produces such a response in GH levels is not known (Bellet *et al.*, 1971). In contrast, growth hormone levels were not significantly changed in six non-obese, non-diabetic, non-alcoholic subjects during a 6 hour period when alcohol was infused at a rate of 236 mg/minute (Bagdade *et al.*, 1972b). Similar results were obtained in another study involving 5 healthy normal subjects given alcohol intravenously at a similar rate for 1 hour (Abramson and Arky, 1968). A more recent study (Leppäluoto *et al.*, 1975) found GH levels to be depressed in healthy males following an oral dose of ethanol of 1.5 g/kg body weight.

Plasma growth hormone response to insulin-induced hypoglycaemia is decreased in healthy volunteers following ethanol consumption (Priem *et al.*, 1976). Peak plasma growth hormone levels in the seven subjects studied were 46.9 ± 26.6 ng/ml following insulin (0.1 U/kg body weight) and 32.9 ± 14.5 ng/ml when the insulin was preceded by 50 ml of alcohol (peak plasma ethanol concentration ranged from 64 to 114 mg/100 ml). The differences in peak growth hormone values for each subject were statistically significant, although the differences between the mean peak values were not. The mechanism by which alcohol impairs growth hormone release in insulin-induced hypoglycaemia is not known. It has been suggested that the decreased response may be due to either diminished sensitivity to growth hormone release-inhibiting hormone or to impaired secretion of growth hormone releasing factor. In contrast, Joffe *et al.*, (1975) have reported elevated serum levels of growth hormone in hypoglycaemic patients.

7.7.2 Prolactin

Prolactin promotes breast development in pregnancy and lactation. Its role in males is still under investigation.

Plasma prolactin levels are moderately increased in men with alcoholic liver disease (Van Thiel *et al.*, 1975), although normal levels have also been reported (Turkington, 1972). In cirrhotics the incidence of hyper-prolactinaemia was higher in cirrhosis associated with alcohol abuse than in non-alcoholic varieties (Wernze and Schmitz, 1977). Enhanced pituitary prolactin reserve after a thyrotropin-releasing hormone (TRH) stimulation test has been noted in male patients with alcoholic cirrhosis (Zanoboni and Zanoboni-Muciaccia, 1975). Basal levels of prolactin were slightly raised but, following TRH, levels were significantly higher than in controls. An unexplained diminution in prolactin response to TRH occurs in male subjects during hangover (Ylikahri *et al.*, 1976b).

Acute administration of ethanol appears to be without effect on serum prolactin levels (Nader *et al.*, 1974).

7.7.3 Follicle-Stimulating Hormone (FSH)

FSH stimulates spermatogenesis in males, whilst in females it stimulates the development of ovarian follicles and, together with luteinising hormone, promotes oestrogen secretion by the follicle.

A study of 40 male alcoholics with liver disease found 7 patients with raised and 3 with lowered values of plasma follicle-stimulating hormone. Two-thirds of the patients showed an abnormal response to a clomiphene stimulation test (i.e. increase in plasma FSH > 50% following clomiphene), and this was interpreted in terms of a suppression of the hypothalmic-pituitary axis by ethanol (Van Thiel *et al.*, 1974).

In contrast, ethanol has also been shown to be without effect on FSH levels in healthy males (Leppäluoto *et al.*, 1975).

7.7.4 Luteinising Hormone (LH)

LH stimulates androgen production by the testis in males, whilst in females it promotes oestrogen secretion and ovulation in the prepared follicle.

Elevated levels of LH have been reported in chronic alcoholics (Wright *et al.*, 1975). Basal levels in the 13 male chronic alcoholics investigated were 9.2 ± 3.6 mU/ml compared with 5.4 ± 1.3 mU/ml in healthy controls. Six of the alcoholics had basal LH levels in excess of 12 mU/ml. An unexplained exaggerated response to luteinising hormone releasing hormone (LHRH) occurred in six of the patients. A low incidence of elevated plasma LH levels (22.5%) has been found in patients with alcoholic liver disease. In 19 out of 26 male patients tested there was an inadequate LH response to clomiphene stimulation which was attributed to hypothalamic-pituitary suppression and to primary gonadal failure (Van Thiel *et al.*, 1974).

Decreased levels of LH have been found in healthy male subjects given ethanol (1.5 g/kg) (Leppäluoto *et al.*, 1975), and elevated and depressed levels in normal males given larger doses of ethanol (Gordon *et al.*, 1976). A more recent study, however, in which blood alcohol, plasma LH and testosterone levels were determined at 20 minute intervals one hour prior to and 5 hours after an oral dose of ethanol (2.4 ml 100 proof beverage/kg), has revealed that at peak blood alcohol levels LH is significantly elevated whilst testosterone levels are depressed. During the descending phase of the blood alcohol/time curve plasma LH levels returned to base-line values. The variation in LH levels was attributed to an enhanced secretory release of LH due to feedback mechanisms associated with the low plasma levels of testosterone (Mendelson *et al.*, 1977).

7.7.5 Adrenocorticotropin (ACTH), Thyrotropin (TSH) and Melanocyte Stimulating Hormone (MSH)

There is little information of the effect of ethanol on any of these hormones. Ethanol is reported not to affect ACTH and TSH levels (Leppäluoto *et al.*, 1975).

NEUROHYPOPHYSEAL HORMONES

7.7.6 Antidiuretic Hormone (ADH)

ADH acts on the distal renal tubule and the collecting ducts to increase permeability to water. Large doses of ethanol (> 0.5 ml/kg) and high blood ethanol levels (> 200 mg/100 ml) are reported to block the release of ADH thus promoting diuresis (Cobo and Quintero, 1969; Merzon and Khorunzhaya, 1970).

7.7.7 Oxytocin

Oxytocin stimulates milk secretion and produces uterine contractions during parturition. An inhibition of oxytocin release has been demonstrated following oral or intravenous administration of ethanol (Cobo and Quintero, 1969; Gibbens and Chard, 1976). This property of ethanol has been utilised in obstetrics for the prevention of premature onset of labour.

THYROID AND PARATHYROID HORMONES

7.7.8 Thyroid Hormones, Parathyroid Hormone and Calcitonin

Conflicting results have been presented regarding the effect of alcohol on thyroid hormones and this may be a consequence of variations in dietary iodine intake, nutrition, liver function and levels of carrier proteins in serum (Marks and Chakraborty, 1973; Wartburg and Papenberg, 1970). Hyper-, hypo- (Augustine, 1967; Murdock, 1967), and euthyroid states have been described in alcoholics (Farmer and Fabre, 1975; Wright et al., 1975). Thyroidal hypo- function (low estimated free thyroxine index) has been reported in both in- toxicated and non-intoxicated alcoholics (Kolakowska and Swigar, 1977).

There appears to be very little information available regarding the effect of ethanol on parathyroid hormone or calcitonin, although whiskey has been utilised in a provocative test for stimulation calcitonin release in patients at risk of developing medullary carcinoma of the thyroid (Dymling et al., 1976).

PANCREATIC HORMONES

7.7.9 Insulin

The actions of insulin are to promote entry of glucose into cells, protein synthesis, glycogenesis, lipogenesis and to inhibit gluconeogenesis and lipolysis. Insulin secretion is stimulated by elevated blood glucose levels, amino-acids (especially leucine and arginine), and glucagon. Low glucose levels and adrenaline inhibit insulin secretion.

In healthy males who had been fasted overnight, ethanol (1.4 ml/kg) was found to be without effect on serum insulin levels (Bellet et al., 1971). Similar results have been obtained in patients given smaller doses of ethanol (Abramson and Arky, 1968).

A study by Taskinen and Nikkila (1977) has shown, however, that doses of ethanol (1.5 g/kg) cause plasma insulin levels to rise, both during the night and during the morning following administration of ethanol to healthy subjects.

After a prolonged fast ethanol produces hypoglycaemia which is accompanied by decreased insulin levels (Bagdade *et al.*, 1972a, 1972b; Turner *et al.*, 1973; Joffe *et al.*, 1975), presumably in response to the low glucose levels rather than to any direct effect of ethanol.

An enhancement of the glucose-stimulated release of insulin has been reported by O'Keefe and Marks (1977). Changes of insulin levels in relation to alcohol changes in glucose levels are considered further in Section 7.11.

7.7.10 Glucagon

The actions of the polypeptide hormone glucagon are to stimulate gluconeogenesis, glycogenolysis in the liver, and insulin secretion. Secretion of glucagon is inhibited by hyperglycaemia and stimulated by hypoglycaemia.

Elevated levels of glucagon have been found in a patient with alcoholic hypoglycaemia (Joffe *et al.*, 1975), although this is probably a consequence of the low glucose level rather than a specific effect of ethanol.

GASTROINTESTINAL TRACT HORMONES

7.7.11 Secretin

Secretin is a polypeptide hormone which stimulates the secretion of pancreatic juices and the flow of bile from the liver. Two separate studies of the effect of oral ethanol on secretin levels in healthy males have reported significant elevation in the plasma levels of this hormone (Straus *et al.*, 1975; Llanos *et al.*, 1977). The latter group of workers also studied the effect on secretin levels of intraduodenal ethanol. Administration of ethanol by this route did not effect secretin levels, a result which provides strong evidence that alcohol does not release secretin directly *via* contact with duodenal mucosa. The mechanism of release is not clear but it may be mediated by alcohol stimulated gastric acid secretion (see next Section).

7.7.12 Gastrin

Gastric acid production by parietal cells is stimulated by the hormone gastrin which is released into the blood in response to decreased gastric acid concentration.

Ethanol has been shown to stimulate the release of gastrin in normal healthy male volunteers. Serum gastrin levels rose from a basal level of 13 ± 5.6 pg/ml to 27 ± 16.3 pg/ml ($p = 0.15$) ten minutes after oral ingestion of 10 grammes of alcohol (Korman *et al.*, 1971). Other workers (Becker *et al.*, 1974; Llanos *et al.*, 1977) have found small, but significant increases in serum gastrin levels following either oral or intravenous administration of ethanol to healthy volunteers. The response to ethanol was dependent upon the mass of alcohol administered. Two factors are believed to be involved in the ethanol mediated rise in gastrin levels, firstly a direct action on parietal cells and secondly release of gastrin from the antrum after local contact. The route(s) by which intravenous alcohol stimulates gastrin secretion are not known. Likewise the significance of ethanol-mediated changes in gastrin and secretin levels in the development of gastro-intestinal tract disorders in alcoholics is not established.

7.8 STEROID HORMONES, PRECURSORS AND METABOLITES

There have been few studies reported on the effects of alcohol on the hypothalamic–pituitary–adrenal/gonadal axis in man. Several authors have reviewed alcohol-endocrine relationships. (Stokes, 1971; Gordon and Southern 1977).

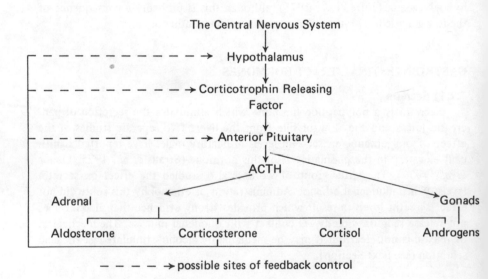

Fig. 7.6 – The Hypothalamic-Pituitary-Adrenal/Gonadal Axis.

The control of adrenal and gonadal hormone release and synthesis is affected by feedback mechanisms (Figure 7.6). The effect of alcohol on these controls is unclear. As well as the functioning of the hypothalamic–pituitary–adrenal/gonadal axis, the degree of protein binding and rate of catabolism will also affect blood levels of the steroids. These may all be affected by alcohol.

THE ADRENAL CORTEX

7.8.1 Glucocorticoids

A detailed description of cortisol metabolism can be found in most endo-crinology textbooks (Butt, 1976) (Figure 7.7). Cortisol is a glucocorticoid synthesized from cholesterol in the *zona fasciculata* of the adrenal cortex. This hormone is mostly protein bound to a specific cortisol binding α_1- globulin

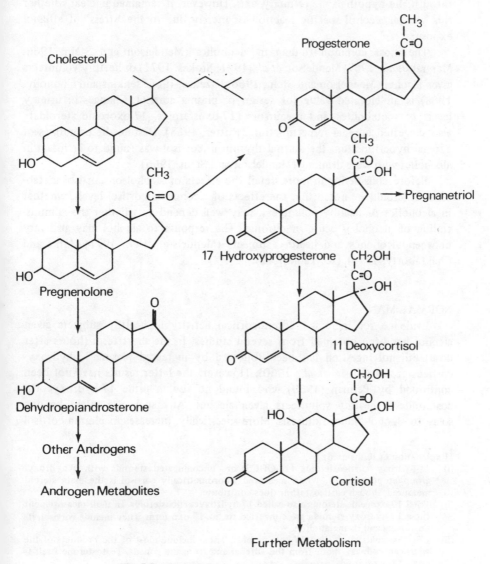

Fig. 7.7 – Pathways of adrenal steroid synthesis.

(cortisol binding globulin, transcortin) and to albumin. The unbound fraction is biologically active. Cortisol is metabolised in the liver and it is conjugated with glucuronic acid and excreted in the urine. Much of the earlier work on the effects of alcohol was carried out on animals and studied the ascorbate and cholesterol content of the adrenals. Urinary metabolites were also measured. This early work is reviewed by Stokes (1971) and Gordon and Southren (1977) and much of it showed that ethanol did affect the adrenal gland, probably through the hypothalamic pituitary axis. However, it remained unclear whether this was an alcohol specific reaction or merely due to the 'stress' of ethanol exposure.

The most common finding in alcoholics (Mendelson and Stein, 1966; Margraf *et al.*, 1967; Mendelson *et al.*, 1971; Stokes, 1971) or healthy volunteers given alcohol (Mendelson and Stein, 1966; Fazekas, 1966; Jenkins and Connolly, 1968) is an elevated value for serum or plasma cortisol. Changes in urinary levels of metabolites and precursors (17-oxosteroids, 17-oxogenic steroids)[†] also suggested adrenal hyperfunction (Rutter, 1968). Despite these findings of adrenal hyperfunction, the diurnal rhythm in cortisol was found to be intact in alcoholics who were drinking (Mendelson and Stein, 1966).

Before considering in more detail the effects of alcohol on cortisol metabolism it should be noted that the effects of alcohol on cortisol levels, whether in alcoholics or healthy volunteers, may well depend on whether the administration of alcohol is acute or chronic. The response to alcohol may also vary between alcoholics and healthy subjects (Mendelson *et al.*, 1971; Marks and Chakraborty, 1973). (see Table 7.12).

NORMAL MAN

Evidence for increased adrenocortical activity in healthy subjects given alcohol has been obtained from several studies. In the short term (hours after dose) ethanol ingestion has been followed by increased plasma 17-hydroxycorticosteroids (Kissin *et al.*, 1960). However, the latter results have not been confirmed by Perman (1960) who found no rise in urine 17-hydroxycorticosteroids in healthy volunteers given alcohol. Any such rise might be due soley to alcohol-induced diuresis. More specifically, increases in plasma cortisol

[†]Explanation of terms used:
(i)   11-hydroxy corticosteroids (11-OHCS) are unconjugated steroids with a hydroxyl group at position 11. When measured fluorometrically cortisol is the main steroid measured, though corticosterone does contribute.
(ii)   Total 17-oxogenic steroids also called 17-hydroxycorticosteroids. In their measurement these 17-hydroxy steroids are converted to the 17-oxo form. They include cortisol, its precursors and its metabolites.
(iii)   17-oxosteroids also called 17-ketosteroids. These include most of the products of the androgen pathway, both from the adrenal and from the gonads. Testosterone itself is not a 17-oxosteroid.

Table 7.12

Cortisol Levels in Plasma and Urine of Alcoholics and Normals given Alcohol.

	Range	Control	Number of subjects	Clinical details	Reference
Plasma	22 ± 7 μg/100 ml	8 ± 1	7	alcoholics with hypoglycaemia	Joffe et al., 1975
Plasma Urine	12.06 ± 0.62 μg/100 ml (S.E.) 260.12 ± 68.20 ng/min	16.85 ± 2.30 161.12 ± 39.87	8	social drinkers given 2ml/kgbw gin	Muir et al., 1973
Plasma (a.m.)	21.8 ± 4.35 μg/100 ml (S.D.)	12.9 ± 4.2	20	chronic alcoholic	Margraf et al., 1967
**Urine	19.2 (11–24) mg/24h	20.5 (12–28)	50		
*Plasma	29.8 ± 11.4 μg/100 ml	15.2 ± 3.9	9	healthy volunteers given alcohol 1.5 ml/kgbw	Bellet et al., 1970
Plasma	71.4–115 [+] μg/100 ml 57.5–74.8 [++] μg/100 ml		5	chronic alcoholic	Levy et al., 1973
Serum (a.m.)	13.9 ± 6.1 μg/100 ml (S.D.) 12.5 ± 5.6 16.9 ± 6.7 19.2 ± 7.9	11.9 ± 3.8 13.2 ± 4.8 	4 4 4 4	non-alcoholic non-alcoholic in withdrawal alcoholic given alcohol 4g/kgbw alcoholic in withdrawal	Mendelson and Stein, 1966
***Urine	9.7–12.9 mg/24h	8.2	5	alcoholic	Rutter 1968
Serum	elevated		4	alcoholic given alcohol	Mendelson et al., 1971
Plasma	elevated		13	healthy controls given i.v. alcohol	Jenkins and Connolly, 1968

Table 7.12 (*continued*)

Plasma (a.m.)	elevated	30	chronic alcoholic abstinent	Merry and Marks, 1972
	decreased	30	alcoholic given alcohol c/f rise in cortisol in normals given alcohol	
Plasma	elevated	15	healthy volunteer given alcohol 1–1.5 g/kgbw	Fazekas, 1966
*Plasma	elevated	11	healthy volunteer	Bellet *et al.*, 1971
Urine	0.57 ± 0.079 mg/h	0.50 ± 0.049	7	healthy volunteers given alcohol 0.5–0.7 g/kgbw	Perman, 1961

*11-OHCS +competitive displacement ++double isotope dilution *17-hydroxycorticosteroids ***17-oxogenic steroids following ethanol ingestion in non-alcoholic volunteers have been shown by several workers (Mendelson and Stein, 1966; Jenkins and Connolly, 1968; Merry and Marks, 1969; Bellet *et al.*, 1970; Bellet *et al.*, 1971). Jenkins and Connolly (1968) found increases in blood cortisol in both male and female subjects, but only when blood alcohol levels were greater than approximately 100 mg/100 ml. Similar results were obtained by Merry and Marks (1969), except that no increase was found in those apparently healthy subject who admitted to heavy drinking in the past. An increase in plasma cortisol was found only in those subjects who suffered gastrointestinal (GIT) symptoms (Mendelson and Stein, 1966). Their subjects, however, did not attain high blood alcohol levels and hence the increase in plasma cortisol may be a stress response to a GIT disturbance.

ALCOHOLICS

Studies of adrenocortical activity in alcoholics have yielded confusing results. Preliminary studies indicated that blood and urine 17-hydroxycorticosteroids are increased in alcoholics who are drinking (Krusius, 1958; Kissin *et al.*, 1960). However this increased excretion may result from an ethanol induced diuresis which allows enhanced clearance of the metabolite. Blood cortisol levels have been found to be both elevated (Mendelson and Stein, 1966) and normal (Merry and Marks, 1969) in drinking alcoholics. Some studies correlate this increase in blood cortisol with the peak in blood alcohol concentration (Mendelson *et al.*, 1971), whilst other workers (Stokes, 1973) have found increased blood cortisol levels during the withdrawal phase.

In summary, the mechanism by which ethanol stimulates adrenocortical secretory activity is not fully understood and three theories have been advanced to explain increased cortisol levels: (Mendelson and Stein, 1966; Margraf *et al.*, 1967; Mendelson *et al.*, 1971; Merry and Marks, 1973).

(i) Increased ACTH secretion due to stress, induced or exacerbated by alcohol.

(ii) Impaired catabolism of cortisol due to hepatic dysfunction secondary to alcohol abuse.

(iii) Increased secretion of corticotrophin (CRF) *via* activation of neural pituitary circuits by ethanol.

In contrast there have been however suggestions of pituitary-adrenocortical insufficiency in chronic alcoholics. Here again the literature is confusing. Early workers found a lack of eosinophilic response to ACTH and epinephrine in chronic alcoholics which was thought to support this. However, it is now known that this is not a good index of adrenal function (Gordon and Southren, 1977).

Later Kissin *et al.*, (1969) by measuring urinary 17-hydroxycorticosteroids and by measuring removal of a non-tracer steroid, concluded that the decrease in adrenocortical responsiveness they found in alcoholics was due to liver disease. Liver disease is known to alter both cortisol clearance by the liver and its metabolism (Gordon and Southren, 1977). This approach was confirmed by Margraf *et al.*, (1967) who studied adrenocortical function in alcoholics. Their findings are summarised in Table 7.13.

Table 7.13

Adrenocortical Activity in Alcoholics

Test	Response
Cortisol Secretion Rate	Normal
Plasma cortisol (fasting 8 a.m.)	Elevated
Total 17-hydroxycorticosteroids	Normal
Urinary 'Porter-Silber' chromogens-cortisol metabolites	Lowered
Plasma corticosterone	Elevated
Urinary 17-oxosteroids	Lowered
Response to ACTH Stimulation	Lowered
Metabolism of Exogenous Hydrocortisone	Lowered
Urinary Metabolites of Corticosterone	Elevated

From these findings and results of cortisol-^{14}C tracer studies in cirrhotics (Zumoff *et al.*, 1967) it was concluded that alterations in steroid metabolism and not adrenocortical function are found in alcoholics.

There remains the possibility of adrenocortical hypofunction due to hypothalamic-pituitary insufficiency. Studies in patients with pituitary lesions, but a normal response to ACTH, show that there is no increase in plasma cortisol after alcohol administration (Jenkins and Connolly, 1968). From this the authors conclude that the normal ethanol effect on cortisol levels is mediated through the pituitary. Merry and Marks (1969, 1972, 1973) have studied the effect of ethanol on the hypothalamic-pituitary-adrenal axis. They found that in acutely withdrawn alcoholics the plasma cortisol level at 0900 hrs. was higher than normal after about 12 hours without alcohol and fell after the ingestion of moderate amounts of alcohol. This contrasts with normal volunteers whose cortisol levels rose on drinking. Thirty per cent of the drinking subjects showed subnormal plasma cortisol response to insulin induced hypoglycaemia. This response returned to normal on abstinence. From these results it is suggested that, in normal subjects, alcohol stimulates the adrenocortical axis, whilst in chronic alcoholics, alcohol reduces the initially elevated cortisol levels, reflecting suppression of the increased hypothalamic-pituitary-adrenal axis activity. It was suggested that this suppression of adrenocortical activity was due to the sedative effects of alcohol or due to a direct effect on the neuroendocrine regulatory centres of the central nervous system.

Finally, the increase in cortisol levels in the blood due to alcohol discussed previously is also reflected in the appearance of Cushingoid features in some patients. Smals *et al.*, (1976) Paton (1976) and Rees *et al.*, (1977) have described an 'alcohol-induced pseudo-Cushing's Syndrome'. The abnormalities of this pseudo-Cushing's Syndrome revert to normal on ethanol withdrawal. Thus a history of alcohol intake should be obtained where Cushing's Syndrome is suspected.

An interesting variation of this syndrome was reported by Frajna and Angeli (1977). They describe two cases with the clinical features of alcohol-induced Pseudo-Cushing's Syndrome. However, these patients had normal to low plasma cortisol levels, normal urinary excretion of hydroxycorticosteroids and 17-oxosteroids, and showed a normal response to Synacthen stimulation. They were however found to have decreased cortisol binding capacity. This might reflect a decrease in cortisol binding globulin due to decreased hepatic synthesis, to enhanced metabolism of the globulin or to the interference by other compounds in binding, e.g. lipoproteins.

There has also been a report of an alcoholic patient with low plasma cortisol and low urinary 17-hydroxycorticosteroids. This patient, admitted with alcohol-induced hypoglycemic coma, was found to be suffering from an isolated corticotrophin-deficiency. This is however a rare occurrence (Baba *et al.*, 1976).

7.8.2 Mineralocorticoids

The main mineralocorticoid synthesized by the adrenal cortex is aldosterone. Its main physiological actions are in water, sodium and potassium homeostasis.

Whilst many earlier workers had observed the effects of alcohol on water and electrolyte balance, and whilst alcohol was known to stimulate glucocorticoid release, there has not until recently been much investigation into the effect of alcohol on mineralocorticoid secretion.

Fabre *et al.*, (1977) studied urinary levels of aldosterone in alcoholics. The levels of aldosterone in urine rose whilst the subjects were drinking, though on prolonged consumption they began to fall again. There are several possible modes of action for ethanol to bring about these changes. *Firstly,* changes in the control of aldosterone synthesis might occur (see Figure 7.8). Alcohol may affect aldosterone synthesis by bringing about pressure or volume changes. *Secondly,* alcohol might have a direct effect on aldosterone synthesis in the adrenal cortex. The first mechanism seems the more likely when considering the results of various animal experiments and the fact that in humans antidiuretic hormone is inhibited by ethanol. This might lead to the change in whole blood volume necessary to alter aldosterone production and excretion.

Studies by Linkola (1975) and Linkola *et al.*, (1976) involving healthy male volunteers support this view. They showed that ethanol had a stimulatory effect on the renin-aldosterone axis. Plasma renin activity increased by 100% when

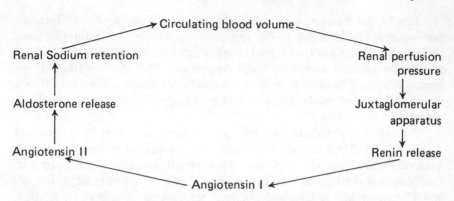

Fig. 7.8 – Renin-angiotensin-aldosterone System.

ethanol was ingested and by 200% during hangover. Plasma aldosterone, on the other hand, decreased during alcohol intoxication but increased greatly during hangover. The authors suggest that the stimulation of the renin-aldosterone axis during alcohol intoxication and hangover is due to dehydration and to increased activity of the sympathetic nervous system.

7.8.3 Sex Hormones

The androgens, C_{19} steroids, are synthesized by a wide variety of tissues: the adrenal, the gonads and the foetoplacental unit (Rudd, 1977). Whilst the synthesis of the adrenal androgens is under the control of ACTH, the hormones, follicle stimulating hormone (FSH) and luteinizing hormone (LH) regulate androgen synthesis in the gonads. Little is known about the control of their synthesis in the foetoplacental unit. There are also differences in the pathways of biosynthesis at these different sites. The adrenal and gonadal androgens will be considered here. The effect of alcohol ingestion on the foetoplacental synthesis of androgens remains unknown, though it may be relevant in the development of the Foetal-Alcohol-Syndrome. The adrenal androgens are chiefly dehydro-epiandrosterone (DHA) and its sulphate (DHAS) and Δ ^{4}-androstenedione. These steroids have an anabolic function. Testosterone is the main androgen of the gonads. For a comprehensive discussion of androgen metabolism see Rudd (1977).

The effects of alcohol on the hypothalamic-pituitary axis have been reviewed (Van Thiel and Lester, 1976). These authors emphasise that there are two effects (1) hypogonadism i.e. gonadal failure and (2) hyperoestrogenisation. From clinical observation it has been known for some time that alcohol affects gonadal function. This is seen as impotence, loss of libido, testicular atrophy, abnormal distribution of body and pubic hair, and gynaecomastia (Distiller *et al.*, 1976). Histological studies in animals and humans also indicate that alcohol has an adverse effect on gonadal structure (Gordon and Southren, 1977). However it is only since the development of radioimmunoassays that the mechanism of alcoholic hypogonadism and feminisation has in any way been understood. Several abnormalities may account for it: changes in hormone production and clearance rates, interconversion of hormones, changes in protein binding and abnormal liver function. Studies have concentrated on two main areas (A) testosterone metabolism (B) oestrogen metabolism, which will now be discussed.

A TESTOSTERONE

Alcohol is known to influence serum and urinary testosterone levels. In healthy volunteers a decrease in plasma testosterone has been found, (Ylikahri et al., 1974c,d; Dotson et al., 1975; Mendelson et al., 1977). In some cases testosterone levels only fell on withdrawal, or 12–20h after intoxication during hangover (Ylikahri et al., 1974c,d; Huttunen et al., 1976) whilst some studies have shown a fall during normal social drinking (Dotson et al., 1975). Acute alcohol ingestion in normals has also been shown to have no effect on plasma testosterone either during intoxication or during withdrawal (Toro et al., 1973; Farmer and Fabre, 1975). A more detailed study has been made by Gordon and Southren (1977) who showed that normally testosterone is secreted episodically, and that when alcohol is given there is a loss of secretory episodes and a fall in the mean plasma testosterone.

Plasma testosterone levels are low in alcoholics, either abstinent or drinking (Liegel et al., 1972; Mendelson and Mello, 1974; Distiller et al., 1976; Persky et al., 1977), whilst urinary excretion of testosterone glucuronide is also increased in alcoholics (Fabre et al., 1973). Studies on testosterone and 17β-hydroxyandrogen levels suggest that there may be an increase in plasma testosterone in the post-drinking phase. This may represent a 'rebound' reaction (Mendelson and Mello, 1974; Wright et al., 1975).

There are several possible mechanisms for these changes in androgen levels. They are (1) altered hypothalamic-pituitary-gonadal function (2) altered androgen metabolism (3) changes in plasma protein binding.

Hypothalamic-pituitary-gondal function. Gonadotrophin and testosterone levels have been studied in male alcoholics (Distiller et al., 1976). These workers found that whilst basal testosterone levels were low, the response of LH/FSH to luteinising hormone releasing hormone (LHRH) and of testosterone to human chorionic gonadotrophin (HCG) were normal. A suppressive effect of alcohol on the pituitary was therefore excluded as a cause for hypogonadism in alcoholic cirrhosis. They suggest that there is evidence of some testicular reserve and also that the low plasma testosterone levels are not due to Leydig cell dysfunction.

Van Thiel et al., (1974), studying the hypothalamic-pituitary axis in alcoholic men, found contrasting results. Plasma testosterone was found to be low, plasma

FSH and LH were normal to elevated, plasma oestradiol was normal, whilst sex steroid-binding globulin was raised. Clomiphene responses were diminished in the majority as shown by there being no increase in either gonadotrophin on Clomiphene stimulation. The alcoholics also failed to show an increase in plasma testosterone after administration of chorionic gonadotrophin. These results indicate that there is primary gondal failure (reduced testicular steroidogenesis) and hypothalamic suppression in men with alcoholic liver disease.

Altered androgen metabolism. Alcohol has been shown to have several effects on androgen metabolism. Firstly, it has been shown to cause a shift from oxidative to reductive metabolism (Cronholm and Sjöval, 1968, 1970; Fabre *et al.*, 1973), see Figure 7.9. Secondly, normal males given alcohol show a 40% increase in the clearance of testosterone during withdrawal (Gordon and Southren, 1977). This may be explained by the increase in liver testosterone reductase which is the rate limiting enzyme for testerone metabolism, and which has been found both in alcoholics and volunteers given alcohol (Rubin *et al.*, 1976). The increase in this enzyme may enhance the removal of testosterone and other Δ^4-3-ketosteroids in the liver. Increased hepatic blood flow is also found and would contribute to the increased clearance of testosterone.

Thirdly, a decreased production rate of testosterone has been demonstrated in normal volunteers given alcohol for 24 days (Gordon *et al.*, 1976).

androst-5-ene-3β, 17β-diol ⟵⎯⎯⎯⟶ dehydroepiandrosterone

5-α-androstan-3α, 17β-diol ⟵⎯⎯⎯⟶ androsterone

5-α-androstane-3β, 17β-diol ⟵⎯⎯⎯⟶ 3β-hydroxy-5 α-androstane-17-one

Fig. 7.9 – Effect of decreased NAD/NADH ratio on androgen metabolism.
(Cronholm and Sjövall 1968 and 1970)

Plasma protein binding. Sex hormone binding globulin (SHBG) is the transport protein for testosterone. Two disturbances may occur due to alcohol: an increase in the level of the protein itself and a decrease in its binding capacity.

Increases in SHBG in alcoholics have been reported (Van Thiel *et al.*, 1974). This may accentuate the low levels of plasma testosterone found in alcoholics because it would diminish the amount of free active hormone. This increase in SHBG may be due to the hyperoestrogenaemia found in alcoholics.

In contrast to the above findings, decreased binding capacities have been found in normals and alcoholics (Gordon and Southren, 1977). No change in binding capacity was found in acute alcohol ingestion or when alcohol was added to the serum.

Thus in those alcoholics without cirrhosis, there is a decrease in plasma testosterone partly due to a direct effect on the gonads and partly, though perhaps more chronically, due to central nervous system effects. Further variations are brought about by changes in metabolism. In alcoholics with cirrhosis a similar picture is seen, except that there is a decrease in protein binding and decreased clearance. These changes may reflect liver dysfunction (Gordon and Southren, 1977).

B. OESTROGENS

As well as changes in androgen metabolism, changes in oestrogen metabolism are thought to contribute to some of the clinical findings in alcoholics (see Figure 7.10).

Whilst there have been conflicting reports as to whether plasma oestradiol is raised in alcoholics, plasma oestrone levels have been found to be increased (Van Thiel *et al.*, 1975), as have urinary oestrone and oestriol (a metabolite of oestrone). Total plasma oestriol has been shown to be normal or reduced in

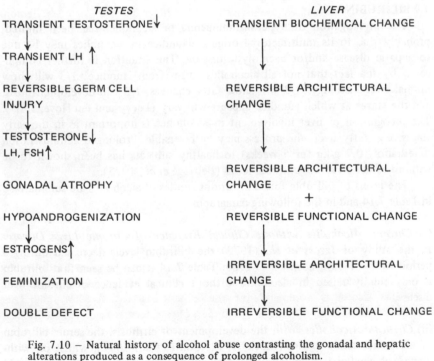

Fig. 7.10 – Natural history of alcohol abuse contrasting the gonadal and hepatic alterations produced as a consequence of prolonged alcoholism.
Reproduced with permission from Van Thiel and Lester, 1976, *Gastroenterology*.
The Williams and Wilkins Co., Baltimore

alcoholics (Van Thiel *et al.*, 1974). There have also been reports of increased conversion of adrenal androgens to oestrogens. Other hormonal changes reflect this hyperoestrogenemia, e.g. increased levels of prolactin and neurophysin in alcoholic men (Pentikäinen *et al.*, 1975; Van Thiel and Lester, 1976). Although hyperoestrogenaemia has been demonstrated in alcoholics, its mechanism remains unclear.

Reduced biliary excretion, decreased hepatic uptake of oestrogens, changes in plasma binding proteins and other causes have been suggested (Pentikäinen *et al.*, 1975).

In conclusion, the symptoms of feminization in alcoholics reflect changes in the hypothalamic-pituitary gondal function and in testosterone metabolism. Such changes are further aggravated by changes in hepatic clearance, protein binding and by hyperoestrogenaemia, whose aetiology remains unknown. It should always be remembered, when considering these studies, that is difficult to separate the direct effects of alcohol from the effects of alcoholic liver disease. Worthy of note is the fact that little if anything is known of the effect of alcohol on the sex hormones in women.

7.9 BILIRUBIN

The investigation of hyperbilirubinaemia in alcoholics has been limited, probably due to its multifactorial origins. Jaundice in alcoholics may be due to hepatic disease and/or haemolytic disease. The situation is further complicated by the fact that not all alcoholics suffer from jaundice: 1/3 will show normal liver histology, 1/3 will show fatty changes, 1/3 will develop cirrhosis, and the stages at which jaundice appears will vary (Leevy and ten Hove, 1967). The recognition of liver involvement in alcoholics is important as in the early stages, e.g. fatty liver, the process may be reversible. Prolonged administration of ethanol (0.9 g/kg for 5 weeks) to healthy subjects has been shown to be without effect on serum bilirubin levels (Belfrage *et al.*, 1973).

The levels of bilirubin found in various studies of alcoholics are summarized in Table 7.14 and in the following paragraphs.

(i) *Chronic Alcoholics without Clinical Evidence of Chronic Liver Disease.* In the study of Jaross *et al.*, (1972) the bilirubin levels decreased during a period of 7–14 days abstinence. From Table 7.14 it can be seen that bilirubin is only mildly raised in alcoholics without clinical evidence of chronic liver disease.

(ii) *Cirrhotic Alcoholics.* With the development of cirrhosis, the serum bilirubin of alcoholics tends to rise (Block, 1972; Conti *et al.*, 1972), whilst on withdrawal of alcohol it may fall. This is exemplified by a study of a 39 year old alcoholic reported by Block (1972). The serum total bilirubin level of this

Table 7.14
Serum Bilirubin Levels in Alcoholics

Specimen	Reference interval (normal range) or control values	Mean ± SD	Number of subjects	Clinical details	Reference
Serum (total)	0.8–1.3 mg/100 ml	< 1	6	chronic alcoholic	Nair et al., 1971
Serum (total)	1.2–2.1 mg/100 ml	< 1	25	chronic alcoholic	Mezey and Tobon, 1971
Serum		0.87 ± 0.45 mg/100 ml	41	chronic alcoholic	Jaross et al., 1972
Serum (total)		0.45 ± 0.11	22	alcohol intoxicated patient	Redetzki et al., 1972
Serum (direct)		0.78 ± 0.52 mg/100 ml	21		
		0.31 ± 0.24 mg/100 ml			

patient fell from 3.9 mg/100 ml to 0.45 mg/100 ml (Direct bilirubin from 1.9 to 0.05 mg/100 ml) during the course of hospitalization and abstinence. Conversely, as the bilirubin rises the prognosis becomes worse.

(iii) *Alcoholic Hepatitis.* Total bilirubin levels of 11.5–35 mg/100 ml have been found in cases of fatal alcoholic hepatitis, unassociated with cirrhosis, but with a long history of alcoholism (Jewell *et al.,* 1971). Almost all the bilirubin was direct reading. It would seem that a high bilirubin carried a poor prognosis.

(iv) *Haemolytic Jaundice.* Alcoholic patients may suffer from anaemia due to many factors, of which haemolysis is one. The recognition of haemolytic disease is complicated by other results of hepatic dysfunction, though the indirect/total bilirubin ratio has been found to be useful (Sherwood, 1972). However, in a case of transient intravascular haemolysis associated with alcoholic liver disease and hyperlipidaemia, the ratio of total/direct bilirubin was not found to reflect the haemolytic nature of the disease as shown by the absence of plasma hapto-globin (Powell *et al.,* 1972). This may result from the stimulation of glucuronid-ation of bilirubin by ethanol (Waltman *et al.,* 1969). In other haematological disorders in alcoholics e.g. sideroblastic anaemia, megaloblastic anaemia and leukopenia, the bilirubin is only mildly raised (Hines and Cowan, 1970; Pezzimenti and Lindenbaum, 1972; Liu, 1973).

(v) *Miscellaneous.* Total bilirubin has been found to be moderately raised in alcoholics with delirium tremens (Irsigler *et al.,* 1971) and in non-alcoholic patients with hypertriglyceridaemia which is ethanol dependent (Kudzma and Schonfeld, 1971).

Finally, it has been suggested (Orten and Sardesai, 1971) that alterations in the distribution and availability of NAD, due to ethanol metabolism, might cause changes in porphyrin metabolism. Conversion of coproporphyrinogen to protoporphyrin requires NAD.

7.10 PORPHYRINS AND RELATED COMPOUNDS

The pophyrias, a complex group of disorders of porphyrin metabolism, have long been known to be affected by the ingestion of ethanol. Franke and Fimkemtscher (1935) were the first to show that the administration of ethanol to alcoholics and to healthy men resulted in an increased urinary excretion of coproporphyrin. Ethanol has been shown to be a precipitating factor in some types of porphrias, e.g. acute intermittent porphyria and cutaneous hepatic porphyria. Many studies support the role of ethanol as a precipitating factor of cutaneous hepatic porphyria. Eales (1963) showed that the clinical relationship of ethanol intake to porphyria cutanea tarda in South Africa is suggested by the almost invariable finding of chronic alcoholism in patients with this disease. An interesting paper of Ferguson *et al.*, (1970) presents the cases of identical twins who both suffered from acute intermittent porphyria. In both cases, though there were complicating factors, ethanol was thought to be the precipitating factor. Urinary porphobilinogen, uroporphyrin and coproporphyrin were raised in both twins.

Many studies in alcoholics and normals have shown that ethanol causes an increased urinary excretion of porphyrins (Orten *et al.*, 1963). The response seems to be dose dependent, but independent of the degree of liver dysfunction. The main porphyrin to be excreted is coproporphyrin III (Watson *et al.*, 1951). Increases in other intermediates δ-amino-laevulinic acid (ALA), porphobilinogen (PBG), coproporphyrin, and uroporphyrin III have been found in the urine of alcoholics (Orten *et al.*, 1963; Orten and Sardesai, 1971). Also red blood cell protoporphyrin and coproporphyrin levels are reported to be elevated in acute alcoholics (Ali and Sweeney, 1974).

In considering the mechanisms of these changes the normal synthesis of the porphyrins should be considered (Figure 7.11). Many theories have been put forward to account for the increase in porphyrin excretion in alcoholics. Increased production could occur due to:

(a) increased formation of ALA from succinyl-CoA and glycine

(b) a block or partial block in the conversion of coproporphyrinogen to protoporphyrin

(c) the action of congeners present in alcoholic beverages

(d) deficiency of cellular NAD which is required for the oxidation of coproporphyrinogen to protoporphyrinogen (Orten and Sardesai, 1971).

The finding of elevated ALA synthetase levels following administration of ethanol suggest that increased formation of ALA may be the cause of the increased porphyrin excretion (Krasner *et al.*, 1974). However Nair *et al.*, (1971) concluded that the effect of ethanol was not due to the induction of this enzyme. They showed that Vitamin E induces a significant depression in the urinary excretion of porphyrins and their precursors in porphyria, whereas the vitamin has no effect on similar changes in chronic alcoholism. They suggest that Vitamin E acts by blocking the induction of hepatic ALA synthetase in porphyria, but not in alcoholics.

Elevated urinary levels of coproporphyrin following ethanol administration may point to ethanol interference with the coproporphyrinogen to protoporphyrin conversion. It seems unlikely that the congeners in alcoholic beverages interfere with porphyrin metabolism changes, but some disruption in the regulation of metabolism through ethanol is possible.

Finally it has been suggested (Orten and Sardesai, 1971) that alterations in the distribution and availability of NAD, due to ethanol metabolism, might cause changes in porphyrin metabolism. Conversion of coproporphyrinogen to protoporphyrin requires NAD. Competition between ethanol and this metab-

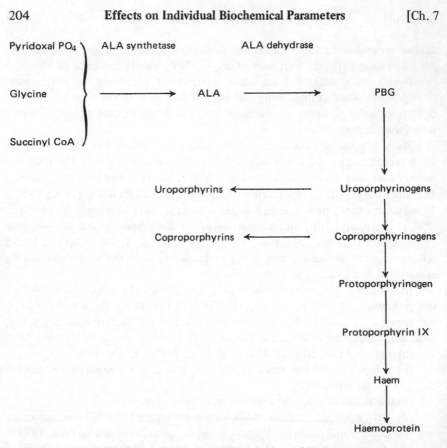

Fig. 7.11 – Biosynthesis of Porphyrins and Haem.

olite for available NAD could lead to an accumulation of coproporphyrinogen and a backing-up of earlier metabolites. Alternatively, increased levels of NADH arising from excessive and/or prolonged ethanol oxidation could compete with succinate in the electron transport chain, and so lead to increased succinate levels and consequent increased porphyrin production.

7.11 CARBOHYDRATE METABOLISM

7.11.1 Introduction

Although there have been numerous studies and reviews (e.g. Badawy, 1977; Isselbacher, 1977) of the effects of ethanol on carbohydrate metabolism, the mechanisms of those disturbances are, so far, incompletely understood. Many factors complicate studies of carbohydrate metabolism following ethanol ingestion including:

1. Nutritional status.
2. Diet.
3. Dose of ethanol.
4. Degree of physical activity.
5. Acute *versus* chronic alcohol abuse.
6. Experience of alcohol (alcohol naive, social drinker, *etc.*).
7. Presence of malabsorption.
8. Effects of ethanol on endocrine systems.
9. Increased hepatic levels of NADH.

Generally, ethanol affects carbohydrate metabolism *via* (i) the ethanol metabolite, acetate, (ii) the change in the balance of the NAD/NADH redox pair during ethanol metabolism, (iii) the actions of ethanol on other metabolic systems.

7.11.2 Biochemistry

The basic biochemical effects will be reviewed briefly (for a fuller discussion see Hawkins and Kalant, 1972; Badaway 1977) before discussion of their clinical relevance.

(a) METABOLISM OF ACETATE

Ethanol is metabolised to acetaldehyde, and the latter to acetate, both in the liver. Acetate (or its active form, acetyl CoA) can be used by many tissues to produce energy by metabolism through the TCA (Krebs) cycle. Acetyl CoA levels have been shown to be affected by ethanol metabolism (Hawkins and Kalant, 1972).

(b) THE TRICARBOXYLIC ACID (TCA OR KREBS) CYCLE

The mitochondrion carries out the functions of (a) oxidation of pyruvate to carbon dioxide coupled with NADH formation, (b) reoxidation of NADH to NAD by the electron transport chain, and (c) coupling of NADH oxidation to ATP formation. These are dependent on the functioning of the tricarboxylic acid cycle and the electron transport chain. Ethanol may have several effects, though it has been shown that the overall effect is inhibition of the TCA Cycle (Forsander, 1970). One possible mechanism for this inhibition is that NADH produced during ethanol metabolism may decrease pyruvate levels and hence levels of oxaloacetate, the first component of the TCA Cycle. In addition, the altered redox state may alter the malate/oxaloacetate ratio, and thus inhibit the cycle (see Figure 7.12).

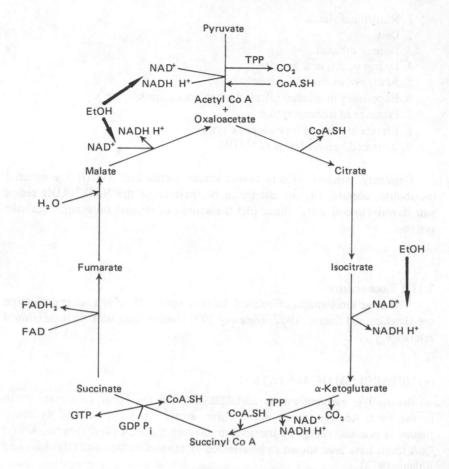

Fig. 7.12 – The Tricarboxylic acid cycle:
Sites of action of ethanol.

(c) GLUCONEOGENESIS

Ethanol inhibits hepatic gluconeogenesis and again several possible mechanisms have been proposed. Firstly, the change in the NADH/NAD ratio decreases pyruvate levels and thus limits the action of pyruvate carboxylase and hence the formation of phosphoenolpyruvate. Secondly, the increase in the above ratio inhibits the conversion of some amino-acids into intermediates utilized in the gluconeogenic pathway, which has important implications for the generation of alcohol-induced hypoglycaemia (Madison, 1968).

(d) GLYCOLYSIS

Ethanol inhibits hepatic glycolysis by inhibiting the step:

3-glyceraldehyde phosphate $+ NAD^+ + P_i \longrightarrow 1,3 -$ diphosphoglycerate

$$+ NADH + H^+$$

This may be due to the increase in the ratio NADH/NAD or, less likely, to inhibition of the enzyme aldehyde dehydrogenase.

Little is known of the effect of ethanol on brain glycolysis, though it may well similarly be inhibited.

(e) GLYCOGENOLYSIS

Glycogenolysis is the complex metabolic pathway by which the storage carbohydrate glycogen is converted into an easily transportable and usable form, glucose. Glycogenolysis is controlled by variations in phosphorylase activity, an enzyme which exists in muscle in an active and an inactive form. The secretion of adrenaline stimulates the formation of active phosphorylase through c–AMP, and since ethanol stimulates the release of catecholamines it may thus influence glycogenolysis.

(f) THE PENTOSE PHOSPHATE PATHWAY

Glucose may also be degraded by the pentose phosphate pathway (Hexose monophosphate shunt, 6-phosphogluconate pathway). Although it is not known whether ethanol affects this pathway in humans, animal experiments suggest that ethanol metabolism, possibly *via* the MEOS, may affect the ratio $NADP^+/NADPH$ and hence the pentose phosphate pathway (see Figure 7.13).

(g) GALACTOSE METABOLISM

Ethanol has been found to decrease the rate of conversion of galactose to carbon dioxide and of its removal from the circulation in the normal subject. It has been suggested (Segal and Blair, 1961) that this is due to the increase in NADH inhibiting the enzyme uridine diphosphate-galactose-4-epimerase (see Figure 7.14).

(h) FRUCTOSE AND SORBITOL METABOLISM

Evidence suggests that, through the increase of NADH, ethanol increases conversion of fructose to sorbitol. There may also be an inhibition of sorbitol oxidation by the NAD-dependent enzyme sorbitol dehydrogenase (Hawkins and Kalant, 1972; Badaway, 1977) (see Figure 7.15).

7.11.3 Clinical Aspects

Clinically two types of carbohydrate disturbance due to ethanol have been described. The first is a diabetic-like glucose intolerance with hyperglycaemia and the second an alcohol-induced hypoglycaemia.

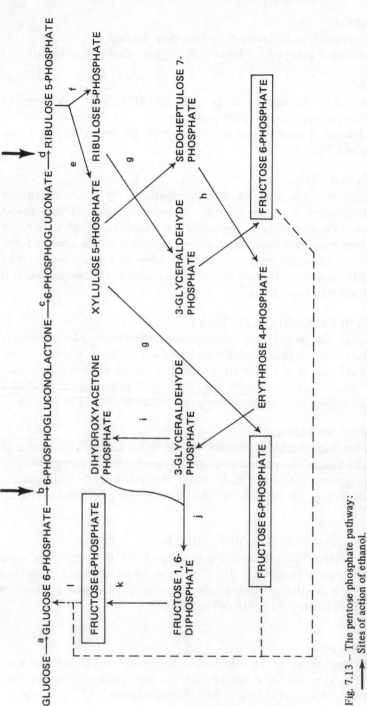

Fig. 7.13 – The pentose phosphate pathway:

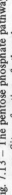 Sites of action of ethanol.

(a) hexokinase (b) glucose-6-phosphate dehydrogenase (c) gluconolactonase (d) 6-phosphogluconate dehydrogenase (e) phosphopentose epimerase (f) phosphopentose isomerase (g) transketolase (h) transaldolase (i) triose phosphate isomerase (j) aldolase (k) fructose 6-phosphatase (l) phosphoglucoisomerase.

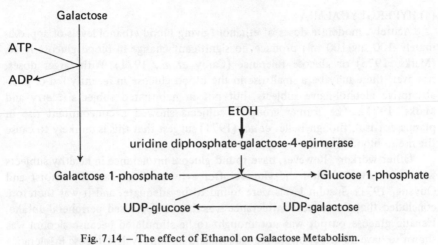

Galactose

ATP

ADP

EtOH

uridine diphosphate-galactose-4-epimerase

Galactose 1-phosphate ——————————→ Glucose 1-phosphate

UDP-glucose �←—————————— UDP-galactose

Fig. 7.14 – The effect of Ethanol on Galactose Metabolism.
——→ Site of action of ethanol

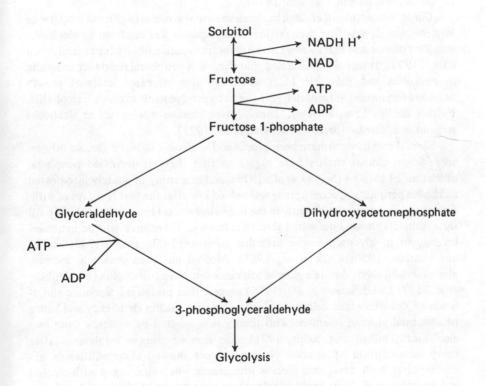

Sorbitol

NADH H$^+$

NAD

Fructose

ATP

ADP

Fructose 1-phosphate

Glyceraldehyde   Dihydroxyacetonephosphate

ATP

ADP

3-phosphoglyceraldehyde

Glycolysis

Fig. 7.15 – Fructose and sorbitol metabolism.

(a) HYPERGLYCAEMIA

Acutely, moderate doses of ethanol (giving blood ethanol levels of approximately 100 mg/100 ml) produce no significant change in blood glucose levels (Marks, 1975) or glucose tolerance (Carey et al., 1971). With larger doses, however, there may be a small rise in the blood glucose in recently fed or post-absorptive alcohol-naive subjects, but not in habituated subjects (Merry and Marks, 1971). The former group of subjects showed a concomitant rise in plasma cortisol, though Bellet et al., (1971) suggest that this is unlikely to cause the rise in blood glucose.

Other workers, however, have found glucose intolerance in healthy subjects who were given alcohol and glucose after a twelve hour fast (Dornhorst and Ouyang, 1971). Insulin levels were found to be adequate, and it was therefore concluded that the glucose intolerance was due to decreased peripheral uptake. Hepatic glucose output was not thought to be stimulated because alcohol was shown to have no effect on fasting glucose and insulin levels. Glucose intolerance was demonstrated in normal subjects who were given moderate doses of alcohol daily for a week and this intolerance was thought to be due to tissue resistance to insulin (Nikkilä and Taskinen, 1975).

Chronic ingestion of ethanol has been shown to give rise to glucose intolerance in alcoholics. It was first thought that this response was confined to alcoholics with liver disease and that there was some defect in hepatic carbohydrate metabolism (Arky, 1971). It was also postulated that there was peripheral resistance to insulin in cirrhotics and that this, in combination with increased levels of growth hormone (an insulin antagonist), gave rise to hyperglycaemia in chronic alcoholics. Further studies have, however, demonstrated glucose intolerance in alcoholics without liver disease (Sereny et al., Had et al., 1975).

Several mechanisms have been proposed for alcohol induced glucose intolerance. Some animal studies have suggested that there is decreased peripheral utilisation of glucose (Sereny et al., 1975), and in a study of acutely intoxicated alcoholics peripheral glucose uptake was indeed low after the first few days of withdrawal and increased significantly in the following weeks (Erikson et al., 1974). All these subjects showed decreased glucose tolerance. There may also be increased breakdown of glycogen in the liver due to ethanol (Matunaga, 1942; Forbes and Duncan, 1950; Clark et al., 1961). Alcohol has been shown to increase plasma insulin levels during a glucose tolerance test in non-alcoholics (Freidenberg et al., 1971), and Sereny et al., (1975) suggest that prolonged alcoholic stimulation of the pancreatic cells could lead to relative insulin deficiency and hence to abnormal glucose tolerance. This theory is supported by evidence from two alcoholics (Phillips and Safrit, 1971) who showed glucose intolerance after heavy consumption of alcohol. Neither subject showed abnormalities on abstinence but both developed glucose intolerance when challenged with alcohol and carbohydrate. Four healthy volunteers were similarly challenged and one developed glucose intolerance. Glucose intolerance was associated with increased insulin levels and a delay in the attainment of peak insulin concentration. Because the subjects did not all show glucose intolerance, a personal predisposition to alcohol-induced glucose intolerance was proposed. Similar experiments were performed by Friedenberg *et al.*, (1971), and subjects with ethanol priming showed a larger early insulin response to the first of 3 glucose loads. This may indicate that the initially augmented secretory response had resulted in depletion of a finite supply of immediately available insulin. However, other studies of insulin levels during glucose tolerance tests after alcohol ingestion shown no change in insulin levels compared with a control period (see Hed *et al.*, 1975).

It is also possible that gluose intolerance arises in alcoholics due to carbohydrate restriction (Hed *et al.*, 1975) because healthy subjects may show a diabetic type of glucose tolerance curve following carbohydrate restriction (Joplin and Wright, 1968). This may be due to delayed hepatic uptake of the load rather than to decreased peripheral glucose uptake (Jackson *et al.*, 1973). In a study of glucose metabolism in six chronic alcoholics on a carbohydrate-poor diet, glucose tolerance was found to be decreased after alcohol (Hed *et al.*, 1975).

It is also worthy of note that alcoholic hyperglycaemia may be blocked by adrenalectomy in dogs and by β-adrenergic blockade (Ammon and Estler, 1968) indicating that an intact adrenal medullary sympathetic nervous system is needed for this response.

An epidemiological study of 100,000 people (Gerard *et al.*, 1977) has shown an association between alcohol drinking habits and serum glucose one hour after a 75 g dose of glucose. Serum glucose was found to be highest in those who drank 6–8 alcoholic drinks a day, though the effect was diminished at more than 9 drinks a day. This association was found to hold even when subjects were controlled for age, sex, race, adiposity, time since last food, time of day, diabetes, and liver disease. The mechanism of this association is unknown, though these results are of importance as this study, unlike others, was concerned with the habitual use of alcohol.

Whilst the glucose intolerance of alcoholics is not severe and does not require insulin treatment, frank diatetes is still found in alcoholics (Cadoret *et al.*, 1975). A drinking problem in diabetes may complicate their management. Not only do alcoholic beverages add more calories to the diet, but if the patient is taking phenformin lactic acidosis is more likely to develop on alcohol consumption. Alcohol consumption may also interfere with the actions and metabolism of sulphonylurea oral hypoglycaemic agents (e.g. tolbutamide).

Finally, Shanely *et al.*, (1972) considered that, in their experience, oral glucose tolerance is often impaired in patients admitted with alcohol-induced hypoglycaemia but may improve on abstinence. However, with fairly low alcohol doses they could show no effect on glucose tolerance in normal subjects.

(b) HYPOGLYCAEMIA

Alcohol-induced hypoglycaemia was first described by Brown and Harvey in 1941 (see Madison, 1968 for a review of earlier work). This response has subsequently been reported in healthy individuals (Arky and Freinkel, 1969; Moss, 1970; Bagdade et al., 1972a,b; Turner et al., 1973; O'Keefe and Marks, 1977), diabetics (Arky et al., 1968; Bagdade et al., 1972; Turner et al., 1973), and alcoholics (Forsander et al., 1958; Field et al., 1963; Freinkel et al., 1963; De Moura et al., 1967; Ibragimov, 1967; Steer et al., 1969; Joffe et al., 1975). Alcohol induced hypoglycaemia has also been reported in a single patient with isolated adrenocorticotrophic hormone deficiency (Steer et al., 1969), and is thought to occur in other states such as decompensated diabetes and thyrotoxicosis (Arky and Freinkel, 1969). Various workers have distinguished types of alcoholic hypoglycaemia based on the different mechanisms involved (Cohen, 1976; Marks and Wright, 1977). Essentially the hypoglycaemia may be drug-induced but potentiated by ethanol, or it may be a reactive hypoglycaemia.

Potentiation by ethanol of drug-induced hypoglycaemia may be particularly severe. In five insulin-dependent diabetics, who gave themselves insulin with a dose of ethanol, fatal hypoglycaemia developed (Arky et al., 1968); alcohol was thought to interfere with hepatic gluconeogenesis and hence to induce hypoglycaemia whenever gluconeogensis was needed to maintain normal glucose levels.

Hypoglycaemia induced by other factors such as exercise may also be potentiated by the ingestion of alcohol. Studies in chronic alcoholics suggested that this response is not due to defects in cortisol and growth hormone response. However, Marks and Wright (1977) conclude that since alcohol affects catecholamine metabolism, it is possible that delayed recovery from induced hypoglycaemia caused by alcohol is due directly or indirectly to interference with adrenergic mechanisms.

In malnourished or fasting individuals hypoglycaemia may develop 6-36 hours after the ingestion of alcohol. Most non-experimental cases are in adult chronic alcoholics or alcohol-naive children. This is illustrated by the work of Arky and Freinkel (1969) who demonstrated alcohol-induced hypoglycaemia in alcoholics but not in healthy volunteers (see Figure 7.16).

There have, however, been reports of alcohol-induced hypoglycaemia in healthy volunteers (O'Keefe and Marks, 1977). These subjects were given (a) alcohol and sucrose (equivalent to a gin and tonic) (b) alcohol and a very small dose of sucrose (gin and 'slimline' tonic) (c) dose of sucrose (tonic). Their behaviour, symptoms, blood glucose and plasma insulin were monitored for 5 hours. Gin and 'slimline' tonic had no significant effect on glucose or plasma insulin levels. Tonic alone gave rise to mild hypoglycaemia and hyperinsulinaemia. However, gin and tonic gave rise to a greater degree of hypoglycaemia and hyperinsulinaemia. The conditions of the experiment simulated lunch-time drinking and the authors suggest that ethanol-induced hypoglycaemia may have

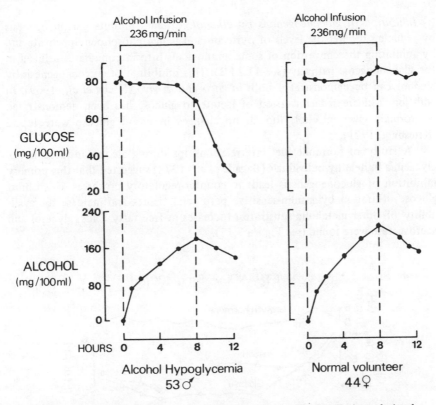

Fig. 7.16 – Glucose response to alcohol after an overnight fast. Patient admitted with alcohol hypoglycaemia and a normal volunteer. Each infusion of 15% alcohol v/v was administered at the ratio of 2 ml/min for 8 hours.
From Arky and Freinkel, Biochemical and Clinical Aspects of Alcohol Metabolism (Sardesai, V. M. *ed.*) 1969. Courtesy of Charles C. Thomas, Publisher, Springfield, Illinois

serious consequences for car drivers. The cause of the hyperinsulinaemia was thought to be alcohol stimulation of the release of one or more intestinal insulin-releasing-polypeptides which augment glucose-stimulated insulin secretion but which do not themselves stimulate insulin secretion except in the presence of hyperglycaemia.

Several mechanisms have been proposed for alcohol-induced hypoglycaemia:
(i) inhibition of gluconeogenesis by ethanol
(ii) inappropriate insulin response
(iii) decreased glycogenolysis
(iv) increased conversion of glucose to a-glycerophosphate
(v) hypothalamic-pituitary-adrenal insufficiency
These mechanisms will now be discussed more fully.

(i) *Inhibition of gluconeogenesis by ethanol.* Ethanol inhibits gluconeogenesis by reducing the hepatic levels of pyruvate and hence phosphoenolpryuvate and by inhibiting the conversion of some amino-acids into intermediates utilized in the gluconeogenic pathway (see 11.11.2). This inhibition of gluconeogenesis by alcohol can be demonstrated both *in vitro* and *in vivo* (Krebs *et al.*, 1969). In addition, a decreased conversion of lactate to glucose has been demonstrated in normals given alcohol, though no changes in blood glucose were found (Kriesberg, 1971).

A study of hormone/fuel interrelationships during alcohol-induced hypoglycaemia in healthy individuals (Bagade *et al.*, 1972) suggested that this primary inhibition of gluconeogenesis leads to counter-regulatory processes which limit glucose utilisation by insulin-sensitive peripheral tissues and increase the availability of other metabolic substrates. Increases in free fatty acids, glycerol and acetoacetate were found (see Figure 7.17).

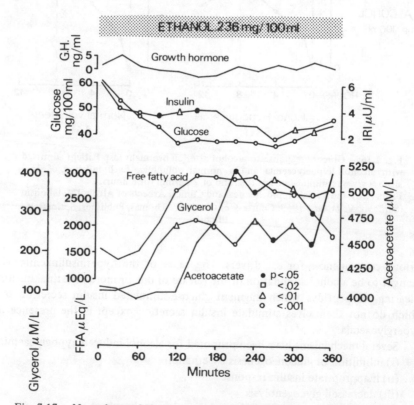

Fig. 7.17 – Mean changes in immunoreactive insulin (IRI), growth hormone (GH) glucose and other substrates in six male subjects during alcohol hypoglycaemia. Reproduced with permission from Bagdade *et al.*, Proceedings of the Society of Experimental Biology and Medicine (1972b)

(ii) *Inappropriate insulin response.* Increased plasma levels of insulin have been found in alcohol-induced hypoglycaemia (Metz *et al.,* 1969; Nikkilä and Taskinen, 1975; O'Keefe and Marks, 1977). O'Keefe and Marks (1977) suggest that the hyperinsulinaemia is due to alcohol stimulation of one or more intestinal insulin releasing polypeptides.

The relationships between ethanol, glucose and insulin levels were examined by Nikkilä and Taskinen (1975) in normal, obese and diabetic subjects. Three experiments were carried out:

(i) Glucose tolerance and insulin levels were studied during ethanol infusion in all three groups of subjects.
(ii) Following moderate meals and an evening drink, overnight glucose and insulin, and glucose tolerance in the morning, were studied in healthy volunteers.
(iii) Glucose tolerance and insulin levels were studied during one week of regular intake of alcohol.

Their results showed that ethanol accelerates the utilisation of glucose, increases the early insulin response to glucose loading, and also increases the second phase response of insulin. In normal subjects this increase in insulin output accentuates the reactive hypoglycaemia which follows glucose loading. Nikkilä and Taskinen (1975) suggested that ethanol-induced hypoglycaemia could occur even without prolonged fasting, and proposed that ethanol influences the secretion of insulin, possibly by affecting the pancreatic β-cell membranes, rather than by influencing hepatic uptake and degradation of insulin.

In contrast to ethanol hypoglycaemia, the subjects given alcohol for a week showed glucose intolerance, with normal insulin levels. This intolerance was thought to be due to insulin resistance of the tissues.

Decreased plasma insulin levels have also been found in alcohol-induced hypoglycaemia (Bagdade *et al.,* 1972; Turner *et al.,* 1973; Joffe *et al.,* 1975). The decreased plasma insulin and increase in other hormones found by Joffe *et al.,* (Table 7.15) indicate that the compensatory mechanisms are appropriate. When the patients were given glucose, some developed hyperglycaemia and this may reflect defective insulin production from slowly-responding pancreatic β-cells. The authors suggest that ethanol might inhibit glucose stimulated insulin secretion after prolonged exposure.

Table 7.15
Hormone/Glucose Interrelationships in Alcohol Induced Hypoglycaemia.

	Glucose mg/100 ml	Insulin μU/ml	Somatropin ng/ml	Hydrocortisone μg/100 ml	Glucagon ng/ml
Patients	22 ± 2	12 ± 1.5	14.9 ± 7.3	22 ± 7	0.67
Controls	84 ± 3	20 ± 2.5	2.3 ± 0.5	8 ± 1	0.20 ± 0.01

(iii) *Decreased glycogenolysis.* Alcohol-induced hypoglycaemia may occur in the fasted individual where liver glycogen is low. Thus glycogenolysis is not effective in counteracting the hypoglycaemia. Ethanol may also affect glycogenolysis through affecting phosphorylase activity.

(iv) *Increased conversion of glucose to α-glycerophosphate.* Studies of extrasplanchnic metabolism (Wolfe *et al.*, 1976) have indicated that in addition to inhibition of hepatic gluconeogensis, enhanced formation of α-glycerophosphate from glucose occurs and accentuates the alcohol-induced hypoglycaemia.

(v) *Hypothalamic-pituitary-adrenal insufficiency.* There is evidence that hypothalamic-pituitary-adrenal insufficiency secondary to chronic alcoholism may also contribute to ethanol-induced hypoglycaemia.

The diagnosis of ethanol-induced hypoglycaemia can be difficult as this condition may be confused clinically with ethanol intoxication itself and other causes of spontaneous hypoglycaemia (De Moura *et al.*, 1967). The subject may present stuporose, comatose or in a confused state. A clinical history of alcohol abuse and fasting, presence of ethanol in the blood, low plasma insulin levels in the presence of hypoglycaemia, and metabolic acidosis with a high lactate/pyruvate ratio may all point to the diagnosis of alcohol-induced hypoglycaemia. Treatment consists of intravenous glucose and hydrocortisone. Mortality has been reported as 10–20% despite treatment and, therefore, hypoglycaemia may well be a cause of unexpected death in alcoholics, remaining undetected at post-mortem.

7.12 LIPIDS AND LIPOPROTEINS

A relationship between alcoholism and hyperlipidaemia was first described by Feigl in 1918 and since then this has been confirmed by many workers. However, it is only within recent years that the biochemical mechanisms involved have been studied, though not fully elucidated. The literature is extensive, but has been reviewed by many authors.[†]

Many conflicting results have been reported and hence further studies are necessary to clarify the effects of ethanol on lipid metabolism. The main areas of interest have been the pathogenesis of the hyperlipidaemia and the fatty liver associated with alcohol abuse (Lieber and DeCarli, 1977), and the role which ethanol may play as a 'risk-factor' in atherogenesis (Castelli *et al.*, 1977).

Interpretation of the literature on plasma lipids is complicated by the terminology employed. Serum triglyceride and cholesterol measurements only serve as a useful guide to blood lipids because in blood, lipids are present in the

[†]Brunt 1971; Hoensch, 1972; Hoyumpa *et al.*, 1975; Kaffarnik and Schneider, 1976; Lieber, 1965b, 1966, 1967a, 1967b; Leiber *et al.*, 1971; Lieber, 1973, Lieber, 1974; Lieber *et al.*, 1975; Lieber and De Carli, 1971; Nordmann and Nordmann, 1971; Porta *et al.*, 1970; Wartburg and Papenberg, 1970.

form of complex lipoproteins. These older and purely chemical measures are being replaced by electrophoretic and ultracentrifugal analyses of lipoproteins. Table 7.16 presents a comparison of lipoprotein classifications obtained by these two techniques together with chemical composition of the lipoprotein classes.

7.12.1 Lipoproteins

The hyperlipidaemia of alcoholism, as reflected by an increase in serum lipoproteins, may result from increased production and release of hepatic lipoproteins (Lieber et al., 1971). Decreased peripheral uptake of lipoproteins due to decreased lipoprotein lipase activity may also contribute to the alcoholic hyperlipoproteinaemia (Jones et al., 1963; Losowsky et al., 1963). As well as generalised hyperlipoproteinaemia, several workers (Johansson and Laurell, 1969; Johansson and Medhus, 1974; Belfrage et al., 1973, 1977) have found an increase in alpha-lipoprotein in alcoholics, which was not correlated with other lipid changes. Usually a Fredrickson type IV or V hyperlipoproteinaemia is found (Mendelson and Mello, 1974; Simons et al., 1975, Wallerstedt, et al., 1977). In a group of 40 acute and chronic alcoholics subjects and 15 patients with delirium studied by Sirtori et al., (1973), a large proportion (15/55) had a Fredrickson type IV, 1/55 a type V, 1/55 a type IIa, and 1/55 a type IIb lipoproteinaemia.

A large dose of ethanol (180 g during 6h) has been shown to cause an increase in the pre-betalipoprotein in plasma specimens taken from habituated heavy drinkers. In five of the subjects studied chylomicra were detected in plasma 3–6h post-ethanol but these had disappeared by 24h. The pre-betalipoprotein fraction was shown to have a density intermediate between VLDL and LDL. It was suggested that this fraction was an intermediate lipoprotein (ILDL), a catabolic product in the conversion of VLDL to LDL, and that the appearance of this lipoprotein was a manifestation of endogenous lipid mobilization by ethanol (Avogãro and Cazzolato, 1975).

Studies of the chemical composition of individual lipoprotein fractions are presented in the next section.

7.12.2 Blood Lipids

The effect of ethanol on blood lipid levels has been studied primarily in order to elucidate the mechanism of alcoholic hyperlipidaemia. However, an understanding of these effects might explain ambiguous results of clinical chemistry tests on subjects who have ingested ethanol. As with all studies of lipid metabolism, the overall state of the patient must be considered before interpreting results. This is especially true in alcoholics where lipid concentrations after ethanol are related to dose, diet (Verdy and Gattereau, 1967; Anon., 1970), stress, and length of abstinence (Jones, 1969). Other factors affecting

Table 7.16

Lipoprotein Classes and Chemical Composition of Lipoproteins

Ultracentrifuge (density)	Particle size	Electrophoresis (mobility)	Chemical Composition*			
			Protein	Triglyceride	Cholesterol	Phospholipid
Chylomicra	5000 Å	Origin	1	90	5	4
VLDL	800 Å	pre-β	10	60	15	15
LDL	350 Å	β	25	10	45	20
HDL	150 Å	α	45	3	32	20

*all figures expressed as a percentage of dry weight

lipid status will be intercurrent illness and associated disorders. It has been suggested that the hyperlipidaemia of alcohol abuse is secondary to alcohol-induced pancreatitis (Jones, 1969; Tasman-Jones and Abraham, 1973). Hyperlipidaemia may occur with pancreatitis, and similarly pancreatitis has been associated with alcoholism. However, it should be noted that alcohol can cause hyperlipidaemia in the absence of pancreatitis. Similarly Zieve's Syndrome (hyperlipidaemia, icterus and haemolytic anaemia) has been associated with alcoholism (Albahary et al., 1968; Paloheimo and Louhija, 1968; Jones, 1969; Rudiger et al., 1970; Thämig, 1970; Powell et al., 1972). There may also be a genetic predisposition to alcoholic hyperlipidaemia (De Gennes et al., 1972; Mendelson and Mello, 1973).

FREE FATTY ACIDS

The effect of ethanol on free fatty acids in serum is variable and depends particularly on the dose of ethanol (Wartburg and Pappenberg, 1970). Large doses of ethanol cause a rise in circulating free fatty acids (Lieber et al., 1963; Schapiro et al., 1965; Liebhardt and Gostomzyk, 1968). This is probably due to enhanced peripheral fat mobilisation, through stimulation of the sympathetic nervous system, and also due to decreased breakdown of free fatty acids in the liver. Initially elevated free fatty acid levels fall rapidly during withdrawal (Wallerstedt et al., 1977b). In patients fasted for either 15 or 69h, hepatic venous and arterial catheterization studies have shown ethanol to cause a reduction in the splanchnic uptake and metabolism of free fatty acids (Wolfe et al., 1976).

Ethanol, when metabolised, generates NADH and this increases the synthesis of free fatty acids in vitro (Wartburg and Pappenberg, 1970). However, ethanol in small doses causes a fall in free fatty acids (Jones et al., 1965). This might be due to increased uptake of free fatty acids by the liver or muscle, or to decreased release of free fatty acids from peripheral adipose tissue. Evidence presented by Crouse et al., (1968) suggests that ethanol decreases adipose tissue lipolysis and hence the concentration of plasma free fatty acids through the action of its metabolite, acetate.

TRIGLYCERIDES

Ethanol causes a rise in plasma triglycerides (Friedman et al., 1965; Kallio et al., 1969; Lepoire et al., 1970; Uzunalimoglu, 1970; Fry et al., 1973). This increase in triglycerides is even greater if the subject was hypertriglyceridaemic previous to ethanol intake (Ginsberg et al., 1974; Taskinen and Nikkilä, 1977).

Population studies, such as the Framingham study, have revealed modest positive correlations between ethanol consumption and plasma triglycerides (Table 7.17), although the correlations were weaker than those between ethanol consumption and HDL cholesterol (Castelli et al., 1977). Table 7.17 illustrates the general trend of increasing mean plasma triglyceride level with increasing weekly ethanol consumption. Long-term intake of moderate amounts of ethanol by healthy normolipaemic volunteers leads to an increase in triglyceride levels. In a study by Barboriak and Hogan (1976), fasting plasma triglyceride levels rose progressively throughout a 7 consecutive day period during which ethanol

Table 7.17
Mean Blood Levels of Lipids in Relation to Alcohol Consumption in Subjects aged 50-69
Reproduced by permission from Castelli *et al.*, Lancet (1977)

Alcohol (oz/wk)	No. of subjects	Mean Level (mg/dl)				Plasma- triglycerides
		Total	Plasma-cholesterol H.D.L.	L.D.L.	V.L.D.L.	
Albany:						
Total	923	219.69	49.55	153.48	16.65	139.36
0	201	215.44	46.28	152.94	16.22	131.89
1-3	372	220.05	47.35	155.18	17.51	140.02
4-9	260	221.21	53.25	152.58	15.38	139.75
10-19	80	224.35	54.57	151.40	18.38	153.49
20+	10	215.00	60.60	141.60	12.80	141.54
Framingham men:						
Total	393	219.77	45.69	140.32	33.76	137.77
0	111	221.21	41.40	143.68	36.13	134.51
1-3	112	213.93	44.78	136.35	32.80	132.02
4-9	111	220.14	47.43	144.70	28.01	126.86
10-19	44	225.98	50.14	136.66	39.18	162.38
20+	15	231.87	58.40	123.33	50.13	213.36
Honolulu:						
Total	1713	220.85	45.11	142.82	32.92	176.73
0	849	221.95	42.18	147.00	32.77	168.72
1-3	320	224.81	44.82	148.53	31.46	167.12
4-9	354	220.25	48.28	138.64	33.32	182;33
10-19	166	213.89	52.20	125.83	35.85	218.55
20+	24	186.08	56.71	97.67	31.71	216.58
San Francisco:						
Total	277	231.04	46.57	149.70	34.77	172.71
0	133	229.25	44.38	151.66	33.21	153.78
1-3	90	236.44	45.75	156.45	34.26	166.32
4-9	40	227.60	51.72	133.92	41.95	252.59
10-19	12	234.00	57.75	145.58	30.67	162.99
Framingham women:						
Total	500	235.96	58.60	149.82	27.55	115.31
0	242	238.80	54.77	155.08	28.95	120.86
1-3	169	232.90	61.38	145.51	26.00	105.23
4-9	82	234.87	63.53	144.45	26.89	121.38
Correlation of Lipids with Alcohol Consumption						
Men:						
Albany		0.06	0.28	−0.04	−0.01	0.04
Framingham		0.05	0.30	−0.09	0.05	0.12
Honolulu		−0.12	0.28	−0.24	0.04	0.11
San Francisco		−0.11	0.25	−0.23	0.05	0.13
Women:						
Framingham		0.06	0.16	−0.12	−0.03	−0.02

(0.75/kg) was consumed each evening before an evening meal. Levels rose by 25% and returned to normal when ethanol was withdrawn. A different triglyceride response has been elicited from a group of 5 healthy volunteers given a total of 75 g ethanol in 5 daily doses over a period of 5 weeks such that blood ethanol levels did not exceed 0.04% (w/v) (40 mg/100 ml). In these subjects, plasma triglycerides exhibited a transient rise and then returned to basal levels (Figure 7.18) (Belfrage *et al.*, 1973, 1977). A single dose of ethanol (1.5 g/kg) given in the evening to 24 healthy normolipaemic volunteers has been shown to cause a marked nocturnal hypertriglyceridaemia which persisted into the next morning. The mean maximal blood alcohol level was 100 mg/100 ml and the mean maximal increase in triglycerides was 1.0 mmol/l. A larger increase, 3.65 mmol/l, was obtained in 10 subjects with endogenous hypertriglyceridaemia. (Taskinen and Nikkilä, 1977).

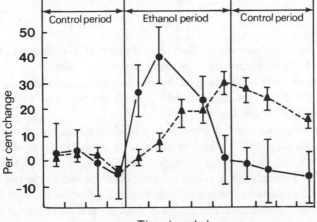

Fig. 7.18 – Effect of Ethanol intake on Plasma Triglyceride (●) and α-lipoprotein (▲). (All points are mean ± S. E. M. for 8 or 9 subjects. The changes are expressed relative to the individual average value during the first control period).
Reproduced by permission from Belfrage *et al.*, European Journal of Clinical Investigation (1977)

Considerably elevated plasma triglyceride levels have been demonstrated in chronic alcoholics, in subjects with acute signs of intoxication, and in alcoholics with delirium tremens (Sirtori *et al.*, 1973). Acute doses of ethanol (180 g during 6h) given to 21 subjects habituated to heavy drinking caused an hypertriglyceridaemia. The response varied from a 26% to 377% increase over basal values (30 mg/100 ml to 506 mg/100 ml, mean increase 257.1 ± 31.2 mg/100 ml). Peak response was evident by the sixth hour of the test in most of the subjects (15/21) but in the remaining 6 subjects the peak was not reached until a further six hours (Avogãro and Cazzolato, 1975).

The mechanism of the increase in triglycerides after ethanol intake is unclear, though increased hepatic synthesis of pre-betalipoproteins (Kudzma and Schonfeld, 1971) and changes in ATP availability (Walker and Gordon, 1970) have been suggested. Chait *et al.*, (1972) found that alcohol did not decrease peripheral uptake of triglycerides from plasma. They suggest that ethanol causes an increased hepatic secretion of lipoproteins. This induces hyperlipidaemia in individuals predisposed by having a low ability to clear triglycerides from plasma. Other workers (Belfrage *et al.*, 1977) have also attributed the hypertriglyceridaemia following ethanol ingestion to increased hepatic secretion of lipoproteins (VLDL).

The finding of a positive correlation between serum GGT activities and serum triglyceride levels in a group of 109 patients submitted for routine lipid and lipoprotein screening has pointed to the possibility that the elevated triglyceride levels may be due to microsomal enzyme induction of enzymes involved in hepatic triglyceride production (Martin *et al.*, 1975).

CHOLESTEROL

Ethanol has been shown to increase cholesterol synthesis (Lieber and De Carli, 1964) through an effect on the microsomes. There may also be accumulation of cholesterol in the liver due to decreased cholesterol catabolism. This is reflected by a reduction in bile acid production and turnover after ethanol intake (Lefevre and Lieber, 1969).

Generally, an acute dose of ethanol or a moderate intake over several days or weeks is without effect on plasma cholesterol levels (Belfrage *et al.*, 1973, 1977; Barboriak and Hogan, 1976, Avogaro and Cazzolato, 1977; Taskinen and Nikkilä, 1977). Similarly, in a group of alcoholics studied by Sirtori and co-workers (1972), cholesterol levels were either normal or only marginally elevated. Results from five population studies have revealed plasma cholesterol (total) and ethanol consumption to be positively associated, although this correlation was chiefly a reflection of the striking correlation between HDL-cholesterol and ethanol (Castelli *et al.*, 1977). In contrast to the latter finding, moderate intake of ethanol by healthy subjects is without effect on total cholesterol or cholesterol in any of the lipoproteins (VLDL, LDL or HDL) (Taskinen and Nikkilä, 1977).

Alcoholic liver disease may alter cholesterol metabolism. In a study of cholesterol metabolism in chronic liver disease, Sandhofer *et al.*, (1973) found a decreased production rate of cholesterol associated with low plasma cholesterol levels in an alcoholic cirrhotic. Sabesin *et al.*, (1977) have studied four patients with acute alcoholic fatty liver. On admission two of the patients had elevated plasma cholesterol values. Considerably reduced levels of cholesteryl esters and a greatly depressed lecithin cholesterol acyltransferase (LCAT) activity were detected in all four patients. These changes in cholesterol esters and LCAT activity reverted to normal with clinical improvement.

The variety of changes in lipid levels due to ethanol is illustrated in Table 7.18.

Table 7.18

Triglyceride, Free Fatty Acid, Cholesterol, Phospholipid and Total Lipid Levels in Alcoholics.

TRIGLYCERIDES

Specimen	Mean ± SD	Reference interval (normal range) or control values	Number of Subjects	Clinical details	Reference*
serum	173.3 ± 26.9 mg/100 ml 188.4 ± 54.8 148.1 ± 24.9	98.9 ± 5.9	16 14 10	chronic alcoholic acute alcoholic alcoholic with delirium tremens	1
plasma	170.1 ± 22.4 mg/100 ml 167.8 ± 39.7 141.7 ± 17.3	98.9 ± 5.9	20 20 15	chronic alcoholic acute alcoholic alcoholic with delirium tremens	2
plasma	1.02 ± 0.14 g/l 0.95 ± 0.12	1.00 ± 0.09	28 15	alcoholic with cirrhosis alcoholic with cirrhosis and ascites	3
serum	83.09 ± 30.65 mg/100 ml	80.50 ± 33.99	41	chronic alcoholic	4
serum	1.44 ± 0.27 mmol/l 2.06 ± 0.34 2.05 ± 0.49 1.78 ± 0.30 1.47 ± 0.27 1.00 ± 0.04 1.47 ± 0.29	1.29 ± 0.14 1.29 ± 0.09 1.55 ± 0.11 2.11 ± 0.22 1.39 ± 0.08 1.40 1.44 ± 0.13	9 19 26 16 13 2 10	alcoholic age 21–30 male 31–40 41–50 51–60 61–70 70 age 50–78 female	5
plasma	121 ± 14 mg/100 ml	97 ± 11	20	healthy volunteer	6

Table 7.18 (*continued*)

FATTY ACIDS

plasma	0.39 ± 0.06 meq/l	20	chronic alcoholic	2
	0.53 ± 0.04	20	acute alcoholic	
	1.09 ± 0.05	15	alcoholic with delirium tremens	
plasma	604 ± 126 Eq/l	28	alcoholic with cirrhosis	3
	916 ± 246	15	alcoholic with cirrhosis and ascites	
serum	0.60–0.26 meq/l	41	chronic alcoholics	4
plasma	decreased	5	healthy volunteer	7
serum	decreased	10	alcoholic	8
serum	0.28 ± 0.06 mEq/l	16	chronic alcoholic	1
	0.59 ± 0.07	14	acute alcoholic	
	0.98 ± 0.06	10	alcoholic with delirium tremens	

CHOLESTEROL

plasma	196.1 ± 9.3 mg/100 ml	20	chronic alcoholic	2
	182.6 ± 6.9	20	acute alcoholic	
	202.8 ± 7.8	15	acute alcoholic with delirium tremens	
plasma	1.72 ± 0.14 g/l	28	alcoholic with cirrhosis	3
	1.70 ± 0.38	15	alcoholic with cirrhosis and ascites	
serum	194.4 ± 38.9 mg/100 ml	41	chronic alcoholics	4

Sample	Value	n		Condition	Ref
serum (free)	84 ± 14 mg/100 ml	26	62 ± 14	alcoholic	9
serum (total)	245 ± 35 mg/100 ml		178 ± 42		
serum	259 ± 46 mg/100 ml	14	206 ± 57	acute alcoholic	10
serum	233 ± 68.0 mg/100 ml	22		alcohol intoxicated	11
csf	0.09 mg/100 ml	9	0.13	alcoholic after acute abuse	12
serum	220 ± 13.3 mg/100 ml	9	221 ± 9.7	alcoholics age 21–30 male	5
	233 ± 12.1	19	236 ± 8.2	31–40	
	235 ± 9.8	26	248 ± 7.7	41–50	
	246 ± 8.3	16	277 ± 8.2	51–60	
	234 ± 12.7	13	257 ± 7.9	61–70	
	206 ± 16.0	2	258	70	
	280 ± 10.9	10	305 ± 11.7	age 50–78 female	
serum	259 ± 46 mg/100 ml	14	206 ± 57	alcoholic	10
serum	205.2 ± 10.2 mg/100 ml	16	203 ± 5.7	chronic alcoholic	1
	181.6 ± 8.4	14		acute alcoholic	
	214.0 ± 7.9	10		alcoholic with delirium tremens	
plasma	214.0 ± 13 mg/100 ml	20	209 ± 13	healthy individual	6

CHOLESTEROL ESTERS

Sample	Value	n		Condition	Ref
plasma	0.95 ± 0.10 g/l	28	1.23 ± 0.07	alcoholic with cirrhosis	3
	0.92 ± 0.28	15		alcoholic with cirrhosis and ascites	
csf	0.09 mg/100 ml	9	0.18	alcoholic	12

Table 7.18 (*continued*)

PHOSPHOLIPIDS

			n		
plasma	1.60 ± 0.16 g/l	1.57 ± 0.09	28	alcoholic with cirrhosis	3
	1.64 ± 0.26		15	alcoholic with cirrhosis and ascites	
serum	283.7 ± 84.1 mg/100 ml	232.2 ± 48.7	41	chronic alcoholic	4
serum	289 ± 47 mg/100 ml	250 ± 53	14	acute alcoholic	10
csf	0.27 mg/100 ml	0.49	9	alcoholic after acute abuse	12
serum*	115.1 ± 9.8 µg/ml	92.5 ± 4.8	9	alcoholic age 21–30 male	5
(*total lipid phosphorus)	117.0 ± 4.6	100.9 ± 6.8	19	31–40	
	121.5 ± 4.0	101.3 ± 3.9	26	41–50	
	120.3 ± 2.6	116.2 ± 7.2	15	51–60	
	114.8 ± 6.2	115.9 ± 5.2	9	61–70	
	129.1 ± 5.2	121.9 ± 4.1	9	age 50–78 female	
serum	289 ± 47 mg/100 ml	250 ± 53	14	alcoholic	10

TOTAL LIPIDS

			n		
csf	0.89 mg/100 ml	1.03	9	alcoholic	12
serum	753 ± 164 mg/100 ml	627 ± 156	14	alcoholic	10

1. Sirtori et al., 1972   2. Sirtori et al., 1973
3. Guisard et al., 1972   4. Jaross et al., 1972
5. Böttiger et al., 1976   6. Barboriak and Hogan, 1976
7. Arbamson and Arky, 1968   8. Lepoire et al., 1970
9. Kallio et al., 1969   10. Alling et al., 1969

Chemical analysis of lipoprotein fractions has been reported in several studies of the interaction of ethanol and lipid metabolism. Acute doses of ethanol caused a mean increase of about twofold in the triglyceride content, and a decrease in the cholesterol/triglyceride ratio in VLDL, LDL, and HDL. An increase in the triglyceride/protein ratio was found in LDL whilst the converse was found for VLDL (Table 7.19). The changes in triglyceride and phospholipid composition of the lipoprotein fractions may be due to an exchange of these substances between lipoproteins. Alterations in protein composition were attributed to an ethanol stimulation of protein synthesis (Avogaro and Cazzolato, 1975). Other studies have noted the increase in triglyceride content of VLDL and LDL following an acute dose of ethanol (Taskinen and Nikkilä, 1977). Cholesterol concentration in VLDL, LDL or HDL was not markedly altered in the previous study.

Increased levels of HDL-cholesterol and lowered levels of LDL-cholesterol have been reported in subjects consuming more than 20 oz ethanol/week (Castelli *et al.*, 1977). (see Table 7.19).

7.12.3 Alcoholic Fatty Liver

The hyperlipidaemia of alcoholism has been singled out for study by several groups of workers in an attempt to elucidate the mechanisms involved in the pathogenesis of alcoholic fatty liver. There are three main sources of lipids found in the liver: chylomicra absorbed from the gut (exogenous lipids), adipose tissue lipids, and lipids synthesized in the liver itself. An increase in any of these might lead to alcoholic fatty liver.

Lieber has summarised the main events leading to the development of alcoholic fatty liver (Lieber and DeCarli, 1977).

(i)   Ethanol replaces fatty acids as a normal fuel for hepatic mitochondria and this leads to fatty acid accumulation.

(ii) Disposal of excess hydrogen generated by ethanol metabolism is achieved by increased lipid synthesis. Metabolism of ethanol is accompanied by an increase in NADH and decrease in NAD levels. This alteration in cofactor levels depresses the critic acid cycle thus decreasing dietary fatty acid oxidation and increasing α-glycerophosphate levels. This in turn increases triglyceride production, whilst acetyl-CoA arising from ethanol metabolism is converted to fatty acids. The nett result of these transformations is a hepatic deposition of lipid.

(iii) Large amounts of ethanol mobilise fatty acids from adipose tissue and these accumulate in the liver.

(iv) Despite an increase in lipid transport from the liver due to increased lipo-protein release hepatic lipids continue to increase.

The reader is referred to Lieber's account (1977) of the metabolic effects of alcohol on the liver for a more detailed coverage of the various factors in the pathogenesis of alcoholic fatty liver.

Table 7.19

Cholesterol, Triglycerides, Phospholipids, and Protein in Whole Plasma and in Ultracentrifugal Fractions Derived therefrom in 10 subjects During an Ethanol Loading Test

Reproduced by permission from Avogaro and Cazzolato, Metabolism, (1973) 24, 1231–1242.

	Cholesterol		Triglyceride		Phospholipid		Protein	
	Basal	Peak*	Basal	Peak*	Basal	Peak*	Basal	Peak*
Total	206.5 ± 24.1	208.5 ± 21.6 N.S.	135.0 ± 12.8	269.1 ± 24.4 001	210.7 ± 9.6	220.0 ± 10.5 005	6.9 ± 0.2	6.9 ± 0.2 N.S.
VLDL	26.7 ± 5.8	39.5 ± 7.5 005	75.5 ± 8.3	158.9 ± 15.4 001	21.4 ± 1.6	25.2 ± 2.0 001	16.4 ± 3.1	35.9 ± 3.8 001
LDL	123.5 ± 14.3	111.0 ± 11.9 005	35.2 ± 3.4	67.0 ± 6.2 001	63.1 ± 4.6	64.8 ± 4.3 N.S.	55.1 ± 5.9	69.8 ± 6.0 005
HDL	56.3 ± 6.5	58.0 ± 6.5 N.S.	24.3 ± 2.8	43.1 ± 4.3 001	126.0 ± 6.3	129.9 ± 7.7 N.S.		

*6th hour

7.13 ORGANIC ACIDS

7.13.1 Lactate, Acetoacetate, Beta-Hydroxybutyrate and Pyruvate

Alcohol ingestion by both healthy subjects (Carey *et al.*, 1971; Ylikahri *et al.*, 1976a), gouty (MacLachlan and Rodnan, 1967) and alcoholic patients (Jenkins *et al.*, 1971; Levy *et al.*, 1973) leads to an elevation of blood lactate levels and an increased urinary excretion of lactate. In one study of acutely intoxicated alcoholics, their blood lactate levels were 31.0 ± 18.0 mg/100 ml (Mean ± SD; normal range 14.6 ± 2.9) and their urinary excretion of lactate was 65.0 ± 48.0 mg/h (normal excretion 3 mg/h) (Sullivan *et al.*, 1966). Increases in blood lactate were found on ingestion of alcohol in a patient suffering from already raised lactate levels. (Sussman *et al.*, 1970) (see Figure 7.19).

Similarly, blood beta-hydroxybutyrate levels (Lefevre *et al.*, 1970; Jenkins *et al.*, 1971; Levy *et al.*, 1973; Ylikahri *et al.*, 1976) and, to a lesser extent, blood acetoacetate levels (Lefevre *et al.*, 1970; Bagdade *et al.*, 1972b; Levy *et al.*, 1973) are elevated in alcoholics and normal subjects (given a high fat diet and alcohol) (Lefevre *et al.*, 1970). In contrast pyruvate levels are lowered by ethanol ingestion (Sussman *et al.*, 1970; Jenkins *et al.*, 1971) or show no consistent change (Carey *et al.*, 1971). The ratio of lactate/pryuvate levels and beta-hydroxybutyrate/acetoacetate levels in blood are increased following the ingestion of ethanol. These changes reflect the increased hepatic NADH/NAD ratio and may be of diagnostic importance (see Chapter 6).

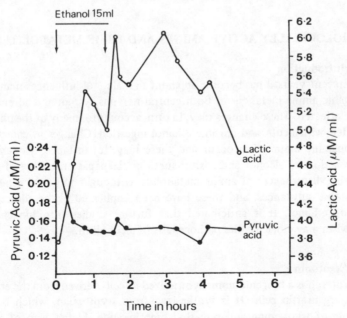

Fig. 7.19 – Changes in blood pyruvate and lactate levels with ethanol ingestion. Patient was given two 15 ml doses of absolute ethanol in orange juice

7.13.2 Acetate

Blood levels of acetate are increased after ethanol consumption, as a consequence of the metabolic conversion of ethanol *via* acetaldehyde to acetate. The extent of the increase is significant, but depends on dose and duration of ethanol intake. This increase may be due to decreased conversion of acetate to acetyl Coenzyme A, either because of decreased availability of CoA, or because of inhibition of the citric acid cycle produced by ethanol ingestion (see Section 7.11).

Although acetate is known to be a central metabolite in intermediary metabolism, the clinical significance of the increase in acetate levels after ethanol metabolism is not clear. Crouse *et al.,* (1968) have suggested that acetate may bring about the decrease in free fatty acids caused by ethanol ingestion (see Section 7.11).

7.13.3 Glucaric acid

Induction of microsomal enzyme systems in the liver by ethanol may be evaluated by measurements of urinary D-glucaric acid (Spencer-Peet and Wood, 1975). Significantly elevated urinary levels of this acid have been found in alcoholic subjects 158.6 ± 21.7 μmol/g creatinine (mean ± S.E.M.) as compared to controls (65.7 ± 4.6) (mean ± S.E.M.). Measurement of the levels of this acid may be diagnostically useful in alcoholism (see Chapter 6).

7.14 BIOLOGICALLY ACTIVE AMINES AND THEIR METABOLITES

7.14.1 Introduction

In recent years it has become apparent that alcohol influences many aspects of biogenic amine metabolism. Both central nervous system and adrenal amines may be affected. These changes may, in turn, account for many of the phenomena associated with acute and chronic ethanol ingestion. Changes in catecholamine and dopamine metabolism occur and these may, for instance, account for the pressor action of alcohol and disturbances in sleep patterns. One of the most interesting disturbances of amine metabolism is thought to be the generation of alkaloid-like substances, and these have been implicated in the addictive properties of ethanol. It is anticipated that further studies into biogenic amine metabolism may elucidate the pathogenesis of alcoholism.

7.14.2 Serotonin

Serotonin is a biogenic amine synthesized by cells derived from the embryonic foregut–argentaffin cells. It is synthesized from tryptophan, which is also the precursor of tryptamine and n-methyl nicotinamide. Metabolism of serotonin may occur by either an oxidative or a reductive pathway. (see Figure 7.20).

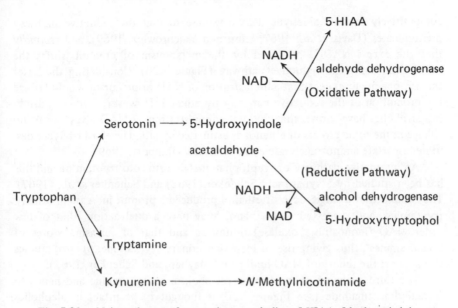

Fig. 7.20 – Main pathways of tryptophan metabolism. 5-HIAA, 5-hydroxyindole 3-acetic acid. NAD, nicotinamide adenine – dinucleotide. NADH, reduced nicotinamide adenine-dinucleotide.

Alcohol was first shown to have an effect on secrotonin metabolism when patients with Carcinoid Disease were found to excrete less 5-hydroxy-3 indole acetic acid (5-HIAA) when given an alcoholic drink (Smith *et al.*, 1957). (As seen from Figure 7.20. 5-HIAA is the oxidative metabolite of 5-hydroxyindole acetaldehyde, a derivative of serotonin). Since then, there have been reports of decreased urinary 5-HIAA excretion in alcoholics (Olsen *et al.*, 1960), and normals given alcohol (Rosenfeld, 1960; Anton 1965). However, these results were not confirmed by Perman (1960) and Murphy *et al.*, (1962) where normal urinary 5-HIAA excretion was found in normals after a dose of ethanol and in alcoholics respectively. Studies using ^{14}C-labelled serotonin have helped to clarify the situation. Feldstein *et al.*, (1964) showed that a dose of ^{14}C-serotonin administered to normal healthy subjects is mainly converted to 5-HIAA and ethanol ingestion blocks this conversion. Davis *et al.*, (1966, 1967e) demonstrated that ethanol ingestion one hour before the administration of ^{14}C-serotonin gave rise to a decreased excretion of ^{14}C-5-HIAA and this was completely accounted for by an increase in tryptophol—so that the ethanol ingestion resulted in a decrease of the oxidative pathway and an increase in the reductive pathway.

The mechanism of the alteration in the pathway to 5-HIAA and tryptophol is uncertain, though two theories have been proposed (Anon., 1972a; Sprince *et al.*, 1972; Lahti, 1975): *firstly* that acetaldehyde, a metabolite of ethanol, competitively inhibits aldehyde dehydrogenase so that the reductive pathway predominates (Davis et al., 1967; Lahti and Majchrowicz, 1969), and secondly that the excess NADH, produced by the metabolism of ethanol, shifts the metabolism along the reductive pathway (Figure 7.20). Considering the latter theory, one might expect that administration of NAD or precursor would reduce the promotion of the reductive pathway by ethanol. However, studies in drinking alcoholics have shown that the oral administration of NAD gives rise to no change in the toxic effects of ethanol as estimated by blood levels of triglycerides, urate, aspartate aminotransferase and cholesterol (Rapport, 1969).

An alternative pathway of tryptophan metabolism is to tryptamine and this has been studied by Maynard and Schenker (1962) and Schenker et al., (1967). They found that a single dose of ethanol produced a prompt increase in urinary tryptamine, and suggested that ethanol 'may have a dual action, that of low order MAO (monoamine oxidase) inhibition and that of releasing stores of bound amines', thus giving rise to increased urinary tryptamine. In vitro studies also support the theory of MAO inhibition (Maynard and Schenker, 1962).

The third pathway of tryptophan metabolism to kynurenine and hence to N-methylnicotinamide (see Figure 7.20) is thought to be intact in alcoholics (Olson et al., 1960).

The changes in these pathways, e.g. pathways leading to 5-HIAA, and tryptamine, may be of diagnostic value. Akhter et al., (1978) have found differences in the ratio of urinary tryptamine/5-HIAA between alcoholics and normals, and between alcoholics and patients with non-alcoholic liver disease.

Whilst these changes in biogenic amines (summarised in Table 7.20) have been noted in blood and urine, the changes in the brain may be different (Wartburg et al., 1975), and their relevance has yet to be understood.

7.14.3 Catecholamines

Catecholamines are biogenic amines derived from cells originating from the embryonic neural crest. These cells are of two types: the chromaffin cells and the nerve cells. Epinephrine (adrenaline) and norepinephrine (noradrenaline) are synthesized from tyrosine in the adrenal medulla in the case of epinephrine and in sympathetic nerve endings in the case of norepinephrine. They are further metabolised either oxidatively or reductively as illustrated in Figure 7.21 for norepinephrine, though the pathways are similar for epinephrine.

There seem to be two different effects of ethanol on catecholamine metabolism. Firstly, ethanol causes an increase in blood and urine catecholamine levels and secondly, the metabolism of these compounds may be altered (findings summarised in Table 7.20).

Ethanol has been shown to give rise to an increase in catecholamine levels in blood and urine, in normal healthy volunteers (Kinzius 1950; Abelin et al., 1958; Perman, 1958; Perman, 1960; Anton, 1965; Jouppila et al., 1970; Gitlow

Table 7.20

Urinary Levels of Biogenic Amines in Alcoholics and Healthy Volunteers Given Alcohol

	Mean ± SD	Reference interval (normal range) or control values	Number of subjects	Clinical details	Reference
5-HIAA					
	decreased		20	healthy volunteer given alcohol 0.71 g/kgbw	Anton, 1965
		4.9 ± 1.2 mg/24h	15	alcoholic	Murphy et al., 1962
		2.5 ± 1.0 mg/24h	34	chronic alcoholic	Olson et al., 1960
	decreased		7	healthy volunteer given alcohol	Feldstein et al., 1964
		238 ± 15.5	7	healthy volunteer given alcohol 0.5–0.7 g/kgbw	Perman, 1960
	decreased	228 ± 12.5 µg/h	5	healthy volunteers given alcohol	Davis et al., 1966
5-HYDROXYTRYPTOPHOL					
	increased		5	healthy volunteers given alcohol	Davis et al., 1966
DOPAMINE					
	normal – increased		20	healthy volunteers given alcohol 0.71 g/kgbw	Anton, 1965

Table 7.20 *(continued)*

normal		4	alcoholic	Ogata et al., 1971
16.78 µg/h	12.74	3	alcoholic	Schenker, 1966
EPINEPHRINE (adrenaline)				
normal		20	healthy volunteers given alcohol 0.71 g/kgbw	Anton 1965
elevated		4	alcoholic	Ogata et al., 1971
elevated		7	healthy volunteer given alcohol 0.3–0.4 g/kgbw	Perman, 1960
9.3 µg/24h	7.4	18	pregnant women given alcohol	Jouppila et al., 1970
1.31 µg/h	0.463	3	alcoholic	Schenker et al., 1966
8.0 ± 1.58 mµg/min	4.8 ± 0.38	43	healthy volunteers given alcohol 0.27–0.54 g/kgbw	Perman, 1958
8.8 ± 0.74 µg/24h	8.7 ± 0.9	40	alcoholic in withdrawal	Segal et al., 1970
NOREPINEPHRINE (noradrenaline)				
elevated		20	healthy volunteers given alcohol 0.71 g/kgbw	Anton, 1965

elevated		4	alcoholic	Ogata et al., 1971
normal		7	healthy volunteer given alcohol 0.3–0.4 g/kgbw	Perman, 1960
48.0 µg/24h	29.6	18	pregnant woman given alcohol	Jouppila et al., 1970
1.02 µg/h	0.88	3	alcoholic	Schenker et al., 1966
17.0 ± 0.82 mµg/min (Mean ± S.E.)	13.5 ± 1.16	43	healthy volunteers given alcohol 0.27–0.54 g/kgbw	Perman, 1958
0.350 ± 0.165 µg/mg creatinine	0.570 ± 0.287	8	social drinkers	Muir et al., 1973
22.8 ± 1.77 µg/24h	27.2 ± 2.7	40	alcoholic in withdrawal	Segal et al., 1970

NORMETANEPHRINE

elevated		20	healthy volunteer given alcohol 0.71 g/kgbw	Anton, 1965
elevated		4	alcoholic	Ogata et al., 1971

TRYPTAMINE

6.03 µg/h	3.43	3	alcoholic	Schenker et al., 1966

VMA

normal		20	healthy volunteer given alcohol 0.71 g/kgbw	Anton, 1965

Table 7.20 (continued)

decreased		4	alcoholic	Ogata et al., 1971
decreased		2	healthy volunteer given alcohol	Davis et al., 1967
	1.266 ± 0.383 µg/mg 3.374 ± 0.745	8	social	Muir et al., 1973

MHPG

elevated		4	alcoholic	Ogata et al., 1971
elevated		2	healthy volunteers given alcohol	Davis et al., 1967

METANEPHRINE

elevated		20	healthy volunteer given alcohol 0.71 g/kgbw	Anton, 1965
elevated		4	alcoholic	Ogata et al., 1971

et al., 1976). The reasons for these increases remain obscure, though several theories have been proposed e.g., diuresis, circulatory changes, metabolic acidosis. There is some evidence, though, that ethanol ingestion may prevent/or obliterate those increase in blood and urinary catecholamines which are due to stressful situations (Garlind *et al.,* 1960).

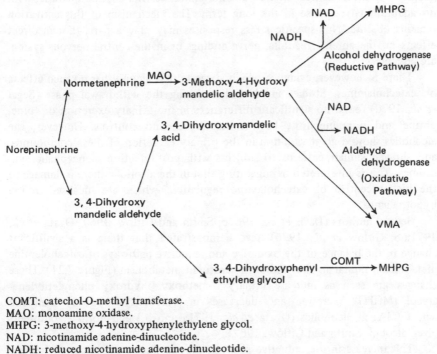

COMT: catechol-O-methyl transferase.
MAO: monoamine oxidase.
MHPG: 3-methoxy-4-hydroxyphenylethylene glycol.
NAD: nicotinamide adenine-dinucleotide.
NADH: reduced nicotinamide adenine-dinucleotide.
VMA: 3-methoxy-4-hydroxymandelic acid.

Fig. 7.21 – Pathways of Norepinephrine Metabolism.

Studies in alcoholics have shown increased urinary excretion of catecholamines during alcohol withdrawal and also during alcohol ingestion by alcoholics (Ogata *et al.,* 1971a,b).

Giacobini *et al.,* (1960) found elevated urinary catecholamines in alcoholics suffering from withdrawal symptoms. The decrease in these symptoms corresponded to a fall in urinary amines. Similarly, increased arterial norepinephrine levels have been found in alcoholics 6h–21 days after alcohol withdrawal (Carlsson and Häggendal, 1967). The highest levels of norepinephrine were found in those patients suffering the more severe withdrawal symptoms. Treatment with a sedative alleviated the patients' symptoms and a reduction in arterial norephinephrine levels was found. The authors suggest that the sympathetic nervous system is activated upon withdrawal of alcohol, and this might lead to increased catecholamine levels.

Increases in urinary epinephrine, metanephrine, norepinephrine and normetanephrine have also been found in drinking alcoholics (Davis *et al.*, 1967a; Davis *et al.*, 1967b; Ogata *et al.*, 1971a,b). These results seem to suggest that in healthy volunteers and alcoholics, alcohol stimulates the adrenal medulla, with no adaptational response in the long term. The mechanism of this activation remains obscure. Non-specific stress responses may play a part, though direct effects on the adrenal medulla, nerve endings or in the central nervous system are possible.

There is, however, evidence which suggests that alcohol has no such effects on catecholamines. Studies in alcoholics during the withdrawal phase (Segal *et al.*, 1970) found no significant differences in the urinary excretion of epinephrine and norepinephrine between alcoholics and controls. However, the alcoholics showed great variation in the urinary excretion of these compounds, and showed similar patterns to subjects with post-infection diencephalic syndromes. This is interpreted as suggesting that in the alcoholic there is damage to the higher centres of catecholamine regulation, which are localised in the hypothalamus.

Several authors (Davis *et al.*, 1967c; Smith and Gitlow, 1967; Ogata *et al.*, 1971a,b; Gitlow *et al.*, 1976) have demonstrated that there is a significant change in the balance of the oxidative and reductive pathways of catecholamine metabolism, similar to that found in serotonin metabolism (Figure 7.21). These changes are seen as increase urinary 3-methoxy-4-hydroxy phenylethyleneglycol (MHPG) excretion and decreases in 3-methoxy-4-hydroxy mandelic acid (VMA) in alcoholics (Ogata *et al.*, 1971a and b,) and normal volunteers given alcohol (Smith and Gitlow, 1967).

This increase in the reductive pathway may be due to an increase in hepatic NADH, generated by the oxidation of ethanol, or it may be due to competitive inhibition of aldehyde dehydrogenase (Davis *et al.*, 1967d; Smith and Gitlow, 1967; Sprince *et al.*, 1972).

These changes may be of diagnostic value (Akhter *et al.*, 1978). Measurement of the ratio VMA/MHPG in urine may be of use in the diagnosis and assessment of alcohol abuse.

7.14.4 Condensation Reactions

One of the most interesting theories to arise from the study of biogenic amine metabolism in alcoholics is that alkaloid-like substances are formed as a result of ethanol ingestion. These compounds may then play a role in the addictive process. (Sprince *et al.*, 1972; Anon., 1972a; Davis, 1973; Caldwell and Sever, 1974; Davis *et al.*, 1975; Deitrich and Erwin, 1975; Rahwan, 1974).

The alkaloid-like products, (Figure 7.22) tetrahydroisoquinolines and tetrahydro-β-carbolines, are thought to arise from the Pictet-Spengler condensation of amines with either acetaldehyde or other intermediate aldehydes. The aldehydes are present in increased amounts due to ethanol metabolism. These 'alkaloids' have been isolated from: brain and liver homogenates, the perfused adrenal gland, and from the urine of Parkinson's patients receiving L-dopa therapy (Sandler *et al.*, 1973). They have, as yet, to be detected in the alcoholic.

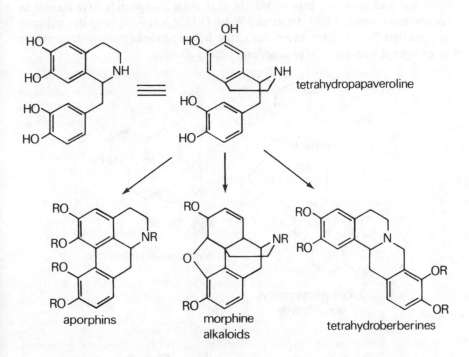

tetrahydropapaveroline

aporphins

morphine
alkaloids

tetrahydroberberines

Fig. 7.22 − Alkaloid − like substances formed following ethanol ingestion. Their
structural similarities to more familiar compounds

Studies in rats, for instance, have shown that dopamine may condense with its aldehyde to form tetrahydropapaveroline (THP). Under normal physiological conditions in the human this may be of little importance. However, following ethanol ingestion, acetaldehyde is generated and may inhibit aldehyde dehydrogenase, leading to a build-up of the aldehyde form of the biogenic amine. These conditions may favour alkaloid synthesis (Davis, 1973). Similar reactions may occur with the catecholamine derived aldehydes.

The condensation products are than probably further metabolised, which may explain the difficulty in their isolation from humans (Davis *et al.*, 1975) (Figure 7.23).

There have been several criticisms of this hypothesis. Firstly, it was noted that the administration of pyrazole, an inhibitor of ethanol metabolism and hence acetaldehyde production, followed by ethanol ingestion, does not prevent all the acute and chronic effects of ethanol (Deitrich and Erwin, 1975). Secondly, it remains unclear whether acetaldehyde can pass the blood-brain barrier (Deitrich and Erwin, 1975). Thirdly, the clinical features of alcohol addiction and withdrawal differ in many respects from the features of alkaloid addiction. This has lead many workers to believe that these compounds have no role in alcoholism (Seever, 1970). Davis and Walsh (1970a,b,c) in reply to this criticism suggest that these differences are due to the diffuse action of exogenous morphine as compared with the local production of these alkaloids.

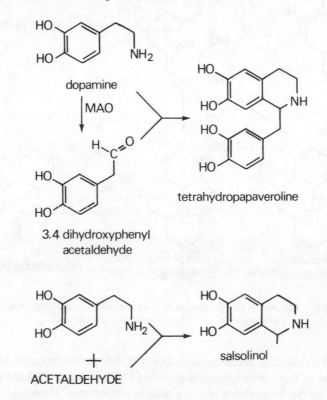

Fig. 2.23 – Synthesis of Alkaloid like substances from Biogenic Amines.

7.14.5 Central Nervous System Amines

There have been few human studies of central nervous system levels of amines and ethanol ingestion. Zarcone et al., (1975) studied csf levels of homovanillic acid (HVA) and 5-HIAA in alcoholics prior to, during, and after alcohol ingestion. They associated increases in their levels on withdrawal in the csf with changes in sleep patterns.

These changes in HVA and 5-HIAA levels in csf were later examined in relationship to cAMP levels (Orenberg *et al.,* 1976). The nucleotide levels were found to parallel the decreases in csf 5-HIAA found on alcohol ingestion. However, there was no significant quantitative correlation of the amount of change and the results were variable. This association between the pattern of change of cyclic AMP and 5-HIAA is interesting because the nucleotide is known to act as a second messenger for a variety of hormones and neurotransmitters. Cyclic-AMP may also be involved in synaptic transmission.

7.15 VITAMINS

Alcoholism is an important cause of vitamin deficiency. Abuse of alcohol may precipitate vitamin deficiency by a number of mechanisms including:

(i) Interference with an intake of a diet adequate in vitamins and protein.

(ii) Reduced absorption of vitamins.

(iii) Reduced storage of vitamins.

(iv) Diminished conversion of vitamins to their metabolically active forms.

The integrity of metabolic pathways involved in the hepatic oxidation of ethanol and re-oxidation of reduced NAD produced during ethanol metabolism, is dependent upon adequate supplies of a number of vitamins. Deficiency of these vitamins may impair ethanol metabolism. Important vitamin-dependent pathways of ethanol metabolism are summarised in Figure 7.24.

Many other metabolic processes are vitamin-dependent and deficiency may lead to impairment of such processes. An important point to note, however, is that in hospitals and clinics, alcoholics are routinely given large doses of multivitamin preparations (e.g Parentrovite) and thus vitamin deficiencies and any biochemical changes due to such deficiencies may not be detectable in such patients.

7.15.1 Vitamin A

Vitamin A is essential for normal mucopolysaccharide synthesis and mucus secretion. It is also a component of the retinal pigment rhodospin. Hepatic stores of Vitamin A are large and clinical signs of deficiency (e.g. 'night blindness', xeroderma, xerophthalmia) only develop after prolonged dietary deficiency. Plasma levels may be low in protein deficiency states, due to lack of the carrier protein retinol binding protein.

Low serum levels of Vitamin A were found in 44% of a group of patients (22 males, 7 females) with alcoholic liver disease investigated by Bollet and Owens (1973). The relative roles of malnutrition, liver disease, malabsorption, and retinol binding protein levels in the genesis of the low Vitamin A levels in these patients was not assessed.

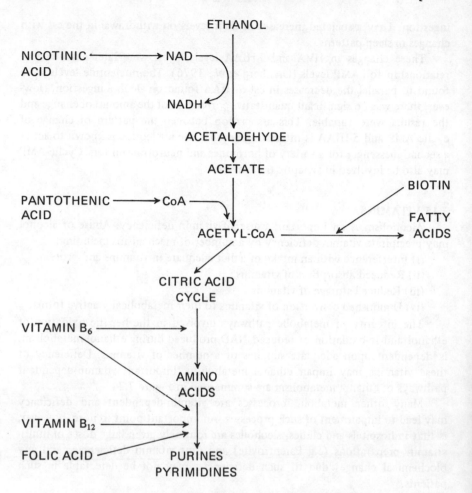

ETHANOL

NICOTINIC ────────→ NAD
ACID

NADH

ACETALDEHYDE

ACETATE

BIOTIN

PANTOTHENIC ────→ CoA
ACID

FATTY
ACIDS

ACETYL-CoA ──────────────────→

CITRIC ACID
CYCLE

VITAMIN B₆ ──────────→

AMINO
ACIDS

VITAMIN B₁₂ ──────→

FOLIC ACID ──────────→   PURINES
PYRIMIDINES

Fig. 7.24 – Vitamin Dependent Pathways of Ethanol Metabolism.

7.15.2 Vitamin B₁ (Thiamine)

Thiamine, as its pyrophosphate is an essential cofactor for decarboxylation of α-oxacids (e.g. pyruvate $\longrightarrow$ acetyl CoA) and also for transketolation reactions. Beri-beri is the best known example of a thiamine deficiency syndrome.

Several investigators have described thiamine deficiency in alcoholics, especially alcoholics with liver disease (Delaney *et al.*, 1966; Dylmer, 1969; Jeffrey and Abelmann, 1971; Banker *et al.*, 1975; Wood *et al.*, 1977). As well as reduced blood levels of thiamine, csf levels may be significantly reduced. This has been found in chronically malnourished alcoholics with peripheral neuropathy with or without mental changes such as disorientation or confusion (Dastur *et al.*, 1976). The relationship between thiamine deficiency and the clinical symptoms is unclear.

Analyses of serum, urine, and stool samples have shown that the absorption of thiamine, following oral or parenteral ^{14}C-(Tomasulo *et al.*, 1968) or ^{35}S-labelled thiamine (Thomson *et al.*, 1970; Thomson and Leevy, 1972) is impaired in alcoholic patients. Factors other than malabsorption may be involved in the development of thiamine deficiency syndromes in alcoholic patients. These factors include decreased conversion of thiamine to thiamine pyrophosphate and decreased hepatic storage of thiamine, both as a consequence of liver damage.

7.15.3 Vitamin B$_2$ (Riboflavin)

In the form of flavin adenine nucleotides (e.g. FMN), riboflavin plays an important role in biological oxidation systems. Clinical symptoms of ariboflavinosis include cheilosis and angular stomatitis.

No significant differences have been reported in urinary levels of Vitamin B$_2$ (Neville *et al.*, 1968), although reduced blood and csf levels have been reported in alcoholics with a history of chronic malnourishment (Dastur *et al.*, 1976).

7.15.4 Vitamin B$_6$ (Pyridoxine)

The active form of Vitamin B$_6$ is pyridoxal-phosphate. The inter-relationship of the various forms of B$_6$, pyridoxine, pyridoxal and pyridoxamine and their 5-phosphorylated derivatives is shown in Figure 7.25. Deficiency of this vitamin causes weight loss, anaemia, and convulsions in infants and confusion, depression, and convulsions in adults.

The incidence of Vitamin B$_6$ deficiency may be as high as 30–50% in alcoholics and 80–100% in those with liver disease (Hines and Love, 1969; Davis and Smith 1974). Inadequate dietary intake is the primary cause of deficiency although acetaldehyde derived from ethanol oxidation, and liver disease also contribute to the development of B$_6$ deficiency.

Low blood, serum and csf levels of pyridoxal phosphate have been reported in alcoholic patients (Hines and Cowan, 1970; Davis and Smith 1974; Lumeng and Li, 1974; Dastur *et al.*, 1976). Several groups of workers (Hines and Cowan, 1970; Lumeng and Li, 1974) have shown that alcohol consumption caused a depression of serum pyridoxal and also impaired phosphorylation of pyridoxine. This latter effect was at first attributed to an inhibition of pyridoxal phosphate synthesis by alcohol. However, the levels of the enzymes required for pyridoxal phosphate synthesis (pyridoxal kinase and phosphatase) in red blood cells from alcoholic patients with low plasma pyridoxal phosphate concentrations and from acutely intoxicated chronic alcoholics have been found to be normal (Lumeng and Li, 1974; Chillar *et al.*, 1976) although decreased levels have also been noted (Hines and Cowan, 1970). Studies with erythrocytes have now indicated that the lowered levels of pyridoxal phosphate in alcoholic patients are due to an acceleration of the degradation of phosphorylated B_6 compounds by acetaldehyde. It appears that acetaldehyde displaces pyridoxal phosphate from its protective binding protein and thus accelarates degradation (Lumeng and Li, 1974; Veitch *et al.*, 1975).

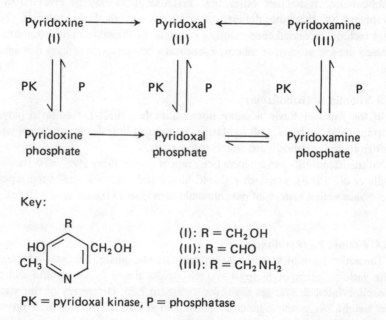

Key:

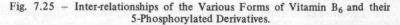

PK = pyridoxal kinase, P = phosphatase

Fig. 7.25 – Inter-relationships of the Various Forms of Vitamin B_6 and their 5-Phosphorylated Derivatives.

Liver disease also affects Vitamin B_6 absorption and metabolism. Chronic alcoholics with liver disease are unable to absorb Vitamin B_6 from food, but are able to absorb the vitamin from synthetic preparations, e.g., brewers yeast (Baker *et al.*, 1975). Degradation of pyridoxal phosphate is increased in alcoholics with liver disease.

Pyridoxal phosphate is an important co-enzyme at several stages in the metabolism of proteins, carbohydrates and fats and this has led to the proposal that a disturbance in its metabolism may contribute to chronic tissue injury, especially in the liver.

7.15.5 Vitamin B_{12} (Cyanocobalamin)

Vitamin B_{12} is absorbed from the terminal ileum in combination with intrinsic factor which is secreted by the stomach. Absence of this factor leads to malabsorption of B_{12} and pernicious anaemia. Megaloblastic anaemia also results from Vitamin B_{12} deficiency.

Generally, the serum levels of Vitamin B_{12} in alcoholic patients have been found to be within the appropriate reference intervals (Cowan and Hines, 1971; Halsted *et al.*, 1971; Pezzimenti and Lindenbaum, 1972; Davis and Smith, 1977), but low values for serum unsaturated B_{12} binding capacity have been reported in a group of chronic alcoholics studied by Liu (1973). Also, alcoholic patients with liver disease had raised serum B_{12} levels and this was attributed to either leakage of B_{12} from damaged cells or to an increase in serum B_{12} binding capacity and hence to an increase in total serum B_{12} (Carney, 1970; Dastur *et al.*, 1976).

Studies in nutritionally-replete chronic alcoholics given ethanol (158–253 g/day) for a period of several weeks have shown that an impaired ileal absorption of Vitamin B_{12} developed (Lindenbaum and Lieber, 1969b). Likewise, 8 out of 29 chronic alcoholics studied by Roggin *et al.*, (1969) had impaired B_{12} absorption.

7.15.6 Folic Acid (Pteroylglutamic acid)

Folate deficiency is one of the most common vitamin deficiency states. The vitamin is absorbed throughout the small intestine, and deficiency occurs in malabsorption syndromes. The active form of the vitamin is tetrahydrofolate (see Figure 7.26) and this plays an important role in purine and pyrimidine biosynthesis.

Although both normal (Williams and Girdwood, 1970; Pezzimenti and Lindenbaum, 1972) and elevated (Carney, 1967, 1970) values have been reported, the predominant finding in alcoholic patients being of a low value for serum folate (Laroche *et al.*, 1969; Hourihane and Weir, 1970; Cowan and Hines 1971; Gardner, 1971; Eichner *et al.*, 1972, Liu, 1973; Davis and Smith, 1974; Wu *et al.*, 1974, 1975).

The less common finding of elevated serum folate levels in alcoholics has been attributed to the high folate content of ingested beer and wines, but this has not been substantiated. An alternative theory suggests that ethanol inhibits the utilisation of folate in haematopoiesis thus leading to an accumulation of folate (Carney, 1970).

Several groups of workers have studied the effect of ethanol on folate in healthy controls and in chronic alcoholics and reported a decline in serum and erythrocyte folate levels (Hines and Cowan, 1970; Eichner and Hillman, 1973; Halsted *et al.*, 1973). The depression of serum folate levels is related to the dose of alcohol. In three normal volunteers investigated by Paine *et al.*, (1973) ingestion of 6, 4, and 3 ounces of 95% ethanol resulted in a 50, 30-35 and 15-20% fall in serum folate, severally.

The mechanism by which ethanol induces a fall in a serum folate levels is not well understood (Anon., 1972b). One component of the mechanism may be an inhibition of intestinal absorption of dietary folate (Thomson *et al.*, 1971; Baker *et al.*, 1975). Studies using tritium labelled folic acid have indicated decreased jejunal uptake in malnourished, actively-drinking alcoholics without liver disease, although this malabsorption could not be demonstrated when the patients were nutritionally replete (Halsted *et al.*, 1971).

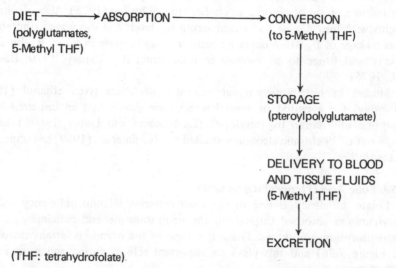

Fig. 7.26 – Folate Metabolism.

Evidence of a direct effect of ethanol on folate metabolism has been presented by Eichner and Hillman (1973). A fasting alcoholic patient developed a low serum folate following an infusion of ethanol. Since the subject fasted throughout the study it was unlikely that the fall in serum folate could have been due to reduced absorption of dietary folate. These authors have also noted that the development of sub-normal folate levels following alcohol ingestion is dependent upon the initial folate status of the patient. In a study of two alcoholic patients with intially high and low serum folate levels respectively, an ethanol induced fall in folate to sub-normal levels was only observed for the patient with initially low serum folate. It was suggested that this was due to differences in folate stores and/or to conversion of absorbed folic acid to 5-methyltetrahydrofolic acid.

More recently, the effect of ethanol on tritium labelled folate and carbon–14 labelled 5-methyltetrahydrofolate has been studied (Lane *et al.*, 1976). Alcohol was found to be without effect on the urinary loss of the labelled vitamin or its labelled breakdown products. Storage and tissue binding of folate were also unaffected, although there was some evidence to indicate that release of tetrahydrofolate from tissue stores was inhibited by ethanol.

Folate status has been assessed indirectly by measurement of urinary formiminoglutamate (FIGLU). This substance is an intermediate in the degradation of histidine to glutamate and its further metabolism is dependent on tetrahydrofolate. Deficiency of tetrahydrofolate decreases metabolism of FIGLU and thus increases its excretion in urine. This test has been used to demonstrate folate deficiency in four acutely intoxicated subjects (Rosenauerova-Ostra *et al.*, 1976).

7.15.7 Vitamin C (Ascorbic Acid)

The functions of Vitamin C in man are not well characterised, but it probably acts as a hydrogen carrier and is also required for normal collagen formation. Deficiency of Vitamin C causes scurvy and many of the symptoms of scurvy can be related to poor collagen formation.

Studies of alcoholic patients (Svirpina, 1971) and alcoholic patients with liver disease (Bollet and Owens, 1973) have shown that 36% and 46%, respectively of the patients studied were Vitamin C deficient. Sub-clinical scurvy is reported to occur commonly in alcoholics with an inadequate dietary intake of Vitamin C. The mean leucocyte ascorbic acid level as 18.18 ± 11.01 $\mu g/10^8$ WBC (range 0–50) in a group of 50 chronic alcoholics, whilst the mean ($\pm$ S.D.) of a control group was 27.41 ± 7.59 $\mu g/10^8$ WBC with a range of 11–46 $\mu g/10^8$ WBC (O'Keane *et al.*, 1972). Vitamin C levels in leucocytes are depressed in alcoholics with liver disease (Dow *et al.*, 1975). This may be of some importance for the metabolism of ethanol in such patients since the activity of alcohol dehydrogenase partially depends on Vitamin C saturation. A highly significant linear correlation has been shown to exist between hepatic alcohol dehydrogenase activity and leucocyte Vitamin C levels (Krasner *et al.*, 1974).

7.15.8 Vitamin D (Cholecalciferol)

Dietary Vitamin D and its precursors (Vitamins D_2 and D_3) are absorbed from the small intestine and stored in the liver. The active form of Vitamin D, 1, 25-dihydroxycholecalciferol, is produced by successive hydroxylations in the liver (25-hydroxylation) and in the kidney (1-hydroxylation). 25-Hydroxycholecalciferol is the main circulating form of the vitamin. The active form of Vitamin D is necessary for intestinal calcium absorption and for deposition and resorption of calcium salts in bone. Deficiency leads to disturbances of calcium metabolism and rickets.

Normal levels of plasma 25-hydroxycholecalciferol have been reported in alcoholics without cirrhosis (Verbanck *et al.*, 1976) although low levels occur in alcoholics with liver disease (Long *et al.*, 1976).

The importance of factors such as diet, hepatic 25-hydroxylation, and malabsorption in the genesis of low Vitamin D levels have not been assessed.

Lund *et al.*, (1977) have reported that alcoholics with fatty liver disease but without cirrhosis, alcoholics with compensated cirrhosis and alcoholics with severely incompensated cirrhosis all exhibited a significant rise in serum 25-hydroxycholecalciferol following either oral or i.v. administration of cholecalciferol, thus indicating that absorption of Vitamin D is not impaired in such patients.

Elevated 25-hydroxycholecalciferol levels have been described in an alcoholic patient with magnesium deficiency (Medalle *et al.*, 1976).

7.15.9 Vitamin E

Vitamin E deficiency is not known to cause disease in man. The vitamin has anti-oxidant properties and is stored in the liver. It may act to stabilise hepatic stores of Vitamins A and D.

In an isolated study, 39% of a group of patients (22 males, 7 females) with alcoholic liver disease were found to have low serum levels of Vitamin E (Bollet and Owens, 1973).

7.15.10 Pantothenic Acid

Pantothenic acid is a component of coenzyme A. To-date no pantothenic acid deficiency states have been described.

Decreased urinary excretion of pantothenic acid occurs in acute alcoholic patients (mean 2.7 mg/day as compared with 3.8 mg/day for normal individuals). In alcoholics undergoing rehabilitation, urinary excretion of pantothenic acid decreases progressively during rehabilitation. It has been suggested that alcoholics are unable to utilise dietary pantothenic acid, but during rehabilitation the vitamin is gradually retained, hence the fall in urinary excretion (Toa and Fox, 1976).

7.15.11 Niacin (Nictonic acid and Nicotinamide)

Nicotinamide, which can be formed in the body from nicotinic acid, is a constituent of the important co-enzymes NAD and NADP. A deficiency of nicotinamide gives rise to pellagra. Although alcoholic beverages have a high nicotinic acid content, deficiency in this substance has been reported in alcoholics (Leevy *et al.*, 1970).

7.16 REFERENCES

Abelin, V. I., Herren, C., and Berli, W. (1958) Uber die erregende Wirkung des Alkohols auf den Adrenalin and Noradrenalinhaushalt des menschlichen Organismus. *Helvet. Med. Acta.*, **25**, 591–600.

Abramson, E. A., and Arky, R. A. (1968) Acute antilipolytic effects of ethyl alcohol and acetate in man. *J. Lab. Clin. Med.,* **72**, 105-117.

Adjarov, D., and Iwanow, E. D. (1973) Neue Aspekte der klinischen Bedeutung der γ-Glutamyl − Transpeptidasebestimmung in Serum. *Acta Hepato-Gastroenterol.* **20,** 315-324.

Agostoni, A., Vergani, C., Stabilini, R., and Marasini, B. (1969) Determination of seven serum proteins in alcoholic cirrhosis. *Clin. Chim. Acta,* **26,** 351-355.

Akdamar, K., Epps, A. C., Maumus, L. T. and Sparks, R. D. (1972) Immunoglobulin changes in liver disease. *Ann. N.Y. Acad. Sci.,* **197,** 101-107.

Akhter, M. I., Clark, P. M. S., Kricka, L. J., and Nicholson, G. (1978) Urinary metabolites of tryptophan, serotonin and norepinephrine. *J. Stud. Alcohol,* **39,** 833-841.

Albahary, C., Auffret, M., and Gland, J. L. Le (1968) Zieve's syndrome alcoholic hyperlipidemia and hemolytic anemia. *Presse Med.,* **76,** 371-375.

Ali, M. A. M., and Sweeney, G. (1974) Erythrocyte coproporphyrin and protoporphyrin in ethanol − induced sideroblastic erythropoiesis. *Blood,* **43,** 291-295.

Alling, C., Dencker, S. J., Svennerholm, L., and Tichy, J. (1969) Serum fatty acid pattern in chronic alcoholics after acute abuse. *Acta Med. Scand.,* **185,** 99-105.

Ammon, H. P. T., and Estler, C. J. (1968) Inhibition of ethanol − induced glycogenolysis in brain and liver by adrenergic β-blockade. *J. Pharm. Pharmacol.,* **20,** 164-165.

Anon. (1970) Effects of dietary fats and ethanol on lipemia. *Nutr. Rev.,* **28,** 162-163.

Anon. (1972a) Alcohol addiction: A biochemical approach. *Lancet,* ii, 24-25.

Anon. (1972b) Alcoholism and Folic acid. *Nutr. Rev.,* **30,** 57-60.

Anton, A. H. (1965) Ethanol and urinary catecholamines in man. *Clin. Pharmacol. Ther.,* **6,** 462-469.

Arky R. A., and Freinkel, N. (1969) Hypoglycaemia action of alcohol. *In* Biochemical and Clinical Aspects of Alcohol Metabolism (Sardesai, V. M. *ed.*) pp. 67-80, Charles C. Thomas, Springfield, Illinois.

Arky, R. A., Veverbrants, E., and Abramson, E. A. (1968) Irreversible hypoglycaemia: a complication of alcohol and insulin. *J. Am. Med. Assoc.,* **206,** 575-578.

Arky R. A. (1971) The effect of Alcohol on Carbohydrate Metabolism. Carbohydrate Metabolism in Alcoholics. *In* The Biology of Alcoholism (Kissin, B., and Begleiter, H. *eds.*) pp. 197-227, Plenum Press, New York.

Augustine, J. R. (1967) Laboratory studies in acute alcoholism. *Canad. Med. Ass. J.,* **96,** 1367-1370.

Avogãro, P., and Cazzolato, G. (1975) Changes in the composition and physicochemical characteristics of serum lipoproteins during ethanol − induced lipaemia in alcoholic subjects. *Metab. Clin. Exp.,* **24,** 1231-1242.

Baba, S., Takase, S., Uenoyama, R., Morita, S., Mizoi, Y., and Hishida, S. (1976) Isolated corticotrophin-deficiency found through alcohol-induced hypoglycemic coma. *Horm. Metab. Res.*, **8**, 274-278.

Badawy, A., A-B (1977) A review of the effects of alcohol on carbohydrate metabolism. *Br. J. Alcohol and Alcoholism*, **12**, 120-136.

Bagdade, J. D., Bierman, E. L., and Porte Jr., D. (1972a) A counter-regulation of basal insulin secretion during alcohol hypoglycaemia in diabetic and normal subjects. *Diabetes*, **21**, 65-70.

Bagdade, J. D., Gale, C. C., and Porte, D. (1972b) Hormone fuel interrelationships during alcohol hypoglycaemia in man. *Proc. Soc. Exp. Biol. Med.*, **141**, 540-542.

Baglin, M. C., Bernot, J. L., Bremond, J. L., Lamy, J., Leroux, M. E., and Weill, J. (1976) Efficacite compares du volume globulinaire moyen (VGM) et de la gamma-glutamyl transferase (γ-GT) serique comme test de triage des buveurs excessifs d' alcohol. *Clin. Chim. Acta,* **68**, 321-326.

Baker, H., Frank, O., Zetterman, R. K., Rajan, K. S., ten Hove, W., and Leevy C. M., (1975) Inability of chronic alcoholics with liver disease to use food as a source of folates, thiamin and vitamin B_6 *Am. J. Clin. Nutr.*, **28**, 1377-1380.

Baraona, E., Leo, M., Berovsky, S. A., and Lieber, C. S. (1975) Alcoholic hepatomegaly: accumulation of protein in the liver. *Science (Wash. D.C.)*, **190**, 794-795.

Barboriak, J. J., and Hogan, W. J. (1976) Preprandial drinking and plasma lipids in man. *Atherosclerosis*, **24**, 323-325.

Beard, J. D., and Knott, D. H. (1968) Fluid and electrolyte balance during acute withdrawal in chronic alcoholic patients. *J. Am. Med. Assoc.*, **204**, 133-139.

Beard, J. D., and Knott, D. H. (1977) The effect of alcohol on fluid and electrolyte metabolism. *In* The Biology of Alcoholism (Kissin, B. and Begleiter, H. *eds.*) Vol. 1. pp. 353-376, Plenum Press, New York.

Becker, H. O., Reeder, D. D., and Thompson, J. C. (1974) Gastrin release by ethanol in man and in dogs. *Ann. Surg.*, **179**, 906-909.

Belfrage, P., Berg, B., Cronholm, T., Elmqvist, D., Hägerstrand, I., Johannson, B., Nilsson-Ehle, P., Norden, G., Sjovall, J., and Wiebe, T. (1973) Prolonged administration of ethanol to young healthy volunteers: Effects on biochemical morphological and neuro-physiological parameters. *Acta Med. Scand., Suppl.*, **552**, 5-43.

Belfrage, P., Berg, B., Hägerstrand, I., Nilsson-Ehle, P., Tornqvist, H., and Wiebe, T., (1977) Alterations of lipid metabolism in healthy volunteers during long-term ethanol intake. *Eur. J. Clin Invest.*, **7**, 127-131.

Bellet, S., Roman, L., DeCastro, O., and Herrera, M. (1970) Effect of acute ethanol intake on plasma 11-hydroxycorticosteroid levels. *Metabolism*, **19**, 664-667.

Bellet, S., Yoshimine, N., DeCastro, O. A. P., Roman, L., Parmar, S. S., and Sandberg, H. (1971) Effects of alcohol ingestion on growth hormone levels: Their relation to 11-hydroxycorticoid levels and serum FFA. *Metab. Clin. Exp.*, **20**, 762–769.

Bendersky, G. (1975) Etiology of hyperuricemia *Ann. Clin. Lab. Sci.*, **5**, 456–467.

Block, R. (1972) Pregnancy in portal cirrhosis *J. Reprod. Med.*, **8**, 143–145.

Bollet, A. J., and Owens, S. (1973) Evaluation of nutritional status of selected hospitalised patients. *J. Clin. Nutr.*, **26**, 931–938.

Boone, D. J., Routh, J. I., and Schrantz, R. (1974) γ-Glutamyl transpeptidase and 5'-nucleotidase. *Am. J. Clin. Pathol.*, **61**, 321–327.

Böttiger, L. E. (1973) Alcohol and the Blood. *Scand. J. Haematol.*, **10**, 321–326.

Böttinger, L. E., Carlson, L. A., Hultman, E., and Romanus, V. (1976) Serum lipids in alcoholics. *Acta Med. Scand.*, **199**, 357–361.

Brewster, A. C., Lankford, H. G., Schwartz, M. G., and Sullivan, J. F. (1966) Ethanol and alimentary lipemia. *Am. J. Clin. Nutr.*, **19**, 255–259.

Brohult, J. and Sundbled, L. (1973) Isoenzyme patterns of serum alkaline phosphatase in ethanol induced liver injury. *Acta Med. Scand.*, **194**, 479–499.

Brunt, P. W., (1971) Alcohol and the liver. *Gut*, **12**, 222–229.

Butt, W. R. (1975) *In* Hormone Chemistry, 2nd *edn*, **Vol. 1**. Ellis Horwood Ltd., Chichester.

Butt, W. R. (1976) Corticosteroids *In* Hormone Chemistry. **Vol. 2**. pp. 147–190, Ellis Horwood Ltd., Chichester.

Cadoret, R. J., Helling, D., Lawhorne, L., Moessner, H., Redlin, J., Widmer, R. B., and Sellers, A. (1975) Alcoholism and diabetes. *J. Family Practice*, **2**, 385–387.

Caldwell, J., and Sever, P. S. (1974) The biochemical pharmacology of abused drugs. II Alcohol and barbiturates. *Clin. Pharmacol. Ther.*, **16**, 737–749.

Callender, S. T., and Malpas, J. S. (1963) Absorption of iron in cirrhosis of the liver. *Br. Med. J.*, **2**, 1516–1518.

Carey, M. A., Jones, J. D., and Gastineau, C. F. (1971) Effects of moderate alcohol intake on blood chemistry values. *J. Am. Med. Assoc.*, **216**, 1766–1769.

Carlsson, C., and Häggendal, J. (1967) Arterial noradrenaline levels after ethanol withdrawal, *Lancet*, **ii**, 889.

Carlsson, C., and Dehlin, O. (1972) Pancreatic exocrine function and D-xylose test in patients with chronic alcoholism. *Acta Med. Scand.*, **191**, 477–480.

Carlsson, C., and Dencker, S. J. (1973) Cerebrospinal uric acid in alcoholics. *Acta Neurol. Scand.*, **49**, 39–46.

Carney, M. W. P. (1967) Serum folate values in 423 psychiatric patients. *Br. Med. J.*, **iv**, 512–516.

Carney, M. W. P. (1970) Serum folate and cyanocobalamin in alcoholics. *Q. J. Stud. Alcohol*, **31**, 816–822.

Castelli, W. P., Doyle, J. T., Gordon, T., Hames, C. G., Hjortland, M. C., Hulley, S. B., Kagan, A., and Zukel, W. J. (1977) Alcohol and blood lipids. *Lancet*, **ii**, 153–155.

Celeda, A., Rudolf, H., and Donath, A. (1977) Influence de l'alcool sur l'absorption du fer. *Schweiz. Med. Wochenschr.*, **107**, 1471.

Chait, A., Mancini, M., February, A. W., and Lewis, B. (1972) Clinical and metabolic study of alcoholic hyperlipidaemia. *Lancet*, **ii**, 62–64.

Champion, H. R., Caplan, Y. H., Baker, S. P., Long, W. B., Benner, C., Cowley, R. A., Fisher, R., and Gill, W. (1975) Alcohol intoxication and serum osmolality, *Lancet*, **ii**, 1402–1404.

Charlton, R. W., Jacobs, P., Seftel, H., and Bothwell, T. H. (1964) Effect of alcohol on iron absorption. *Br. Med. J.*, **2**, 1427–1429.

Chillar, R. K., Johnson, C. S., and Beutler, E. (1976) Erythrocyte pyridoxine kinase levels in patients with sideroblastic anaemia. *N. Engl. J. Med.*, **295**, 881–882.

Chowdhury, A. R., Malmud, L. D., and Dinoso, V. P. (1977) Gastrointestinal plasma protein loss during ethanol ingestion. *Gastroenterology*, **72**, 37–40.

Clark, W. C., Wilson, J. E., and Hulpieu, H. R. (1961) Production of hypoglycemia by Solox and by ethanol. *Q. J. Stud. Alcohol*, **22**, 365–373.

Cobo, E., and Quintero, C. A. (1969) Milk – ejecting and antidiuretic activities under neurohypophyseal inhibition with alcohol and water overload. *Am. J. Obstet. Gynecol.*, **105**, 877–887.

Cohen, S. (1976) A review of hypoglycaemia and alcoholism with or without liver disease. *Ann. N. Y. Acad. Sci.*, **273**, 338–342.

Conti, F., Mandelli, V., Natangelo, R., and Tamassia, V. (1972) Prognosi a breve termine del paziente con cirrosi alcoolica mediante l'uso della fuzione discriminante. *Minerva Med.*, **63**, 949–999.

Cowan, D. H., and Hines, J. D. (1971) Thrombocytopenia of severe alcoholism. *Ann. Int. Med.*, **74**, 37–43.

Cronholm, T., and Sjövall, J. (1968) Effect of ethanol on the concentrations of solvolyzable plasma steroids. *Biochem. Biophys. Acta*, **152**, 230–233.

Cronholm, T., and Sjövall, J. (1970) Effect of ethanol metabolism on redox state of steroid sulphates in man. *Eur. J. Biochem.*, **13**, 124–131.

Crouse, J. R., Gerson, C. D., De Carli, L. M., and Lieber, C. S. (1968) Role of acetate in the reduction of plasma free fatty acids produced by alcohol in man. *J. Lipid. Res.*, **9**, 509–512.

Dastur, D. K., Santhadevi, N., Quadros, E. V., Avari, F. C. R., Wadia, N. H., Desia, M. M., and Bharucha, E. P. (1976) The B-Vitamins in malnutrition with alcoholism. *Br. J. Nutr.*, **36**, 143–159.

Davis, V. E. (1973) Neuroamine-derived alkaloids: A possible common denominator in alcoholism and related drug dependencies. *Ann. N. Y. Acad. Sci.*, **215**, 111–115.

Davis, A. E., and Badenoch, J. (1962) Iron absorption in pancreatic disease. *Lancet,* ii, 6-8.

Davis, V. E., and Walsh, M. J. (1970a) Alcohols, amines and alkaloids: a possible biochemical basis for alcohol addiction. *Science,* 167, 1005-1007.

Davis, V. E., and Walsh, M. J. (1970b) Alcohol addiction and tetrahydropapaveroline. *Science,* 169, 1105-1106.

Davis, V. E., and Walsh, M. J. (1970c) Ans. Morphine and ethanol physical dependence and a critique of a Hypothesis. *Science,* 170, 1114-1115.

Davis, R. E., and Smith, B. K. (1974) Pyridoxal and folate deficiency in alcoholics. *Med. J. Aust.,* 2, 357-360.

Davis, V. E., Cashaw, J. L., Huff, J. A., and Brown, H. (1966) Identification of 5-hydroxytryptophol as a serotonin metabolite in man. *Proc. Soc. Exp. Biol. Med.,* 122, 890-893.

Davis, V. E., Brown, H., Huff, J. A., and Cashaw, J. L. (1967a) Ethanol induced alterations of norepinephrine metabolism in man. *J. Lab. Clin. Med.,* 69, 787-799.

Davis, V. E., Cashaw, J. L., Huff, J. A., Brown, H., and Nicholas, N. L. (1967b) Alteration of endogenous catecholamine metabolism by ethanol ingestion. *Proc. Soc. Exp. Med.,* 125, 1140-1143.

Davis, V. E., Huff, J. A., and Brown, H. (1967c) Alcohol and biogenic amines. *In* Biochemical and Clinical Aspects of Alcohol Metabolism (Sardesai, V. M. *ed.*) pp. 95-104, Charles C. Thomas, Springfield, Illinois.

Davis, V. E., Brown, H. Huff, J. A., and Cashaw, J. L. (1967d) The alteration of serotonin metabolism to 5-hydroxytryptophol by ethanol ingestion in man. *J. Lab. Clin. Med.,* 69, 132-140.

Davis, V. E., Cashaw, J. L., and McMurrey, K. D. (1975) Disposition of catecholamine — derived alkaloids in mammalian systems. *Adv. Exp. Med. Biol.,* 59, 65-78.

De Gennes, J. L., Thompoulos, P., Truffert, J., and Labrousse de Tregomain, B. (1972) Hyperlipémies depédantes de l' alcool. *Nutr. Metab.,* 14, 141-158.

Dehlin, O., Hallgren, B., and Lundvall, O. (1970) Exocrine pancreatic function in porphyria cutanea tarda. *Acta Med. Scand.,* 188, 549-552.

Deitrich, R. A., and Erwin, V. G. (1975) Involvement of biogenic amine metabolism in ethanol addiction. *Fed. Proc.,* 34, 1962-1968.

Delaney, R. L., Lankford, H. G., and Sullivan, J. F. (1966) Thiamine, magnesium and plasma lactate abnormalities in alcoholic patients. *Proc. Soc. Exp. Biol. Med.,* 123, 675-679.

De Moura, M. C., Correia, J. P., and Madeira, F. (1967) Clinical alcohol hypoglycaemia. *Ann. Int. Med.,* 66, 893-905.

De Terok, D., and De Crow, C. A. J. (1976) Quantitative and qualitative plasma protein studies on alcoholics versus non-alcoholics. *Ann. N. Y. Acad. Sci.,* 273, 167-174.

Dettori, A. G., Ponari, O., Civardi, E., Megha, A., Pini, M., and Poti, R. (1977) Impaired fibrin formation in advanced cirrhosis. *Haemostasis*, 6, 137-148.

Devenyi, P., Rutherdale, J., Sereny, G., and Olin, J. S. (1970) Clinical diagnosis of alcoholic fatty liver. *Am. J. Gastroenterol.*, 54, 597-602.

Dillon, E. S., Dyer, W. W., and Smelo, L. S. (1940) Ketone acidosis in non-diabetic adults. *Med. Clin. North Am.*, 24, 1813-1822.

Dimich, A., and Wallace, S. (1969) Magnesium transport in humans with hypomagnesaemia. *J. Clin. Endocrinol. Metab.*, 29, 496-505.

Dinoso, V. P., Chey, W. Y., Padow, D., Rosen, A., Ottenberg, D. and Lorber, S. H. (1971) Gastrointestinal disorders in chronic alcoholics. *Am. J. Gastroenterol.*, 56, 209-215.

Distiller, L. A., Sagel, J., Dubowitz, B., Kay, G., Carr, P. J., Katz, M., and Kew, M. C. (1976) Pituitary-gonadal function in men with alcoholic cirrhosis of the liver. *Horm. Metab. Res.*, 8, 461-465.

Dornhorst, A. and Ouyang, A. (1971) Effect of alcohol on glucose tolerance. *Lancet*, ii, 957-959.

Dotson, L. E., Robertson, L. S., and Tuchfeld, B. (1975) Plasma alcohol, smoking, hormone concentrations and self-reported aggression. *J. Stud. Alcohol*, 36, 578-586.

Dow, J., Krasner, N., and Goldberg, A. (1975) Relation between hepatic alcohol dehydrogenase activity and the ascorbic acid in leucocytes of patients with liver disease. *Clin. Sci. Mol. Med.*, 49, 603-608.

Dymling, J. F., Ljungberg, O., Hillyard, C. J., Greenberg, P. B., Evans, I. M. A., and MacIntyre, I. (1976) Whisky: A new provocative test for calcitonin secretion. *Acta. Endocrinol.*, 82, 500-509.

Dylmer, H. (1969) Wernicke's encephalopathy. *Nord. Med.*, 81, 311-313.

Eales, L. (1963) Porphyria as seen in Cape Town. A survey of 250 patients and some recent studies. *S. Afr. J. Lab. Clin. Med.*, 9, 151-162.

Earll, J. M., Gaunt, K., Earll, L. A., and Djuh, Y. Y. (1976) Effect of ethyl alcohol on ionic calcium and prolactin in man. *Aviat. Space Environ. Med.*, 47, 808-810.

Eichner, E. R., and Hillman, R. S. (1971) The evaluation of anemia in alcoholic patients. *Am. J. Med.*, 50, 218-232.

Eichner, E. R., and Hillman, R. S. (1973) Effect of alcohol on serum folate level. *J. Clin. Invest.*, 52, 584-591.

Eichner, E. R., Buchanan, B., Smith, J. W., and Hillman, R. S. (1972) Variations in the hematologic and medical status of alcoholics. *Am. J. Med. Sci.*, 263, 35-42.

Eriksson, C. E., Hed, R., Lindblad, L. E., Nygren, A. Sundblad, L. (1974) Glucose intolerance and peripheral glucose uptake in acutely intoxicated alcoholics. *Lancet*, i, 811-812.

Estep, H., Shaw, W. A., Watlington, C., Hobe, R., Holland, W., and Tucker, St. G., (1969) Hypocalcaemia due to hypomagnesemia and reversible parathyroid hormone unresponsiveness. *J. Clin. Endocrinol. Metab.*, **29**, 842-848.

Evans, J. G., Prior, I. A. M., and Harvey, H. P. B. (1968) Relation of serum uric acid to body bulk, haemoglobin and alcohol intake in two south pacific polynesian populations. *Ann. Rheum. Dis.*, **27**, 319-325.

Fabre, L. F., Farmer, R. W., and Davis, H. W. (1971) Effect of ethanol on adrenocortical steroid secretion. *In* Biological Aspects of Alcohol. (Roach, M. K., McIsaac, W. M., and Creaven, P. J. *eds.*) pp. 418-445, University of Texas Press, Austin.

Fabre, L. F., Pasco, P. J., Liegel, J. M., and Farmer, R. W. (1973) Abnormal testosterone excretion in men alcoholics. *Q. J. Stud. Alcohol*, **34**, 57-63.

Farmer, R. W., and Fabre, L. F. (1975) Some endocrine aspects of alcoholism. *Adv. Exp. Med. Biol.*, **56**, 277-289.

Fazekas, I. G. (1966) Hydrocortisone content of human blood, and alcohol content of blood and urine after wine consumption. *Q. J. Stud. Alcohol*, **27**, 439-446.

Feigl, J. (1918) Neue Untersuchung zurchemie des Blutes bei akuter Alkohol Intoxication und bei chronische Alkoholismus mit besonderer Berucksichtigung der Fette und Lipoide. *Biochem. Z.*, **92**, 282.

Feinman, L., and Lieber, C. S. (1967) Effect of ethanol on plasma glycerol in man. *Am. J. Clin. Nutr.*, **20**, 400-403.

Feizi, T. (1968) Immunoglobulins in chronic liver disease. *Gut*, **9**, 193-198.

Feldstein, A., Hoagland, H., Wong, K., and Freeman, H. (1964) Biogenic amines, biogenic aldehydes and alcohol. *Q. J. Stud. Alcohol*, **25**, 218-225.

Ferguson, J. C., Beattie, A. D., McAlpine, S. G., and Conway, H. (1970) Acute intermittent porphyria in identical twins. *Postgrad. Med. J.*, **46**, 717-734.

Field, J. B., Williams, H. E., and Mortimore, G. E. (1963) Studies on the mechanism of ethanol induced hypoglycaemia. *J. Clin. Invest.*, **42**, 497-506.

Fisher, A. J. G., Wardle, N., van Oldenborgh, M., and Chips, B. (1965) The effect of acute alcoholism on the serum amylase of normal persons. *S. Afr. Med. J.*, **39**, 673-676.

Flink, E. B. (1971) Mineral Metabolism in Alcoholism. *In* The Biology of Alcoholism (Kissin, B. and Begleiter, H. *eds.*) **Vol. 1**, pp. 277-395, Plenum Press, London.

Flink, E. B., Shane, S. R., Jacobs, W. H., and Jones, J. E. (1969) Some aspects of magnesium deficiency and chronic alcoholism. *In* Biochemical and Clinical Aspects of Alcohol Metabolism. (Sardesai, V. M. *ed.*) pp. 247-258, Charles, C. Thomas, Springfield, Illinois.

Forbes, J. C., and Duncan, G. M. (1950) The effect of alcohol on liver lipids and on liver and heart glycogen. *Q. J. Stud. Alcohol*, **11**, 373-380.

Forsander, O. A. (1970) Influence of ethanol on the redox state of the liver. *Q. J. Stud. Alcohol*, **31**, 550-570.

Forsander, O, Varita, K. O., and Krusius, F. E. (1958) Experimentelle Studien über die Biologische Wirkung von Alkohol. 1 Alkohol Blutzucker. *Ann. Med. Exp. Biol. Fenn.*, **35**, 416–423.

Frajna, R., and Angeli, A. (1977) Alcohol-induced pseudo-Cushing's syndrome. *Lancet*, **ii**, 1050–1051.

Franke, K., and Fimkemtscher, R. (1935) Die Bedeutung der quantitativen Porphyrinbestimmung der Lumineszenzmessung für Ernahrungsfragen. *Muench. Med. Wochenschr.*, **82**, 171–172.

Freer, D. E., and Statland, B. E. (1977a) The effects of ethanol (0.75 g/kg body weight) on the activities of selected enzymes in sera of healthy young adults; 1 Intermediate – term effects. *Clin. Chem.*, **23**, 830–834.

Freer, D. E., and Statland, B. E (1977b) Effects of ethanol (0.75 g/kg body weight) on the activities of selected enzymes in the sera of healthy young adults; 2 Inter-individual variations in response of γ-glutamyltransferase to repeated ethanol challenges. *Clin. Chem.*, **23**, 2099–2102.

Friedenberg, R., Metz, R., Mako, M., and Surmaczynska, B. (1971) Differential plasma insulin response to glucose and glucagon stimulation following ethanol priming. *Diabetes*, **20**, 397–403.

Friedman, M., Rosenman, R. H., and Byers, S. O. (1965) Effect of moderate ingestion of alcohol upon serum triglyceride responses of normo- and hyperlipemic subjects. *Proc. Soc. Exp. Biol. Med.*, **120**, 696–698.

Freinkel, N., Singer, D. L., Arky, R. A., Bleicher, S. J., Anderson, J. B., and Silbert, C. K. (1963) Alcohol hypoglycaemia. I. Carbohydrate metabolism of patients with clinical alcohol hypoglycaemia and experimental reproduction of the syndrome with pure ethanol. *J. Clin. Invest.*, **42**, 1112–1133.

Fry, M. M., Spector, A. A., Connor, S. L., and Connor, W. E. (1973) Intensification of hypertriglyceridemia by either alcohol or carbohydrate. *Am. J. Clin. Nutr.*, **26**, 798–802.

Fulop, M., Katz. S., and Lawrence, C. (1971) Extreme hyperbilirubinemia. *Arch. Intern. Med.*, **127**, 254–258.

Gardner, A. J. (1971) Folate status of alcoholic in-patients. *Br. J. Addict.*, **66**, 183–184.

Garlind, T., Goldberg, L. Graf, K., Perman, E. S., Strandell, T., and Ström, G. (1960) Effect of ethanol circulatory, metabolic and neurohormonal function during muscular work in man. *Acta Pharmacol. Toxicol.*, **17**, 106–114.

Garrod, A. B. (1876) *A Treatise on Gout and Rheumatic Gout*. 3rd *edn.*, Longmans, Green, London.

Gault, M.H., Stein, J., and Aronoff, A. (1966) Serum ceruloplasmin in hepatobiliary and other disorders: significance of abnormal values. *Gastroenterology*, **50**, 8–18.

Gérard, M. J., Klatsky, A. L., Siegelaub, A. B., Friedman, G. D., Feldman, R. (1977) Serum glucose levels and alcohol consumption habits in a large population. *Diabetes*, **26**, 780–785.

Giacobini, E., Izekowitz, S., and Wegmann, A. (1960) The urinary excretion of nor-adrenaline and adrenaline during acute alcohol intoxication in alcoholic subjects. *Experientia*, **16**, 767.

Gibbens, G. L. D., and Chard, T. (1976) Observations on maternal oxytocin release during human labor and the effect of intravenous alcohol administration. *Am. J. Obsts. Gynecol.*, **126**, 243-246.

Ginsberg, H., Olefsky, J., Farquar, J. W., and Reaven, G. M. (1974) Moderate ethanol ingestion and plasma triglyceride levels. A study in normal and hyper-triglyceridemic persons. *Ann. Intern. Med.*, **80**, 143-149.

Gitlow, S. E., Dziedzic, L. M., Dziedzic, S. W., and Wong, B. L. (1976) Influence of ethanol on human catecholamine metabolism. *Ann. N. Y. Acad. Sci.*, **273**, 203-277.

Gleichmann, E., and Deicher, H. (1968) Quantitative Immunoglobulin – Bestümmungen in serum bei entzündlichen Leberkrankenheiten, *Klin. Wochenschr.*, **46**, 793-802.

Goldbarg, J. A., and Altshule, M. D. (1966) Serum aminopeptidase and beta-glucuronidase activities. *Arch. Gen. Psychiatry*, **15**, 341-343.

Goldberg, D. M., and Watts, C. (1965) Serum enzyme changes as evidence of liver reaction to oral alcohol. *Gastroenterology*, **49**, 256-261.

Gordon, G. G., and Southren, A. L. (1977) Metabolic effects of alcohol on the endocrine system. *In* Metabolic Aspects of Alcoholism. (Lieber, C. S. *ed.*) pp. 249-302, M. T. P. Press, Lancaster.

Gordon, G. G., Altman, K., Southren, A. L., Rubin, E., and Lieber, C. S. (1976) Effect of alcohol (ethanol) administration on sex hormone metabolism in normal men. *N. Engl. J. Med.*, **295**, 793-797.

Guisard, D., Bigard, M. A., and Debry, G. (1972) Etude de l'épuration plasmatique des lipides chez des sujets attients de cirrhose hépatique d'origine éthylique avec asite. *Nutr. Metab.*, **14**, 193-202.

Halsted, J. A., Hackley, B., Rudzki, C., and Smith, J. C. (1968) Plasma zinc concentration in liver diseases. *Gastroenterology*, **54**, 1098-1105.

Halsted, C. H., Robles, E. A., and Mezey, E. (1971) Decreased jejunal uptake of labelled folic acid (^{3}H-PGA) in alcoholic patients: Roles of alcohol and nutrition. *N. Eng. J. Med.*, **285**, 701-706.

Halsted, C. H., Robles, E. A., and Mezey, E. (1973) Intestinal malabsorption in folate – deficient alcoholics. *Gastroenterology*, **64**, 526-532.

Hawkins, R. D., and Kalant, H. (1972) The metabolism of ethanol and its metabolic effects. *Pharmacol. Rev.*, **24**, 67-157.

Hed, C., Lundmark, C., Fahlgren, H., and Orell, S. (1962) Acute muscular syndrome in chronic alcoholism. *Acta Med. Scand.*, **171**, 585-599.

Hed, R., Nygren, A., Sundblad, L. (1972) Muscle and liver serum enzyme activities in healthy volunteers given alcohol on a diet poor in carbohydrates. *Acta Med. Scand.*, **191**, 529-534.

Hed, R., Nygren. A., Röjdmark, S., and Sundblad, L. (1975) Decreased glucose tolerance in chronic alcoholics after alcohol ingestion when fed a carbohydrate poor diet. *Horm. Metab. Res.*, **7**, 115-118.

Helwig, H. L. (1969) Zinc levels in serum and urine of alcoholics. *In* Biochemical and Clinical Aspects of Alcohol Metabolism (Sardesai, V. M. *ed.*) pp. 40-44, Charles C. Thomas, Springfield, Illinois.

Helwig, H. L., Hoffer, E. M., Thielen, W. C., Alcocer, A. E., Hotelling, D. R., Rogers, W. H., and Lench, J. (1966) Urinary and serum zinc levels in chronic alcoholism. *Am. J. Clin. Pathol.*, **45**, 156-159.

Hilden, T., and Svendsen, T. L. (1975) Electrolyte disturbances in beer drinkers. *Lancet*, **ii**, 245-246.

Hines, J. D., and Love, D. S. (1969) Determination of serum and blood pyridoxal phosphate concentrations with purified rabbit skeletal muscle apophosphorylase b. *J. Lab. Clin. Med.*, **73**, 343-349.

Hines, J. D., and Cowan, D. H. (1970) Studies on the pathogenesis of alcohol-induced sideroblastic bone-marrow abnormalities. *N. Engl. J. Med.*, **283**, 441-446.

Hobbs, J. R. (1967) Serum proteins in liver disease. *Proc. R. Soc. Med.*, **60**, 1250-1254.

Hoensch, H. (1972) The effects of alcohol on the liver. *Digestion*, **6**, 114-123.

Hourihane, D. O'B., and Weir, D. G. (1970) Suppression of erythropoiesis by alcohol. *Br. Med. J.*, **i**, 86-89.

Hoyumpa, Jr., A. M., Greene, H. L., Dunn., G. D., and Schenker, S. (1975) Fatty liver: Biochemical and clinical considerations. *Dig. Dis.*, **20**, 1142-1170.

Huttunen, M. O., Härkönen, M., Niskanen, P., Leino, T., and Ylikahri, R. (1976) Plasma testosterone concentrations in alcoholics. *J. Stud. Alcohol*, **37**, 1165-1177.

Ibragimov, V. Kh. (1967) Some biochemical blood parameters in cases of chronic alcoholism. *Vrach Delo*, **6**, 134-135.

Irsigler, K., Krypsin-Exner, K., Mildschuh, W., Pointer, H., and Schmidt, P. (1971) Liver morphology and liver functions in delirium tremens. *Dtsch. Med. Wochenschr.*, **96**, 9-13.

Israel, Y. (1970) Cellular effects of alcohol. *Q. J. Stud. Alcohol*, **31**, 293-316.

Israel, Y, Valenzuela, J. E., Salazar, I., and Ugarte, G. (1969) Alcohol and amino acid transport in the human small intestine. *J. Nutr.*, **98**, 222-224.

Isselbacher, K. J. (1977) Metabolic and hepatic effects of alcohol. *N. Eng. J. Med.*, **269**, 612-616.

Itturriaga, H., Pereda, T., Estévez, A. and Ugarte, G. (1977) Serum immunoglobulin A changes in alcoholic patients. *Ann. Clin. Res.*, **9**, 39-43.

Jackson, R. A., Advani, U., Perry, G., Rogers, J., Peters, N., Day, S., and Pilkington, T. R. E. (1973) The influence of a low carbohydrate diet on forearm metabolism in men. *Diabetes*, **22**, 145-159.

Jacobs, P., Bothwell, T. and Charlton, R. W. (1964) Role of hydrochloric acid in iron absorption. *J. Appl. Physiol.*, **19**, 187–188.

Jaross, von W., Hanefeld, M., Schentke, K. U. T., Trübsbach, A., Stötzner, H., Leonhardt, W., Herrmann, V., and Fuchs, R. (1972) Veränderungen von metabolischen Parametern, insbesondere des Fettstoffwechsels bei chronischen Alkoholikern unter klinischer Alkoholkarenz. *Z. Gesamte Inn. Med. Grenzgeb.*, **27**, 311–316.

Jenkins, J. S., and Connolly, J. (1968) Adrenocortical response to ethanol in man. *Br. Med. J.*, **2**, 804–805.

Jenkins, D. W., Eckel, R. E., and Craig, J. W. (1971) Alcoholic ketoacidosis. *J. Am. Med. Assoc.*, **217**, 177–183.

Jeffrey, F. E., and Abelmann, W. H. (1971) Recovery from proven shosin beriberi. *Am. J. Med.*, **50**, 123–128.

Jewell, L. D., Medline, A., and Medline, N. M. (1971) Alcoholic hepatitis. *Can. Med. Assoc. J.*, **105**, 711–713.

Joffe, B. I., Seftel, H. C., and Vanas, M. (1975) Hormonal responses in ethanol-induced hypoglycaemia. *J. Stud. Alcohol*, **36**, 550–554.

Johannson, B. G., and Laurell, C.-B. (1969) Disorders of serum α-lipoproteins after alcohol intoxication. *J. Clin. Lab. Invest.*, **23**, 231–234.

Johansson, B. G., and Medhus, A. (1974) Increase in plasma α-lipoproteins in chronic alcoholics after acute abuse. *Acta Med. Scand.*, **195**, 273–277.

Jones, D. P. (1969) Effects of ethanol on lipid transport in man. *In* Biochemical and Clinical Aspects of Alcohol Metabolism (Sardesai, V. M. *ed.*) pp. 86–94, Charles C. Thomas, Springfield, Illinois.

Jones, D. P., Losowsky, M. S., Davidson, C. S., and Lieber, C. S. (1963) Low plasma lipoprotein lipid activity as a factor in the pathogenesis of alcohol hyperlipemia. *J. Clin. Invest.*, **42**, 945–946.

Jones, D. P., Perman, E. S., and Lieber, C. S. (1965) Free fatty acid turnover and triglyceride metabolism after ethanol ingestion in man. *J. Lab. Clin. Med.*, **66**, 804–813.

Jones, J. E., Shane, S. R., Jacobs, W. H., and Flink, E. B. (1969) Magnesium balance studies in chronic alcoholism. *Ann. N. Y. Acad. Sci.*, **162**, 934–946.

Joplin, G. F., and Wright, A. D. (1968) The detection of diabetes in man. *In* Carbohydrate Metabolism and Its Disorders (Dickens, F., Randle, P. J., and Whelan, A. P. *eds.*) Academic Press, London.

Jouppila, P., Huikko, M., and Järvinen, P. A. (1970) Effect of ethyl alcohol on urinary excretion of noradrenaline and adrenaline in patients with threatened premature delivery. *Acta. Obstet. Gynec. Scand.*, **49**, 359–362.

Kaffarnik, H., and Schneider, J. (1976) Die äthanolinduzierte Hyperlipoproteinämine des Stoffwechselgesunden. *Muench. Klin. Wochenschr.*, **54**, 747–754.

Kallai, L., Keler-Bacoka, M., Blazević, K., and Knezević, S. (1966) The interpretation of haptoglobin values in the diagnosis of liver disease. *Gastroenterologia*, 105, 27-34.

Kallio, V., Saarimaa, H., and Saarimaa, A. (1969) Serum lipids and postprandial lipemia in alcoholics after a drinking bout. *Q. J. Stud. Alcohol*, 30, 565-569.

Kimber, C., Deller, D. J., Ibbotson, R. N., and Lander, H. (1965) The mechanism of anaemia in chronic liver disease. *Q. J. Med.*, 34, 33-64.

Kinzius, H. (1950) Adrenalin und Arbeit, die Beeinfluss und des Blutadrenalin Spiegels durch Pervitin, Luminal und Alkohol. *Arbeits Physiol.*, 14, 243-248.

Kissin, B., Schenker, V. J., and Schenker, A. C. (1960) The acute effect of ethanol ingestion on plasma and urinary 17-hydroxycorticoids in alcoholic subjects. *Am. J. Med. Sci.*, 239, 690-705.

Kissin, B., Schenker, V. J., and Schenker, A. C. (1965) Hyperdiuresis after ethanol in chronic alcoholics. *Am. J. Med. Sci.*, 248, 660.

Kissin, B., Schenker, V. J., and Schenker, A. C. (1969) Adrenal cortical function and liver disease in alcoholics. *Am. J. Med. Sci.*, 238, 344-353.

Knochel, J. P. (1977) The pathophysiology and clinical characteristics of severe hypophosphatemia. *Arch. Intern. Med.*, 137, 203-220.

Kolakowska, T. and Swigar, M. E. (1977) Thyroid function in depression and alcohol abuse. *Arch. Gen. Psychiatry*, 34, 984-988.

Konttinen, A., Louhija, A., and Härtel, G. (1968) Serum guanine deaminase, ornithine carbamoyl transferase, and γ-glutamyltranspeptidase activities in chronic alcoholics. *Ann. Med. Exp. Biol. Fenn.*, 46, 18-22.

Konttinen, A., Härtel, G., and Louhija, A. (1970a) Multiple serum enzyme analysis in chronic alcoholics. *Acta Med. Scand.*, 188, 257-264.

Konttinen, A., Louhija, A., and Härtel, G. (1970b) Blood transketolase in assessment of thiamine deficiency in alcoholics. *Ann. Med. Exp. Biol. Fenn.*, 48, 172-175.

Korman, M. G., Soveny, C., and Hansky, J. (1971) Effect of food on serum gastrin evaluated by radioimmunoassay. *Gut*, 12, 619-624.

Krasner, N., Dow, J., Moore, M. R., and Goldberg, A. (1974) Ascorbic-acid saturation and ethanol metabolism. *Lancet*, ii, 693-695.

Krasner, N., Moore, M. R., Thompson, G. G., McIntosh, W., and Goldberg, A. (1974) Depression of erythrocyte δ-aminolaevulinic acid dehydratase activitity in alcoholics. *Clin. Sci. Mol. Med.*, 46, 415-418.

Krasner, N., Cochran, K. M., Russell, R. I., Carmichael, H. A., and Thompson, G. G. (1976) Alcohol absorption from the small intestine. *Gut*, 17, 245-248.

Krebs, H. A., Cunningham, D. J. C., Stubbs, M., and Jenkins, D. J. A. (1969a) Effect of ethanol on postexercise lactacidemia. *Israel J. Med. Sci.*, 5, 959-962.

Krebs, H. A., Freedland, R. A., Hems, R. and Stubbs, M. (1969b) Inhibition of hepatic gluconeogenesis by ethanol. *Biochem. J.*, 112, 117-124.

Kreisberg, R. A., Siegal, A. M., and Owen, W. C. (1971) Glucose lactate interrelationships: Effect of ethanol. *J. Clin. Invest.*, 50, 175-185.

Krusius, F. E., Vartia, K. O., and Forsander, O. (1958) Experimentelle Studien über die biologische Wirkung von Alkohol. *Ann. Med. Exp. Biol. Fenn.*, **36**, 424.

Kudzma, D. J., and Schonfeld, G. (1971) Alcoholic hyperlipidemia; Induction by ethanol but not by carbohydrate. *J. Lab. Clin. Med.*, **77**, 384-395.

Lafair, J. S., and Myerson, R. M. (1968) Alcoholic myopathy. *Arch. Intern. Med.*, **122**, 417-422.

Lahti, R. A. (1975) Alcohol, aldehydes and biogenic amines. *Adv. Exp. Med. Biol.*, **56**, 239-253.

Lahti, R. A., and Majchrowicz, E. (1969) Acetaldehyde – an inhibitor of the enzymatic oxidation of 5-hydroxyindole acetaldehyde. *Biochem. Pharmacol*, **18**, 535-538.

Lamy, J., Aron, E., Martin, J. C., and Weill, J. (1973) Hyperhaptoglobinemie des alcooliques chroniques. *Clin. Chim. Acta*, **46**, 257-260.

Lamy, J., Baglin, M-C., Ferrant, J-P., and Weill, J. (1975) Emploi de la mesure de la γ-glutamyl transpeptidase serique pour controler le succes descures de desintoxication anti-alcoolique. *Clin. Chim. Acta*, **66**, 103-107.

Lane, F., Goff, P., McGuffin, R., Eichner, E. R., and Hillman, R. S. (1976) Folic acid metabolism in normal, folate deficient and alcoholic man. *Br. J. Haematol.*, **34**, 489-500.

Laroche, C., Navarro, J., Cosson, A., Gregoire, J., and Caquet, R. (1969) Serum folic acid in fatty liver and alcoholic cirrhosis. *Sem. Hop. (Paris)*, **45**, 633-639.

Lee, F. I. (1965) Immunoglobulins in viral hepatitis and active alcoholic liver disease. *Lancet*, **ii**, 1043-1046.

Leevy, C. M., and ten Hove, N. (1967) Pathogenesis and sequelae of liver disease in alcoholic man. *In* Biochemical Factors in Alcoholism (Maickel, R. P. *ed.*) pp. 151-165, Pergamon Press, Oxford.

Leevy, C. M., Tamburro, C. and Smith, F. (1970) Alcoholism drug addiction and nutrition. *Med. Clin.*, **54**, 1567-1575.

Leevy, C. M., Tanribilir, A. K., and Smith, F. (1971) Biochemistry of gastrointestinal and liver disease in alcoholism. *In* The Biology of Alcoholism (Kissin, B., and Begleiter, H. *eds.*) **Vol. 1**, pp. 307-325, Plenum Press, New York.

Lefèvre, A., and Leiber, C. S. (1969) Effect of ethanol on bile acid metabolism. *Clin. Res.*, **17**, 388.

Lefèvre, A., Adler, H., and Lieber, C. S. (1970) Effect of ethanol on ketone metabolism. *J. Clin. Invest.*, **49**, 1775-1782.

Leppäluoto, J., Rapeli, M., Varis, R., and Ranta, T. (1975) Secretion of anterior pituitary hormones in man: Effects of ethyl alcohol. *Acta Physiol. Scand.*, **95**, 400-406.

Lepoire, E., Gelot, M. A., Royer, J., Gonand, J. P., and Debry, G. (1970) Effects of intravenous perfusions of ethanol on the lipid constituents of the serum of man. *C. R. Seances Soc. Biol. Fil.*, **164**, 1339-1343.

Levy, L. J., Duga, J., Girgis, M., and Gordon, E. E. (1973) Ketoacidosis associated with alcoholism in nondiabetic subjects. *Ann. Int. Med.*, **78**, 213-219.

Lieber, C. S. (1965a) Hyperuricemia induced by alcohol. *Arthritis Rheum.*, **8**, 786-798.

Lieber, C. S. (1965b) Alcohol and the liver. *Prog. Liver Dis.*, **2**, 134-154.

Lieber, C. S. (1966) Hepatic and metabolic effects of alcohol. *Prog. Gastroenterology*, **50**, 119-133.

Lieber, C. S. (1967a) Metabolic derangement induced by alcohol. *Annu. Rev. Med.*, **18**, 35-54.

Lieber, C. S. (1967b) Alcoholic fatty liver, hyperlipemia and hyperuricemia. *In* Biochemical Factors in Alcoholism (Maickel, R. P. *ed.*) pp. 167-183, Pergamon Press, Oxford.

Lieber, C. S. (1973) Hepatic and metabolic effects of alcohol (1966 to 1973). *Gastroenterology*, **65**, 821-846.

Lieber, C. S. (1974) Effects of ethanol on lipid metabolism. *Lipids*, **9**, 103-116.

Lieber, C. S. (*ed.*) (1977) *Metabolic Aspects of Alcoholism*, ATP Press Ltd., Lancaster.

Lieber, C. S., and DeCarli, L. M. (1964) Effect of ethanol on cholesterol metabolism. *Clin. Res.*, **12**, 274.

Lieber, C. S., and DeCarli, L. M. (1977) Metabolic effects of alcohol on the liver. *In* Metabolic Aspects of Alcoholism (Lieber, C. S. *ed.*) pp. 31-79, MTP Press Ltd., Lancaster.

Lieber, C. S., Jones, D. P., Losowsky, M. S., and Davidson, C. S. (1962) Interrelation of uric acid and ethanol metabolism in man. *J. Clin. Invest.*, **41**, 1863-1870.

Lieber, C. S., Jones, D. P., Mendelson, J., and DeCarli, L. M. (1963) Fatty liver, hyperlipemia and huperuricemia produced by prolonged alcohol consumption, despite adequate dietary intake. *Trans. Assoc. Am. Physicians*, **76**, 289-301.

Lieber, C. S., Rubin, E., and DeCarli, L. M. (1971) Effects of ethanol on lipid, uric acid, intermediary and drug metabolism, including the pathogenesis of alcoholic fatty liver. *In* The Biology of Alcoholism (Kissin, B. and Begleiter, H. *eds.*) Vol. 1, pp. 266-305, Plenum Press, New York.

Lieber, C. S., Teschke, R., Hasumura, Y., and DeCarli, L. M. (1975) Differences in hepatic and metabolic changes after acute and chronic alcohol consumption. *Fed. Proc.*, **34**, 2060-2073.

Liebhardt, E., and Gostomzyk, J. G. (1968) The determination of glucose and free fatty acids in serum after the administration of alcohol and glucose. *Z. Klin. Chem. Klin. Biochem.*, **6**, 377-379.

Liegel, J., Fabre, L. F., Howard, P. Y., and Farmer, R. W. (1972) Plasma testosterone binding globulin (SBG) in alcoholic subjects. *Physiologist*, **15**, 198 (abstr.).

Lim, P., and Jacob, E. (1972) Magnesium status of alcoholic patients. *Metab. Clin. Exp.*, **21**, 1045-1051.

Lindenbaum, J., and Lieber, C. S. (1969a) Hematologic effects of alcohol in man in the absence of nutritional deficiency. *N. Engl. J. Med.*, **281**, 333-338.

Lindenbaum, J., and Lieber, C. S. (1969b) Alcohol-induced malabsorption of vitamin B_{12} in man. *Nature (Lond.)*, **224**, 806.

Linkola, J. (1975) Natururesis after diluted ethanol solutions. *Lancet*, **ii**, 1157.

Linkola, J., Fyhrquist, F., Nieminen, M. M., Weber, T. H., and Tontti, K. (1976). Renin-aldosterone axis in ethanol intoxication and hangover. *Europ. J. Clin. Invest.*, **6**, 191-194.

Liu, Y. K. (1973) Leukopenia in alcoholics. *Am. J. Med.*, **54**, 605-610.

LoGrippo, G. A., Anselm, K., and Hayashi, H. (1971) Serum immunoglobulins and five serum proteins in extra hepatic obstructive jaundice and alcoholic cirrhosis. *Am. J. Gastroenterol.*, **56**, 357-363.

Long, R. G., Skinner, R. K., Wills, M. R., and Sherlock, S. (1976) Serum 25-hydroxy-vitamin-D in untreated parenchymal and cholestatic liver disease. *Lancet*, **ii**, 650-652.

Losowsky, M. S., Jones, D. P., Davidson, C. S., and Lieber, C. S. (1963) Studies of alcoholic hyperlipemia and its mechanisms. *Am. J. Med.*, **35**, 795-803.

Llanos, O. L., Swierczek, J. S., Teichmann, R. K., Rayford, P. L., and Thompson, J. C. (1977) Effect of alcohol on the release of secretin and pancreatic secretion. *Surgery (St. Louis)*, **81**, 661-667.

Luisier, M., Vodoz, J. F., Donath, A., Courvoisier, B., and Garcia, B. (1977) Carence en 25-hydroxyvitamine D avec diminution de l'absorption intestinale de calcium et de la densité osseuse dans l'alcooholisme chronique. *Schweiz. Med. Wochenschr.*, **107**, 1529-1533.

Lumeng. L., and Li, T-K. (1974) Vitamin B_6 metabolism in chronic alcohol abuse. *J. Clin. Invest.*, **53**, 693-704.

Lund, B., Sorensen, O. H., Hilden, M., and Lund, B. (1977) The hepatic conversion of vitamin D in alcoholics with varying degrees of liver affection. *Acta. Med. Scand.*, **202**, 221-224.

Lundquist, F., Tygstrup, N., Winkler, K., Mellemgaard, K., and Munk-Peterson, S. (1962) Ethanol metabolism and production of free acetate in human liver. *J. Clin. Invest.*, **41**, 955-961.

Lyon, J. L., Gardner, J. W., Klauber, M. R. (1976) Alcohol and cancer. *Lancet*, **i**, 1243.

Maclachlan, M. J., and Rodnan, G. P. (1967) Effects of food, fast and alcohol on serum uric acid and acute attacks of gout. *Am. J. Med.*, **42**, 38-57.

Madison, L. L. (1968) Ethanol induced hypoglycaemia. *Adv. Metabolic Disorders*, **3**, 85-109.

MacSweeney, D. (1975) Body composition in control, alcoholic and depressive individuals using a multiple isotope technique and whole body counting of potassium. *Adv. Exp. Med. Biol.*, **59**, 257-269.

Marasini, B., Agostoni, A., Stabilini, R., and Dioguardi, N. (1972) Serum proteins of hepatic and extrahepatic origin in alcoholic cirrhosis. *Clin. Chim. Acta*, **40**, 501–502.

Margraf, H. W., Mayer, C. A., Ashford, L. E., and Lavalle, L. W. (1967) Adrenocortical function in alcoholics. *J. Surg. Res.*, **7**, 55–62.

Markkanen, T., and Peltola, O. (1971a) Pentose-phosphate pathway of leucocytes. *Acta Haematol. (Basel)*, **46**, 36–44.

Markkanen, T., and Peltola, O. (1971b) Pentose-phosphate pathway in erythrocytes in metabolic diseases. *Acta Haematol. (Basel)*, **45**, 285–289.

Marks, V. (1975) Alcohol and changes in body constituents; glucose and hormones. *Proc. Roy. Soc. Med.*, **68**, 377–380.

Marks, V. and Chakraborty, J. (1973) The clinical endocrinology of alcoholism. *J. Alcohol*, **8**, 94–103.

Marks, V. and Wright, J. W. (1977) Endocrinological and metabolic effects of alcohol. *Proc. Roy. Soc. Med.*, **70**, 337–344.

Martin, P. J., Martin, J. V., and Goldberg, D. M. (1975) γ-Glutamyl transpeptidase, triglycerides and enzyme induction. *Lancet*, **i**, 17–18.

Mata, J. M., Kershenobich, D., Villarreal, E., and Rojkind, M. (1975) Serum free proline and free hydroxyproline in patients with chronic liver disease. *Gastroenterology*, **68**, 1265–1269.

Matunaga, M. (1942) Experimentelle Untersuchungen über der Einfluss des Alkohols auf den Kohlenhydratstoffwechsel I Uber die Wirkung des Alkohols auf den Blutzuckerspiegel und den Glykogenhalt der Leber mit besonderer Berücksichtigung seines Wirkungsmechanismus. *Tohaku J. Exp. Med.*, **44**, 130–157.

Maynard, L. S., and Schenker, V. J. (1962) Monoamine oxidase inhibition by ethanol *in vitro*. *Nature (London)*, **196**, 575–576.

McDonald, J. T., and Margen, S. (1976) Wine versus ethanol in human nutrition 1. Nitrogen and calorie balance. *Am. J. Clin Nutr.*, **29**, 1093–1103.

Medalle, R., and Waterhouse, C. (1973) A magnesium − deficient patient presenting with hypocalcaemia and hypophosphataemia. *Ann. Intern. Med.*, **79**, 76–79.

Medalle, R., Waterhouse, C., and Hahn, T. J. (1976) Vitamin D resistance in magnesium deficiency. *Am. J. Clin.Nutr.*, **29**, 854–858.

Mekhjian, H. S., and May, E. S. (1977) Acute and chronic effects of ethanol on fluid transport in the human intestine. *Gastroenterology*, **72**, 1280–1286.

Mendelson, J. H., and Stein, S. (1966) Serum cortisol levels in alcoholics and non-alcoholic subjects during experimentally induced ethanol intoxication. *Psychosom. Med.*, **28**, 616–626.

Mendelson, J. H., Ogata, M., and Mello, N. K. (1969) Effects of alcohol ingestion and withdrawal on magnesium states of alcoholics. Clinical and experimental findings. *Ann. N. Y. Acad. Sci.*, **162**, 918–933.

Mendelson, J. H., Ogata, M., Mello, N. K. (1971) Adrenal function and alcoholism. 1. Serum cortisol. *Psychosom. Med.*, **33**, 145-157.

Mendelson, J. H., and Mello, N. K. (1973) Alcohol-induced hyperlipidemia and beta lipoproteins. *Science (Wash. D. C.)*, **180**, 1372-1374.

Mendelson, J. H., and Mello, N. K. (1974) Significance of alcohol-induced hypertriglyceridemia in patients with Type IV hyperlipoproteinemia. *Ann. Intern. Med.*, **80**, 270-271.

Mendelson, J. H., and Mello, N. K. (1974) Alcohol, aggression and androgens. *In* Agression (Frazier, S. H. *ed.*) pp. 225-247, Williams and Wilkins, Baltimore.

Mendelson, J. H., Mello, N. K., and Ellingboe, J. (1977) Effects of acute alcohol intake on pituitary — gonadal hormones in normal human males. *J. Pharmacol. Exp. Ther.*, **202**, 676-682.

Merry, J., and Marks, V. (1969) Plasma-hydrocortisone response to ethanol in chronic alcoholics. *Lancet*, **i**, 921-923.

Merry, J., and Marks, V. (1971) Ethanol and cortisol release. *In* Metabolic Changes Induced by Alcohol (Martini, G. A., and Bode, C. H. *eds.*) pp. 199-206, Springer-Verlag, Berlin.

Merry, J. and Marks, V. (1972) The effect of alcohol, barbiturate, and diazepam on hypothalamic/pituitary/adrenal function in chronic alcoholics. *Lancet*, **ii**, 990-992.

Merry, J., and Marks, V. (1973) Hypothalamic pituitary-adrenal function in chronic alcoholics. *Adv. Exp. Med. Biol.*, **35**, 167-179.

Merzon, A. K., and Khorunzhaya, L. V. (1970) A method for studying the hydrouretic component of the osmoregulation system. *Fiziol. Zh. SSSR Im i m Sechenova*, **56**, 288-291 (*Biol. Abs.* (1971) **52**, 77636).

Metz, R., Berger, S., and Mako, M. (1969) Potentiation of the plasma insulin response to glucose by prior administration of alcohol. An apparent islet-priming effect. *Diabetes*, **18**, 517-522.

Meyer, J. G., and Urban, K. (1977) Electrolyte changes and acid base balances after alcohol withdrawal. *J. Neurol.*, **215**, 135-140.

Mezey, E., Jow, E., Slavin, R. E., and Tobon, F. (1970) Pancreatic function and intestinal absorption in chronic alcoholism. *Gastroenterology*, **59**, 657-644.

Mezey, E., and Tobon, F. (1971) Rates of ethanol clearance and activities of the ethanol — oxidising enzymes in chronic alcoholic patients. *Gastroenterology*, **61**, 707-715.

Miller, A. I., Moral, M. D., and Schiff, E. R. (1975) Presence of serum α-l-fetoprotein in alcoholic hepatits. *Gastroenterology*, **68**, 381-383.

Moore, T. L., Kupchik, H. Z., Marcon, N. and Zamcheck, N. (1971) Carcino-embryonic antigen assay in cancer of the colon and pancreas and other digestive tract disorders. *Am. J. Dig. Dis.*, **16**, 1-7.

Moss, M. H. (1970) Alcohol-induced hypoglycaemia and coma caused by alcohol sponging. *Pediatrics*, **46**, 445-447.

Murator, F., Riccardino, N., and Sansalvadore, F. (1971) Observations on the behaviour of the immunoglobulins in severe alcoholic cirrhosis. *G. Batteriol. Virol. Immunol. Ann. Osp. Maria Vittoria Tonino Parte l sez Microbiol.*, **64**, 66-74.

Murdock, H. R. (1967) Thyroidal effects of alcohol. *Q. J. Stud. Alcohol*, **28**, 419-423.

Murphy, G. E., Guze, S. B., and King, L. J. (1962) Urinary excretion of 5-HIAA in chronic alcoholism. *J. Am. Med. Assoc.*, **182**, 167.

Murray-Lyon, I. M., Clarke, H. G. M., McPherson, K., and Williams, R. (1972) Quantitative immunoelectrophoresis of serum proteins in cryptogenic cirrhosis, alcoholic cirrhosis and active chronic hepatitis. *Clin. Chim. Acta*, **39**, 215-220.

Nader, S., Tulloch, B., Blair, C., Vydelingum, N., and Fraser, T. R. (1974) Is prolactin involved in precipitating migraine? *Lancet*, **ii**, 17-19.

Nair, P. P., Mezey, E., Murty, H. S., Quartener, J., and Mendeloff, A. I. (1971) Vitamin E and porphyrin metabolism in man. *Arch. Intern. Med.*, **128**, 411-415.

Neville, J. N., Eagles, J. A., Samson, G., and Olson, R. E. (1968) Nutritional status of alcoholics. *Am. J. Clin. Nutr.*, **21**, 1329-1340.

Nikkilä, E. A., and Taskinen, M. R. (1975) Ethanol-induced alterations of glucose tolerance, postglucose hypoglycaemia and insulin secretion in normal, obese and diabetic subjects. *Diabetes*, **24**, 933-943.

Ning, M., Lowenstein, L. M., and Davidson, C. S. (1967) Serum amino-acid concentrations in alcoholic hepatitis. *J. Lab. Clin. Med.*, **70**, 554-562.

Nordmann, R., and Nordmann, J. (1971) Effects of alcohol on hepatic metabolism. *Rev. Eur. Etudes Clin. Biol.*, **16**, 965-969.

Nygren, A. (1966) Serum creatine phosphokinase activity in chronic alcoholism in connection with acute alcohol intoxication. *Acta Med. Scand.*, **179**, 623-630.

Nygren, A. (1967) Serum creatine phosphokinase in chronic alcoholism. *Acta Med. Scand.*, **182**, 383-388.

Nygren, A. (1971) Studies on alcoholic myopathy with special reference to the occurrence and pathogenesis of sub-clinical myopathy. *Opusc. Med. Suppl.*, **21**, 1-16.

Nygren, A., and Sundblad, L. (1971) Lactate dehydrogenase isoenzyme patterns in serum and skeletal muscle in intoxicated alcoholics. *Acta Med. Scand.*, **189**, 303-307.

Ogata, M., Mendelson, J. H., and Mello, N. K. (1968) Electrolytes and osmolality in alcoholics during experimentally induced intoxication. *Psychosom. Med.*, **30**, 463-488.

Ogata, M., Mendelson, J. H., Mello, N. K., and Majchrowicz, E. (1971a) Adrenal function and catecholamines. *Psychosom. Med.*, **33**, 159-180.

Ogata, M., Mendelson, J. M. Mello, N. K., Majchrowicz, E. (1971b) Adrenal function and alcoholism. *In* Recent Advances in Studies of Alcoholism (Mello, N. K., and Mendelson, J. H., *eds.*) pp. 140-172, NIMM/NIH, Washington, D. C.

O'Keane, M., Russell, R. I., and Goldberg, A. (1972) Ascorbic acid status of alcoholics. *J. Alcohol,* **7**, 6-11.

O'Keefe, S. J. D., and Marks, V. (1977) Lunchtime gin and tonic a cause of reactive hypoglycaemia. *Lancet,* i, 1286-1288.

Olin, J. S., Devenyi, P., and Weldon, K. L. (1973) Uric acid in alcoholics. *Q. J. Stud. Alcohol,* **34**, 463-488.

Oliva, P. B. (1970) Lactic acidosis. *Am. J. Med.,* **48**, 209-225.

Olson, R. E., Gursey, D. and Vester, J. W. (1960) Evidence for a defect in tryptophan metabolism in chronic alcoholism. *N. Engl. J. Med.,* **263**, 1169-1174.

Orenberg, E. K., Zarcone, V. P., Renson, J. F., and Barchas, J. D. (1976) The effects of ethanol injestion on cyclic AMP, homovanillic acid, and 5-hydroxy indoleacetic acid in human cerebrospinal fluid. *Life Sci.,* **19**, 1669-1672.

Orten, A. U. (1963) Intestinal phase of amino acid nutrition. *Fed. Proc.,* **22**, 1103-1109.

Orten, J. M., Doehr, S. A., Bond, C., Johnson, H., and Pappes, A. (1963) Urinary excretion of porphyrins and porphyrin intermediates in human alcoholics. *Q. J. Stud. Alcohol.,* **24**, 598-609.

Orten, J. M., and Sardesai, V. M. (1971) Protein, nucleotide and porphyrin metabolism. *In* The Biology of Alcoholism (Kissin, B., and Begleiter, H. *eds.*) **Vol. 1**, pp. 229-261, Plenum Press, New York.

Ortinians, H., and Eisenberg, K. (1976) Bedeutung biochemscher Messwerte bei Diagnostik und Verlaufs kontrolle alkoholbedingter Lebererkrankung. *Med. Klin.,* **71**, 380-384.

Ott, A., Hayes, J., and Polin, J. (1976) Severe lactic acidosis associated with intravenous alcohol for premature labor. *Obstet. and Gynecol.,* **48**, 362-364.

Ozkan, K., Turkvan, M., and Uzunalimoglu, O. (1968) A study on the determination of serum cholinesterase and its value in clinical chemistry. *Ankara Univ. Tip. Fak. Mecm.,* **21**, 1115-1122 (*Biol. Abs.,* (1970) **51**, 123207).

Paine, C. P., Eichner, E. R., and Dickson, V. (1973) Concordance of radioassay and microbiological assay in the study of the ethanol-induced fall in serum folate levels. *Am. J. Med. Sci.,* **266**, 135-138.

Paloheimo, J. A., and Louhija, A. (1968) Jaundice, hemolysis and hyperlipemia in alcoholics: Zieve's syndrome. *Ann. Med. Intern. Fenn.,* **57**, 129-133.

Patel, S., and O'Gorman, P. (1975) Serum enzyme levels in alcoholism and drug dependency. *J. Clin. Pathol. (Lond.),* **28**, 414-417.

Paterson, Y., and Lawrence, E. F. (1972) Factors affecting serum creatine phosphokinase levels in normal adult females. *Clin. Chim. Acta,* **42**, 131-139.

Paton, A. (1976) Alcohol induced Cushingoid syndrome. *Br. Med. J.,* **2**, 1504.

Pertikäinen, L. A., Azarnoff, D. L., and Dujovne, C. A. (1975) Plasma levels and excretion of estrogens in urine in chronic liver disease. *Gastroenterology*, **69**, 20-27.

Perkoff, G. T., Hardy, P., and Velez-Garcia, E. (1966) Reversible acute muscular syndrome in chronic alcoholism. *N. Engl. J. Med.*, **274**, 1277-1285.

Perman, E. S. (1958) The effect of ethyl alcohol on the secretion from the adrenal medulla in man. *Acta Physiol. Scand.*, **44**, 241-247.

Perman, E. S. (1960) Observations on the effect of ethanol on the urinary excretion of histamine, 5-hydroxyindolacetic acid, catecholamines and 17-hydroxycorticosteroids in man. *Acta Physiol. Scand.*, **51**, 62-67.

Persky, H., O'Brien, C. P., Fine, E., Howard, W. J., Khan, M. A., and Beck R. W. (1977) The effect of alcohol and smoking on testosterone function and aggresion in chronic alcoholics. *Am. J. Psychiatry*, **134**, 621-625.

Pezzimenti, J. F., and Lindenbaum, J. (1972) Megaloblastic anaemia associated with erythroid hypoplasia. *Am. J. Med.*, **53**, 748-754.

Phillips, G. B., and Safrit, H. F. (1971) Alcoholic diabetes. Induction of glucose intolerance with alcohol. *J. Am. Med. Assoc.*, **217**, 1513-1519.

Piccinino, F., daVilla, G., and Giusti, G. (1966) Determinazione dei livelli sierici de haptoglobina ecrso di varie epatopatie. *Minerva Med.*, **57**, 4331-4335.

Pitchumoni, C. S., Lopes, J. D., and Glase, G. B. J. (1975) The prevalence of gastric autoantibodies in chronic alcoholics. *Am. J. Gastroenterol.*, **64**, 187-190.

Plaza de los Reyes, M., Orozco, R., Rosemblitt, M., Rendic, Y., and Espinace, M. (1968) Renal excretion of magnesium and other electrolytes under the influence of acute ingestion of alcohol in normal subjects. *Rev. Med. (Chile)*, **96**, 138-141. (*Biol. Abs.*, (1969) **50**, 98234).

Pojer, J., Radivojevic, M., and Williams, T. F. (1972) Dupuytren's Disease. *Arch. Intern. Med.*, **129**, 561-566.

Porta, E. A., Koch, O. R., and Hortcroft, W. S. (1970) Recent advances in molecular pathology: A review of the effects of alcohol on the liver. *Exp. Mol. Pathol.*, **12**, 104-132.

Powell, L. W., Roeser, H. P., and Halliday, J. W. (1972) Transient intravascular haemolysis associated with alcoholic liver disease and hyperlipidemia. *Aust. N.Z. J. Med.*, **1**, 39-43.

Priem, H. A., Shanley, B. C., and Malan, C. (1976) Effect of alcohol administration of plasma growth hormone response to insulin-induced hypoglycaemia. *Metab. Clin. Exp.*, **25**, 397-403.

Rahwan, R. G. (1974) Speculations on the biochemical pharmacology of ethanol. *Life Sciences*, **15**, 617-633.

Raïha, N. and Mänpää, P. (1964) The influence of ethanol on the acid base balance of the blood in man and rat. *Scand. J. Clin. Lab. Invest.*, **16**, 267-272.

Rapport, M. (1969) NAD effects on the biochemistry and psychological performance of alcoholics under stress. *Q. J. Stud. Alcohol,* **30A**, 570-584.

Redetzki, H. M., Koener, T. A., Hughes, J. R., and Smith, A. G. (1972) Osmometry in the evaluation of alcohol intoxication. *Clin. Toxicol.,* **5**, 343-363.

Rees, L. H., Besser, G. M., Jeffcoate, W. J., Goldie, D. J., and Marks, V. (1977) Alcohol-Induced pseudo-Cushing's syndrome. *Lancet,* **i,** 726-728.

Rinderknecht, H., Goekas, M. C., Carmack, C., and Haverback, B. J. (1970a) The determination of arylsulfatases in biological fluids. *Clin. Chim. Acta,* **29,** 481-491.

Rinderknecht, H., Silverman, P., Haverback, B. J., and Geokas, M. C. (1970b) Serum creatine phosphokinase in acute pancreatitis. *Clin. Biochem.,* **3,** 165-170.

Roberts, D. M., and Taylor, G. (1973) Gastric parietal cell antibodies in young men with alcoholism and with non-ulcer dyspepsia. *Digestion,* **9,** 30-35.

Roggin, G. M., Iber, F. L., Kater, R. M. H., and Tabon, F. (1969) Malabsorption in the chronic alcoholic. *Hopkins Med. J.,* **125,** 321-330.

Rollason, J. G., Pincherle, G., and Robinson, D. (1972) Serum gamma-glutamyl transpeptidase in relation to alcohol consumption. *Clin. Chim. Acta,* **39,** 75-80.

Rosalki, S. B. (1975) Gamma-glutamyl transpeptidase. *Adv. Clin. Chem.,* **17,** 53-107.

Rosalki, S. B., and Rau, D. (1972) Serum γ-glutamyl transpeptidase activity in alcoholism. *Clin. Chim. Acta,* **39,** 41-47.

Rosen, H. M., Yoshimura, N., Hodgman, J. M., and Fischer, J. E. (1977) Plasma amino-acid patterns in hepatic encephalopathy of differing etiology. *Gastroenterology,* **72,** 483-487.

Rosenauerova-Ostra, A., Hilgertova, J., and Sonka, J. (1976) Urinary formiminoglutamate in man: Normal values related to sex and age: Effect of low calorie intake and alcohol consumption. *Clin. Chim. Acta,* **73,** 39-43.

Rosenfeld, G. (1960) Inhibitory influence of ethanol on serotonin metabolism. *Proc. Soc. Exp. Biol. Med.,* **103,** 144-149.

Rosenthal, W. S., Adham, N. F., Lopez, R., and Cooperman, J. M. (1973) Riboflavin deficiency in complicated chronic alcoholism. *Am. J. Clin. Nutr.,* **26,** 858-860.

Roser, H. (1970) Quantitative immunoglobulin determinations in patients with hepatic diseases. *Muench. Med. Wochenschr.,* **122,** 1392-1394.

Rothschild, M. A., Schreiber, S. S., and Oratz, M. (1975) Alcohol inhibition of protein synthesis. *Clin. Toxicol.,* **8,** 349-357.

Rothfeld, B., Carulli, N., Kaihara, S., Reus, I., and Wagner, Jr. H. N. (1970) Serum arginase concentration in acute alcoholism. *Biochem. Med.,* **4,** 36-42.

Rubin, E., Lieber, C. S., Altman, K., Gordon, G. G., and Southren, A. L. (1976) Prolonged ethanol consumption increases testosterone metabolism in the liver. *Science (Wash. D.C.),* **191,** 563-564.

Rudd, B. T. (1977) Androgens *In* Hormone Chemistry, (Butt, W. R., *ed.*) Vol. 2, pp. 118-146, Ellis Horwood Limited, Chichester.

Rüdiger, H. W. von, Blume, K. G., Esselborn, H., Glogner, P., Kaffarnik, H., Finke, J., and Löhr, G. W. (1970) Transitorische Hämolyse, Hyperlipämie und unspezifische Leberveränderung bei Alkohollobuses (Zieve-Syndrome). *Blut*, **20**, 178-184.

Rutter, L. F. (1968) Endocrine disorders and dermatoglyphics in alcoholism. *J. Alcoholism*, **3**, 51-56.

Sabesin, S. M., Hawkins, H. L., Kuiken, L., and Ragland, J. B. (1977) Abnormal plasma lipoproteins and lecithin − cholesterol acyltransferase deficiency in alcoholic liver disease. *Gastroenterology*, **72**, 510-518.

Saker, B. M., Toffer, O. B., Burvill, M. J., and Reilly, K. A. (1967) Alcohol consumption and gout. *Med. J. Aust.*, **i**, 1213-1216.

Samloff, I. M., Liebman, W. M., and Panitch, N. M. (1975) Serum group I pepsinogens by radioimmunoassay in control subjects and patients with peptic ulcer. *Gastroenterology*, **69**, 83-90.

Sandhofer, F., Bolzano, K., Sailer, S., and Braunsteiner, H. (1973) Cholesterol turnover in patients with chronic liver disease. *Europ. J. Clin. Invest.*, **3**, 10-15.

Sandler, M., Carter, S. B., Hunter, K. R., and Stern, G. M. (1973) Tetrahydro-isoquinoline alkaloids: *in vivo* metabolites of L-dopa in man. *Nature, (Lond.).*, **241**, 439-443.

Schapiro, R. H., Scheig, R. L., Drummey, G. D., Mendelson, J. H., and Isselbacher, K. J. (1965) Effects of prolonged ethanol ingestion on the transport and metabolism of lipids in man. *N. Eng. J. Med.*, **272**, 610-615.

Schenker, V. J., Kissin, B., Maynard, L. S., and Schenker, A. C. (1966) Adrenal hormones and amine metabolism in alcoholism. *Psychosom. Med.*, **28**, 564-569.

Schenker, V. J., Kissin, B., Maynard, L. S., and Schenker, A. C. (1967) The effects of ethanol on amine metabolism in alcoholism. *In* Biochemical Factors in Alcoholism. (Maickel, R. P. *ed.*) pp. 39-52, Pergamon Press, Oxford.

Schnaberth, G., Gell, G., and Jaklitsch, H. (1972) Entgleisung des Säure-Basen-Gleichgewichtes in Liquor Cerebrospinalis beim Delerium Tremens. *Arch. Psychiat. Nervenkr.*, **215**, 417-428.

Seevers, M. H. (1970) Morphine and ethanol physical dependence: A critique of a hypothesis. *Science*, **170**, 1113-1114.

Segal, S., and Blair, A. (1961) Some observations on the metabolism of D-galactose in normal man. *J. Clin. Invest.*, **40**, 2016-2025.

Segal, B. M., Kushnarev, V. M., Urakov, I. G., and Misionzhnik, E. U. (1970) Alcoholism and disruption of the activity of deep cerebral structures. *Q. J. Stud. Alcohol*, **31**, 587-601.

Sereny, G., Rapoport, A., and Husdan, H. (1966) The effect of alcohol withdrawal on electrolyte and acid-base balance. *Metab. Clin. Exp.*, **15**, 896-904.

Sereny, G., Endrenyi, L., and Devenyi, P. (1975) Glucose intolerance in alcoholism. *J. Stud. Alcohol*, **36**, 359-364.

Shanley, B. C., Robertson, E. J., Jourbert, S. M., and North-Coombes, J. D. (1972) Effect of alcohol on glucose tolerance. *Lancet*, **i**, 1232.

Shaw, D. M., Camps, F. E., Robinson, A. E., Short, R., and White, S. (1970) Electrolyte content of the brain in alcoholism. *Br. J. Psychiat.*, **116**, 185-193.

Shaw, D. A., Tidmarsh, S. F., MacSweeney, D. A., Johnson, A. L., Godfrey, B. E., Allan, D. J., and Merry, J. (1974) Body composition in alcoholic as compared to control individuals. *Ann. Clin. Biochem.*, **11**, 164-167.

Shaw, S., Stimmel, B., and Lieber, C. S. (1976) Plasma alpha amino-n-butyric acid/leucine ratio: an empirical biochemical marker of alcoholism. *Science, (Wash. D.C.)*, **194**, 1057-1058.

Shaw, S., Stimmel, B., and Lieber, C. S. (1977) Plasma alpha amino-n-butyric acid/leucine; A biochemical marker of alcohol consumption. Application for the detection and assessment of alcoholism. *In* Currents in Alcoholism: Biological, Biochemical, and Clinical Studies (F. A. Seixas *ed.*) **Vol. 1**, pp. 17-31, Grune and Stratton Inc., New York.

Sherwood, W. C. (1972) The recognition of hemolytic disease in patients with cirrhosis. *Am. J. Clin. Pathol.*, **57**, 618-624.

Shishov, V. I., Barybin, A. S., and Khodakov, N. M. (1972) Characteristics of electrolyte metabolism in chronic alcoholic intoxication. *Zh. Nevro. Patol. Psikhiatr. imm s.s. Korsakova*, **72**, 885-888 (*Biol. Abs.*, (1973) **56**, 29065).

Siegel, F. L., Roach, M. K., and Pomeroy, L. R. (1964) Plasma amino acid patterns in alcoholism; The effects of ethanol loading. *Proc. Nat. Acad. Sci.*, **51**, 605.

Simons, L. A., Williams, P. F., and Turtle, J. R. (1975) Type V hyperlipoproteinaemia re-visited: Findings in a Sydney population. *Aust. N.Z. J. Med.*, **5**, 219-223.

Sirton, C. R., Agadi, E., Mariani, C., Canel, N., and Frattola, L. (1972) Alcoholic hyperlipidaemia. *Lancet*, **ii**, 820-821.

Sirtori, C. R., Agradi, E., and Mariani, C. (1973) Hyperlipoproteinemia in alcoholic subjects. *Pharmacol. Res. Commun.*, **5**, 81-85.

Skude, G., and Wadstein, J. (1977) Amylase, hepatic enzymes and bilirubin in serum of chronic alcoholics. *Acta. Med. Scand.*, **201**, 53-58.

Smals, A. G., Kleppenborg, P. W., Njo, K. T., Knoben, J. M., and Ruland, C. M. (1976) Alcohol-induced Cushingoid syndrome. *Br. Med. J.*, **2**, 1298.

Smith, A. N., Nyhus, L. M., Dalgliesh, C. E., Dutton, R. W., Lennox, B., and Macfarlane, P. S. (1977) Further observations on the endocrine aspects of argentaffinoma. *Scott. Med. J.*, **2**, 24-38.

Smith, A. A., and Gitlow, S. (1967) Effect of disulfiram and ethanol on the catabolism of norepinephrine in man. *In* Biochemical Factors in Alcoholism. (Maickel, R. P. *ed.*) pp. 53-59, Pergamon Press, Oxford.

Smith, J. W., Johnson, L C., and Burdick, J. A. (1971) Sleep, psychological and clinical changes during alcohol withdrawal in NAD-treated alcoholics. *Q. J. Stud. Alcohol*, **32**, 982-994.

Smith, J. W., and Layden, T. A. (1972) Changes in psychological performance and blood chemistry in alcoholics during and after hospital treatment. *Q. J. Stud. Alcohol*, **33**, 379-394.

Song, S. K., and Rubin, E. (1972) Ethanol produces muscle damage in human volunteers. *Science (Wash. D.C.)*, **175**, 327-328.

Sorensen, E. W. (1966) Studies on iron absorption. V. The effect of ascorbic acid and ethyl alcohol on the absorption of iron in iron-deficient subjects. *Acta Med. Scand.*, **180**, 241-244.

Souminen, H., Forsberg, S., Heikkinen, E., and Österback, L. (1974) Enzyme activities and glycogen concentrations in skeletal muscle in alcoholism. *Acta Med. Scand.*, **196**, 199-202.

Speck, B. (1970) Die Tagesschwankungen des Serumeisens und der latenten Eisenbindungskapazitat bei Hepatitis, Leberzirrhose, Alkoholismus, Hämo-chromatos und aplastische Anämie. *Schweiz. Med. Wochenschr.*, **100**, 303-305.

Spencer-Peet, J., and Wood, D. C. F. (1975) Urinary D-glucaric acid excretion and serum gamma-glutamyl transpeptidase activity in alcoholism. *Br. J. Addict.*, **70**, 359-364.

Sprince, H., Parker, C. M., Smith, G. G., and Gonzales, L. J. (1972) Alcoholism: Biochemical and nutritional aspects of brain amines, aldehydes and amino-acids. *Nutrition Reports International*, **5**, 185-200.

Steer, P., Marnell, R., and Werk, E. E. (1969) Clinical alcohol hypoglycaemia and isolated adrenocorticotrophic hormone deficiency. *Ann. Int. Med.*, **71**, 343-348.

Stokes, P. E. (1971) Alcohol — endocrine interrelationships. *In* Biology of Alcoholism (Kissin, B. and Begleiter, H. *eds.*) Vol. 1, pp. 397-436, Plenum Press, New York.

Stokes, P. E. (1973) Adrenocortical activation in alcoholics during chronic drinking. *Ann. N. Y. Acad. Sci.*, **215**, 77.

Straus, E., Urbach, H. J., and Yallow, R. S. (1975) Alcohol-stimulated secretion of immunoreactive secretin. *N. Engl. J. Med.*, **293**, 1031-1032.

Sturner, W. Q., and Coe, J. I. (1973) Electrolyte imbalance in alcoholic liver disease. *J. Forensic Sci.*, **18**, 344-350.

Sullivan, J. F., and Lankford, H. G. (1965) Zinc metabolism and chronic alcoholism. *Am. J. Clin. Nutr.*, **17**, 57-63.

Sullivan, J. F., Lankford, H. G., and Robertson, P. (1966) Renal excretion of lactate and magnesium in alcoholism. *Am. J. Clin. Nutr.*, **18**, 231-236.

Sullivan, J. F. (1968) The incidence of low serum zinc in hospitalised patients. *Am. J. Clin. Nutr.*, **21**, 537.

Sullivan, J. F., and Heaney, R. P. (1970) Zinc metabolism in alcoholic liver disease. *Am. J. Clin. Nutr.*, **23**, 170-177.

Sullivan, J., Parker, M., and Carson, S. B. (1968) Tissue cobalt content in 'beer drinkers' myocardiopathy'. *J. Lab. Clin. Med.*, **71**, 893-896.

Sullivan, J. F., Wolpert, P. W., Williams, R., and Egan, J. D. (1969) Serum magnesium in chronic alcoholism. *Ann. N.Y. Acad. Sci.*, **162**, 947-962.

Sussman, K. E., Alfrey, A., Kirsch, W. M., Zweig, P., Felig, P., and Messner, F. (1970) Chronic lactic acidosis in an adult. *Am. J. Med.*, **48**, 104-112.

Sviripa, E. V. (1972) Dynamics of copper metabolism and caeruloplasmin activity in patients with alcoholism and alcoholic psychosis. *Vrach Delo*, **1**, 115-117.

Svirpina, E. V. (1971) Vitamin C metabolism in alcoholic patients and alcoholic psychoses. *Zh. Nervopatol. Psikhiatr. im s.s. Korsakova*, **71**, 422–425.

Taskinen, M-R., and Nikkilä, E. A. (1977) Nocturnal hypertriglyceridemia and hyperinsulinemia following moderate evening intake of alcohol. *Acta Med. Scand.*, **202**, 173-177.

Tasman-Jones, C., and Abraham, A. (1973) Hyperlipemia and pancreatitis *Dig. Dis.*, **18**, 767-772.

Toa, H. G., and Fox, H. M. (1976) Measurements of urinary pantothenic acid excretions of alcoholic patients. *J. Nutr. Sci. Vitaminol.*, **22**, 333-337.

Territo, M.C., and Tanaka, K.R. (1974) Hypophosphatemia in chronic alcoholism. *Arch. Int. Med.*, **134**, 445–447.

Thämmig, R. von. (1970) Das Zieve-syndrom. *Z. Gastroenterol.*, **8**, 339-345.

Thiessen, J. J., Sellers, E. M., Denbeigh, P., and Dolman, L. (1976) Plasma protein binding of diazepam and tolbutamide in chronic alcoholics. *J. Clin. Pharmacol.*, **16**, 345-351.

Thomson, A. D., and Leevy, C. M. (1972) Observations on the mechanism of thiamine hydrochloride absorption in man. *Clin. Sci.*, **43**, 153-163.

Thomson, A. D., Baker, H., and Leevy, C. M. (1970) Patterns of ^{35}S-thiamine hydrochloride absorption in the malnourished alcoholic patient. *J. Lab. Clin. Med.*, **76**, 34–45.

Thomson, A. D., Baker, H., and Leevy, C. M. (1971) Folate-induced malabsorption of thiamine. *Gastroenterology*, **60**, 756 (abstr.).

Tichy, J., Alling, C., Dencker, S. J., and Svennerholm, L. (1970) Fatty acid profiles in cerebrospinal fluid lipids in normals and chronic alcoholics. *Scand. J. Clin. Lab. Invest.*, **25**, 192-197.

Tomasulo, P. A., Kater, R. M. H., and Iber, F. L. (1968) Impairment of thiamine absorption in alcoholism. *Am. J. Clin. Nutr.*, **21**, 1340-1344.

Toro, G., Kolodny, R. C., Jacobs, L. S., Masters, W. H., and Daughaday, W. H. (1973) Failure of alcohol to alter pituitary and target organ hormone levels. *Clin. Res.*, **21**, 505.

Turkington, R. W. (1972) Serum prolactin levels in patients with gynacomastia. *J. Clin. Endocrinol.*, **34**, 62–66.

Turner, R. C., Oakley, N. W., and Nabarro, J. D. N. (1973) Changes in plasma insulin during ethanol-induced hypoglycaemia. *Metab. Clin. Exp.*, **22**, 111–121.

Uzunalimoglu, O. (1970) Alcoholic hyperlipemia. *Ankara Univ. Tip. Fak. Mecm.*, **23**, 719–724 (*Biol. Abs.*, (1971) **52**, 98926).

Vanha-Perttula, T., and Kalliomäki, J. L. (1973) Comparison of dipeptide arylamidase I and II, amino-acid arylamidase and acid phosphatase activities in normal and pathological human sera. *Clin. Chim. Acta*, **44**, 249–258.

Van Thiel, D. H., and Lester, R. (1976) Alcoholism: its effect on hypothalamic pituitary gonadal function. *Gastroenterology*, **71**, 318–327.

Van Thiel, D. H., Lester, R., and Sherins, R. J. (1974) Hypogonadism in alcoholic disease: Evidence for a double defect. *Gastroenterology*, **67**, 1188–1199.

Van Thiel, D. H., Gavaler, J. S., Lester, R., Loriaux, D. L., and Braunstien, G. D. (1975) Plasma estrone, prolactin, neurophysin and sex steroid-binding globulin in chronic alcoholic man. *Metab. Clin. Exp.*, **24**, 1015–1019.

Veitch, R. L., Lumeng, L., and Li, T. K. (1975) Vitamin B_6 metabolism in chronic alcohol abuse: The effect of ethanol oxidation on hepatic pyridoxal 5'-phosphate metabolism. *J. Clin. Invest.*, **55**, 1026–1032.

Verbanck, M., Verbanck, J., Brauman, J., and Mullier, J. P. (1976) Bone histology and 25-OH vitamin D plasma levels in alcoholics without cirrhosis. *Calcd. Tiss. Res. Suppl.*, **22**, 538–541.

Verdy, M., and Gattereau, A. (1967) Ethanol, lipase activity, and serum-lipid level. *Am. J. Clin. Nutr.*, **20**, 997–1003.

Vetter, W. R., Cohn, L. H., and Reichgott, M. (1967) Hypokalaemia and electrocardiographic abnormalities during acute alcohol withdrawal. *Arch. Intern. Med.*, **120**, 536–541.

Vier, V. G., and Karapina, T. N. (1967) Protein fractions in the blood plasma in alcoholism. *Zdra. Vookhr. Beloruss*, **13**, 44–46.

Vodoz, J. F., Luisier, M., Donath, A., Courvoisier, B., and Garcia, B. (1977) Dimminution de l'absorption intestinale de 47-calcium dans l'alcoolisme chronique. *Schweiz. Med. Wochenschr.*, **107**, 1525–1529.

Vogelberg, K. H., Gries, F. A., Miss, H. D., and Jahnke, K. (1971) Die Hyperlipämie bei chronischem Alkoholabusus. *Dtsh. Med. Wochenschr.*, **96**, 13–21.

Walker, J. E. C., and Gordon, E. R. (1970) Biochemical aspects associated with an ethanol induced fatty liver. *Biochem. J.*, **119**, 511–516.

Wallerstedt, S., Cederblad, G. Korsen-Bengtsen, K., and Olsson, R. (1977a) Coagulation factors and other plasma proteins during abstinence after heavy alcohol consumption in chronic alcoholics. *Scand. J. Gastroenterol.*, **12**, 649–655.

Wallerstedt, S., Gustafson, A., and Olsson, R. (1977b) Serum lipids and lipo-
    proteins during abstinence after heavy alcohol consumption in chronic
    alcoholics. *Scand. J. Clin. Lab. Invest.,* **37,** 599-604.
Walshe, J. M., and Briggs, J. (1962) Caeruloplasmin in liver disease. A diagnostic
    pitfall. *Lancet,* **ii,** 243-265.
Waltman, R., Bonura, F., Nigrin, G., and Pipet, C. (1969) Ethanol and neonatal
    bilirubin levels. *Lancet,* **ii,** 108.
Wartburg, J. P. von. and Papenberg, J. (1970) Biochemical and enzymatic
    changes induced by chronic ethanol intake. *In* International Encyclopedia
    of Pharmacology and Therapeutics (Tremolieres, J. *ed.*) Vol. 2, pp. 301-343,
    Pergamon Press, Oxford.
Wartburg, J. P. von, Berger, D., Ris, M. M., and Tabakoff, B. (1975) Enzymes of
    biogenic aldehyde metabolism. *Adv. Exp. Med. Biol.,* **59,** 119-138.
Waters, A. H., Morley, A. A., and Rankin, J. G. (1966) Effect of alcohol on
    haemopoiesis. *Br. Med. J.,* **2,** 1565-1568.
Watson, C. J., Sutherland, D., and Hawkins, V. (1951) Studies on coproporphyrin
    V. The isomer distribution and *per diem* excretion of urinary coproporphyrin
    in cases of cirrhosis of the liver. *J. Lab. Clin. Med.,* **37,** 8-28.
Wernze, H., and Schmitz, E. (1977) Plasma prolactin and prolactin release in
    liver cirrhosis. *Acta Hepato-Gastroenterol.,* **24,** 97-101.
Whitby, L. G., Percy-Robb, I. W., and Smith, A. F. (1975) *Lecture Notes on
    Clinical Chemistry.* p. 214, Blackwell Scientific Publications, Oxford.
Wietholtz, H. and Colombo, J. P. (1976) Das Verhalten der γ-glutamyl-trans-
    peptidase und anderer Leberenzyme in Plasma während der Alkohol-
    Entziehungskur. *Schweiz. Med. Wochenschr.,* **106,** 981-987.
Williams, I. R., and Girdwood, R. H. (1970) The folate status of alcoholics.
    Scott. Med. J., **15,** 285-288.
Williams, R. R. (1976) Breast and thyroid cancer and malignant melanoma
    promoted by alcohol-induced pituitary secretion of prolactin, T. S. H.,
    and M. S. H. *Lancet,* **i,** 966-999.
Wilson, I, D., Onstad, G. R., Williams, R. C., and Carcy, J. B. (1968) Selective
    immunoglobulin A (IgA) deficiency in two patients with alcoholic cirrhosis.
    Gastroenterology, **54,** 253-259.
Wilson, I. D., Onstad, G., and Williams, R. C. (1969) Serum immunglobulin
    concentrations in patients with alcoholic liver disease. *Gastroenterology,*
    57, 59-67.
Wilson, B. E., Schreibman, P. H., Brewster, A. C., and Arky, R. A. (1970)
    The enhancement of alimentary lipemia by ethanol in man. *J. Lab. Clin.
    Med.,* **75,** 264-274.
Wilson, I. D. (1972) Human serum antibodies specific for secretory IgA.
    Immunology, **22,** 1001-1011.
Wiseman, S. M., and Spencer-Peet, J. (1977) The effect of drinking patterns on
    enzyme screening tests for alcoholism. *Practitioner,* **219,** 243-245.

Wolfe, S. M., and Victor, M. (1976) The relationship of hypomagnesemia and alkalosis to alcohol withdrawal. *Ann. N.Y. Acad. Sci.*, 162, 973–984.

Wolfe, B. M., Havel, J. R., Marliss, E. B., Kane, J. P., Seymour, J., and Ahuja, S.P. (1976) Effects of a 3-day fast and of ethanol on splanchnic metabolism of FFA, amino-acids and carbohydrates in healthy young men. *J. Clin. Invest.*, 57, 329–340.

Wood, B., Breen, K. J., Penington, D. G. (1977) Thiamine status in alcoholism. *Aust. N.Z. J. Med.*, 7, 475–484.

Wright, J., Merry, J., Fry, D., and Marks, V. (1975) Pituitary function in chronic alcoholism. *Adv. Exp. Med. Biol.*, 59, 253–255.

Wu, A., Chanarin, I., Levi, A. J. (1974) Macrocytosis of chronic alcoholism. *Lancet*, i, 829–831.

Wu, A., and Levi, A. J. (1975) Effect of alcohol on total urinary hydroxyproline excretion. *Am. J. Gastroenterology*, 64, 217–220.

Wu, A., Chanarin, I., Slavin, G., and Levi, A. J. (1975) Folate deficiency in the alcoholic — its relationship to clinical and haematological abnormalities, liver disease and folate stores. *Br. J. Haematol.*, 29, 469–478.

Wu, A., Slavin, G., and Levi, A. J. (1976) Elevated serum gamma-glutamyl-transferase (transpeptidase) and histological liver damage in alcoholism. *Am. J. Gastroenterol.*, 65, 318–323.

Ylikahri, R. H., Poso, A. R., Huttunen, M. O., and Hillbom, M. E. (1974) Alcohol intoxication and hangover: Effects on plasma electrolyte concentrations and acid-base balance. *Scand. J. Clin. Lab. Invest.*, 34, 327–336.

Ylikahri, R. H., Huttunen, M. O., Eriksson, C. J. P., and Nikkita, E. A. (1974b) Metabolic studies on the pathogenesis of hangover. *Eur. J. Clin. Invest.*, 4, 93–100.

Ylikahri, R., Huttunen, M., Härkönen, M. and Adlercreutz, H. (1974c) Letter to the editor: Hangover and testosterone. *Br. Med. J.*, 2, 445.

Ylikahri, R. Huttunen, M., Härkönen, M., Seuderling, U., Onikki, S., Karoner, S-L., and Adlercreutz, H. (1974d) Low plasma testosterone values in man during hangover. *J. Steroid Biochem.*, 5, 655–658.

Ylikahri, R. H., Lein, T., Huttunen, M. O., Posö, A. R., Eriksson, C. J. P. and Nikkilä, E. A. (1976a) Effects of fructose and glucose on ethanol-induced metabolic changes and on the intensity of alcohol intoxication and hangover. *Europ. J. Clin. Invest.*, 6, 93–102.

Ylikahri, R. H., Huttunen, M. O., and Härkönen, M. (1976b) Effect of alcohol on anterior-pituitary secretion of trophic hormones. *Lancet*, i, 1353.

Zakharov, V. N. (1968) Clinical and functional condition of the liver in chronic alcohol poisoning. *Sov. Med.*, 31, 57–62.

Zanoboni, A., and Zanoboni-Mucciaccia, N. (1975) Gynaecomastia in alcoholic cirrhosis. *Lancet*, ii, 876.

Zanoboni, A. and Zanoboni-Mucciaccia, W. (1976) Alcohol and Cancer. *Lancet*, i, 1408.

Zanoboni, A., and Zanoboni-Mucciaccia, W. (1977) Elevated basal growth hormone levels and growth hormone response to TRH in alcoholic patients with cirrhosis. *J. Clin. Endocrinol. Metab.*, **45**, 576–578.

Zarcone, V., Barchas, J., Hoddes, E., Montplaisir, J., Sack, R., and Wilson, R. (1975) Experimental ethanol ingestion: sleep variables and metabolites of dopamine and serotonin in the cerebrospinal fluid. *Adv. Exp. Med. Biol.*, **59**, 431–451.

Zazgornik, J. (1973) Über die Zinkausscheidung im Schweiss und Harn bei chronischen Alcoholikern während Wärme exposition. *Res. Exp. Med.*, **160**, 252–254.

Zazgornik, J., Schnack, H., Wessely, P., and Kotzaurek, R. (1970) Serum zinc content in hepatic damage due to alcoholism. *Z. Gastroenterol.*, **8**, 346–350.

Zazgornik, J., Irsigler, K., Kline, E., and Kryspin-Exner, K. (1972) The eccrine sweat-gland function of chronic alcoholics. *Nutr. Metab.*, **14**, 307–312.

Zein, M., and Discombe, G. (1970) Serum gamma-glutamyl transpeptidase as a diagnostic aid. *Lancet*, **ii**, 748–750.

Zumoff, B., Bradlow, H. L., Gallagher, T. F., and Hellman, L. (1967) Cortisol metabolism in cirrhosis. *J. Clin. Invest.*, **46**, 1735–1743.

Appendix

Conversion Scales for S.I. and Conventional Units
(see Bold and Wilding, 1975)

	Conversion
	S.I. $\longrightarrow$ Conventional

Albumin $\quad\dfrac{g/l}{10} = g/100\ ml$

Bicarbonate $\quad mmol/l = mEq/l$

Bilirubin $\quad\dfrac{\mu mol/l}{17.1} = mg/100\ ml$

Calcium $\quad mmol/l \times 4 = mg/100\ ml$
$\qquad\qquad$ or
$\qquad mmol/l \times 2 = mEq/l$

Cholesterol $\quad mmol/l \times 38.7 = mg/100\ ml$

Cortisol $\quad\dfrac{nmol/l}{27.6} = \mu g/100\ ml$

Creatinine $\quad\dfrac{\mu mol/l}{88.4} = mg/100\ ml$

Carbon dioxide $\quad kPa \times 7.5 = mm\ Hg$

Globulin $\quad\dfrac{g/l}{10} = g/100\ ml$

Glucose $\quad mmol/l \times 18 = mg/100\ ml$

Hydrogen Ion
pH $\quad$ 7.02 $\quad$ 7.07 $\quad$ 7.12 $\quad$ 7.19 $\quad$ 7.26 $\quad$ 7.35 $\quad$ 7.46 $\quad$ 7.60
nmol/l $\quad$ 95 $\quad\quad$ 85 $\quad\quad$ 75 $\quad\quad$ 65 $\quad\quad$ 55 $\quad\quad$ 45 $\quad\quad$ 35 $\quad\quad$ 25

Iron $\quad\mu mol/l \times 5.6 = \mu g/100\ ml$

Magnesium $\quad mmol/l \times 2 = mEq/l$
$\qquad\qquad$ or
$\qquad mmol \times 2.4 = mg/100\ ml$

Oxygen	kPa × 7.5 = mm Hg
Phosphate	mmol/l × 3.1 = mg/100 ml
Potassium	mmol/l = mEq/l
Protein-bound iodine	$\dfrac{\text{nmol/l} = \text{ug/100 ml}}{78.8}$
Sodium	mmol/l = mEq/l
Thyroxine	$\dfrac{\text{nmol/l} = \mu\text{g/100 ml}}{12.87}$
Triglycerides	mmol/l × 88.6 = mg/100 ml
Urate	$\dfrac{\mu\text{mol/l} = \text{mg/100 ml}}{59.5}$
Urea	mmol/l × 6 = mg/100 ml
VMA	$\dfrac{\mu\text{mol/period} = \text{mg/period}}{5.05}$
Metanephrines	$\dfrac{\mu\text{mol/period} = \text{mg/period}}{5.46}$

Bold, A. M., and Wilding, P. (1975) Clinical Chemistry, Blackwell Scientific Publications, London.

Index

A

acetaldehyde, 30, 35, 66–74
  biogenic amine metabolism and, 71
  blood levels, 67–70
  catecholamine release, 71
  disulfiram (Antabuse), 74
  metabolic effects, 70
  metabolism, 66–67
  organ effects, 72
  oxidative phosphorylation, 70–71
  porphyrins, 73
  tetrahydro-β-carbolines, 72
  tetrahydroisoquinolines, 71
  teratology, 74
acetate, 30, 230
  metabolism, 205
acetoacetate, 214, 229
acetyl coenzyme A, 30
acid-base status, 152–154
acid phosphatase, 155
adenohypophyseal hormones, 182–185
adrenal cortex, 189
  activity, 194
adrenaline (see epinephrine)
adrenocorticotrophin (ACTH), 185, 194
alanine aminotransferase, 155, 163
albumin, 168, 172
alcohol
  absorption, 30–45
    factors influencing, 32–33
    retardation of, 33
    rates of, 32
    sites of, 31
  abuse
    biochemical tests for, 111–132
      detection of, 111–132
      assessment of, 111–132
    diseases and, 22–29, 102
    incidence of, 22–29
  blood levels of, 111–113
  cancer and, 180–182

alcohol (*contd.*)
  clearance of, 41
  consumption statistics, 23–25
  dependence, 19
    dependence syndrome, 19
  distribution in body fluids of, 35–37
  endocrine effects of, 101–102
  endogenous, 35
  elimination of, 40–45
  excretion of, 30–45
  historical aspects of, 22–23
  irritant properties of, 32
  metabolism, 30–45
    chronopharmacogenetics, 44, 45
    effect of exercise on, 33, 44
    effect of food on, 33, 34, 44
    effect of fructose on, 42–43
    genetic influence on, 45
    hepatic, 37–40
    menstrual cycle and, 44
    racial variation, 44
  solubility and solvent effects of, 97–99
  related disabilities, 19–20
alcohol dehydrogenase (ADh), 30, 38–39,
    42
alcoholic
  beverages, 96–97
    chemical constituents, 97
    congener content, 54, 55
alcoholics
  death rate, 27
  definitions, 15–21
  mortality, 27, 28
alcoholism
  alpha, 20
  beta, 20
  definitions, 15–21
  delta, 20
  diseases and, 26–28, 102
  economic cost, 22
  epsilon, 20

alcoholism (*contd.*)
  gamma, 20
  incidence, 23–26
    methods of estimation, 23–26
aldehyde dehydrogenase, 30
aldosterone, 195
alkaline phosphatase, 155, 166
alkaloids, 239, 240
alpha amino–n–butyric acid/leucine ratio,
  116–118
alpha – amylase, 155
alpha$_1$ – antitrypsin, 168
alpha$_1$ – easily precipitable glycoprotein,
  168
alpha – foetoprotein, 174
alpha$_1$ – globulin, 168
alpha$_2$ – globulin, 168
alpha$_2$ – group component, 168
alpha – glycerphosphate, 216
alpha$_2$ – macroglobulin, 168
amino acids, 177–179
  catabolism, 87
amino acid arylamidase, 155
aminopyrine breath test, 130–131
anaemia, 150–152
  megaloblastic, 151, 245
androgens, 196
  metabolism, 198
antidiuretic hormone (ADH), 138, 139,
  186
arginase, 155
ascorbic acid (*see* vitamin C)
aspartate aminotransferase, 95, 126, 127,
  156, 163
aryl sulphatase A and B, 156

B
beta – globulins, 169
beta – glucoronidase, 156
beta – hydroxybutyrate, 229
bilirubin, 200–202
biochemical
  parameters, 84–105, 138–248
    analytical interferences on, 103–
      104
    congeners and, 96
    disease and, 102
    genetic factors and, 102–103
    nutritional status and, 99–101
    stress and, 102
    time of testing and, 93–96
    type of beverage, 96
  profiling, 124–128
biogenic amines, 88, 230–241
  metabolites, 114–116

C
caeruloplasmin, 174
calcitonin, 186
calcium, 147
candida albicans, 35
carbohydrate metabolism, 204–216
carcino embryonic antigen (CEA), 174
carcinoid disease, 231
carotene (*see* vitamin A)
catalase, 40
catecholamines, 232–238
central nervous system amines, 240–241
chloride, 139–146
cholecalciferol
    1,25–dihydroxycholecalciferol, 147,
      247
    25–hydroxycholecalciferol, 247
cholesterol, 222–227, 228
    esters, 225
cholinesterase, 156
chylomicra, 218
cirrhosis (*see* liver)
    mortality rates, 25
congeners, 54–74, 96–97
    acute lethal dose, 62
    analysis of, 55
    blood levels of, 56
    definitions of, 54
    origins of, 55
    pathology, 60
    pharmacology and toxicity of, 57–59
    threshold limit values, 58
    urine levels, 56
condensation reactions, 238–240
convictions
    drinking and driving, 22
    drunkeness, 22
copper, 148
coproporphyrin, 203
cortisol, 189, 191–192
C–reactive protein, 169
creatine phosphokinase, 156, 166–167
creatinine, 179
cultures
    abstinent, 16
    ambivalent, 16
    over permissive, 16
    permissive, 16
cyanocobalamin (*see* vitamin B$_{12}$)
cyclic AMP, 241
cysteine, 178

D
delta aminolaevulinic acid dehydratase,
    124, 157
dehydroepiandrosterone, 189, 196

dopamine, 233-234
dipeptidyl arylamidase I, 157
dipeptidyl arylamidase II, 157
discriminant function analysis, 127
drinking
  heavy, 18, 20
  moderate, 17, 20

E

electrolytes, 138-154
enzymes, 119-124, 154-167
  of alcohol metabolism, 38-40
  multiple analyses of, 154, 163
epinephrine, 232, 234
ethanol (see alcohol)

F

fatty acids, 214, 219, 224
feminization and hypogonadism syndrome, 196-199
fibrin, 176
foetal alcohol syndrome, 196
folic acid (folate), 245, 247
  metabolism, 246
follicle stimulating hormone, 184-185, 196
forminoglutamate (FIGLU), 247
Framingham study, 219
fructose
  effects on alcohol metabolism (see alcohol)
  metabolism, 43, 207, 209
fructose-6-phosphate kinase, 157
fusel oils (see congeners)

G

galactose
  metabolism, 207, 209
  tolerance test, 114
gamma globulins, 169
gamma glutamyl transferase (transpeptidase), 119-123, 126, 127, 129, 157, 163-166
gastric antibodies, 173-174
gastrin, 187-188
gastrointestinal tract
  alcohol absorption, 31
  hormones, 187
globulins, 169, 172-174
glucagon, 187, 215
D-glucaric acid, 130, 131, 230
glucocorticoids, 189-195
  alcoholism, in, 193-195
  normal man, in, 190-193

gluconeogenesis, 206
  inhibition, 214
glucose, 87, 214-215
  intolerance, 210-211
glucose-6-phosphate dehydrogenase, 157
glucose-6-phosphogluconate dehydrogenase, 157
glutamate (glutamic acid), 178
glutamate dehydrogenase, 124, 125, 158
glutathione reductase, 158
glycine, 178
glycogenolysis, 207, 216
glycolysis, 207
gout, 179
growth hormone, 182-184, 214, 215
guanase, 158

H

haemochromatosis, 152
haemolytic jaundice, 202
haemopexin, 169
hangover, 60, 154
haptoglobin, 169, 175
hepatitis, 202
hexokinase, 158
high density lipoprotein (HDL), 222, 227
higher alcohols, 61-63
  absorption, 61
  metabolic effects, 61-62
  metabolism, 61
  pharmacology, 62-63
  toxicity, 62-63
histidine, 178
hydrocortisone, 215
hydroxybutyrate dehydrogenase, 158
5-hydroxyindole-3-acetic acid (5-HIAA), 231, 233
5-hydroxytryptophol, 233
hyperglycaemia, 210-211
hyperuricaemia, 179
hyperlipidaemia, 217
hypoglycaemia, 212-216
  drug induced, 212
  reactive, 212
hypothalmic – pituitary – adrenal insufficiency, 216
hypothalmic – pituitary – gonadal function, 188, 197-198

I

IgA, 170, 172-173
IgG, 170, 173
IgM, 170, 173
Immunoglobulins, 172-174

insulin, 186–187, 214, 215
    inappropriate response, 215
intermediate low density lipoprotein
    (ILDL), 217
iron, 150–152
isocitrate dehydrogenase, 158

K

ketones, 88
kynurenine, 232

L

lactate, 88, 229
lactate/pyruvate ratio, 113
lactate dehydrogenase, 158, 167
lecithin cholesterol acyltransferase, 222
leucine aminopeptidase, 159
lipase, 217
lipids, 87, 216–228
    blood, 217, 220
    metabolism, 86
    total, 226
lipoproteins, 216–228
    classes, 218
liver
    cirrhosis, 26, 200
    disease, 28
    dysfunction, 28
    fatty, 227
    redox state, 86
low density lipoprotein (LDL), 217, 222,
    227
luteinising hormone (LH), 185
lysozyme, 159

M

magnesium, 146–147
malabsorption, 99
mean corpuscular volume, 126, 129–130
Meiteisho, 35
melanocyte stimulating hormone, 185
metabolic clearance rate, 38
metanephrine, 236, 238
methanol, 63–66
    absorption, 63–65
    blood levels, 65–66
    metabolism, 63–65
3–methoxy–4–hydroxymandelic acid
    (VMA), 235–236, 238
3–methoxy–4–hydroxyphenylethylenegly-
    col, 236, 238
5–methyltetrahydrofolic acid, 246
microsomal ethanol oxidising system
    (MEOS), 30, 40

mineral deficiency, 101
mineralocorticoids, 195–196

N

$(Na^+ + K^+)$ – activated ATP ase activity,
    99
NAD/NADH ratio, 113
    alcoholic fatty liver and, 227
    androgens, 198
    lactate and, 88
    lipids and, 86
    porphyrins and, 203
neurohypophyseal hormones, 186
niacin, 248
nicotinamide, 248
nicotinic acid, 248
noradrenaline (*see* norepinephrine)
norepinephrine, 232, 234–235, 237
    metabolism 237
normetanephrine, 235
5'–nucleotidase, 159
nutritional status, 99–101

O

oestrogens, 199–200
oestradiol, 199
oestriol, 199
oestrone, 199
organic acids, 229–230
orosomucoid, 169
ornithine carbamoyl transferase, 159
osmolality, 111–113, 146
oxytocin, 186

P

pancreatic hormones, 186–187
pancreatitis, 27
pantothenic acid, 248
parathyroid, hormone, 147, 186
pattern analysis, 124–128
pentose phosphate pathway, 207, 208
pepsinogen, 159
peptide hormones, 180–188
pH, 153
phosphate, 148–150
3–phosphoglyceromutase, 159
phospholipids, 226, 228
porphobilinogen, 203
porphyrias, 202
porphyrins, 131, 202–204
potassium, 139–146
prealbumin, 172
prolactin, 184
protein 9, 169

proteins, 167–177
    metabolism, 176–177
pseudo Cushing's syndrome, 195
psychosis, 27
pteroylglutamic acid (*see* folic acid)
pyridoxal, 243
pyridoxal phosphate, 243
pyridoxal phosphokinase, 159
pyridoxine (*see* vitamin B_6)
pyridoxine phosphate oxidase, 160
pyruvate, 229

R

renin-angiotensin-aldosterone system, 196
riboflavin (*see* vitamin B_2)
rhythms, 93
    circadian, 93
    infradian, 93
    ultradian, 93

S

secretin, 187
serological markers, 128–129
serotonin, 230–232
sex hormones, 196–200
sex hormone binding globulin, 169, 198
sodium, 139–146
somatotropin (*see* growth hormone)
sorbitol
    metabolism, 207, 209
steroids, 88, 116
    hormones, 188–200
    17–hydroxycortico steroids, 190, 193
    17–oxo steroids, 190
    17–oxogenic steroids, 190
    precursors and metabolites, 189
stress, 102

T

TCA (Krebs) cycle, 205–206
testosterone, 197
thiamine (*see* vitamin B_1)
thyroid hormones, 186
thyroid stimulating hormone, 185

thyroxine binding pre-albumin, 168
transferrin, 169, 176
transketolase, 160
triglycerides, 219–222, 223, 228
triose-phosphate isomerase, 160
trypsin, 160
tryptamine, 232, 235
tryptophan, 178, 232
    metabolism, 231
tyrosine, 178

U

urate (uric acid) 88, 179–180, 181
urea, 179
uroporphyrin, 203

V

very low density lipoprotein (VLDL),
    217, 222, 227
vitamins, 241–248
    A, 241
    allowances, 100
    B_1, 242–243
    B_2, 243
    B_6, 243–244
    B_{12}, 244–245
    C, 247
    D, 247–248
    E, 248
VMA (*see* 3–methoxy–4–hydroxy man-
    delic acid)

W

water, 138–139
    extra-cellular, 139
    intra-cellular, 139
    total body, 138–139

Z

Zieve's syndrome, 219
zinc, 147–148
    serum levels, 147–148, 149
    urinary excretion, 131

NOTES

NOTES

NOTES